Contributors

FREDERICK BURKLE, Jr., M.D., M.P.H.

Dr. Burkle came to the psychiatry residency program of Dartmouth Medical School after a practice in pediatrics. He has since left chilly New England and is now in private psychiatric practice and a consultant in adolescent health care in Maui.

Adolescents, Chapter 10

ROBERT CHAPMAN, M.D.

Dr. Chapman is an Associate Professor of Clinical Psychiatry and Community and Family Medicine, Dartmouth Medical School. He had been the Director of the Dartmouth-Hitchcock Mental Health Center Comprehensive Alcohol Services Program and has been involved with the training of Medex, Physician's Assistants. His lectures have been incorporated in this handbook.

Medications, Chapter 9

STUART COPANS, M.D.

Dr. Copans was formerly a Fellow in Child Psychiatry, Dartmouth Medical School. The material on the effects of alcohol abuse on the family has been drawn largely from his lectures to the counselor trainees. He presently is an assistant professor of clinical psychiatry at Dartmouth and works with long-term adolescent inpatients and outpatients at the Brattleboro Retreat. He occasionally provides coverage for the adult and adolescent alcohol treatment units at the Retreat, but states that he is better at drawing cartoons about alcoholism than at treating it, and so leaves that to his more skillful colleagues.

Illustrator

RICHARD GOODSTEIN, M.D.

Suicide prevention, Chapter 9;
The elderly, Chapter 10

Dr. Goodstein is Deputy Medical Director and Director of Education at Carrier Foundation, Belle Mead, New Jersey, and Clinical Associate Professor of Psychiatry at Rutgers Medical School.

PETER HAURI, Ph.D.

Sleep disturbances, Chapter 5

Dr. Hauri is a Professor of Psychiatry and Director of the Sleep and Dreaming Laboratory at the Dartmouth Medical School. His lectures on sleep have been edited for this book.

SUSAN McGRATH

Chapter 1;
Sociological aspects, Chapter 4

Susan McGrath was a Research Assistant with the Alcohol Counselor Training Program of the Dartmouth Medical School. Intimately involved with the training program from its beginning, her contributions here evolved from a series of lectures she gave to the counselor trainees. She is presently affiliated with the Public Affairs Center of Dartmouth College.

THOMAS MacKENZIE, M.D.

Psychiatric diagnosis, Chapter 9

Dr. MacKenzie is currently an Assistant Professor of Psychiatry and Medicine at the University of Minnesota Medical School. He is a consultation liaison psychiatrist and is interested in psychiatric diagnosis.

HUGH MacNAMEE, M.D.

Adolescents, Chapter 10

Dr. MacNamee is an Associate Professor of Clinical Psychiatry in the Division of Child Psychiatry, Dartmouth Medical School, and is Medical Director of West Central New Hampshire Community Mental Health Services. His lectures on adolescents were edited for inclusion here.

TREVOR PRICE, M.D.

Alcohol and the Body,
Chapter 2
Medical complications,
Chapter 5

Dr. Price is an Associate Professor of Psychiatry and an Assistant Professor of Medicine, Dartmouth Medical School, and Co-Director of the In-patient Service of the Dartmouth-Hitchcock Mental Health Center. He entered psychiatry after training in internal medicine. He has been responsible for the bulk of the material available here.

The material from these contributors was originally derived from lectures and presentations given at the Alcohol Counselor Training Program, conducted by the Dartmouth Medical School between 1972-1978.

UNDERSTANDING ALCOHOL

UNDERSTANDING ALCOHOL

JEAN KINNEY, M.S.W.

Assistant Professor, Department of Psychiatry, and Associate Director,
Alcohol Counselor Training Program, Dartmouth Medical School,
Hanover, New Hampshire

GWEN LEATON

Formerly Research Assistant, Department of Psychiatry, Alcohol Counselor
Training Program, Dartmouth Medical School, Hanover, New Hampshire;
formerly Director of Education, Edgehill Newport;
Private consultant in alcohol education

Illustrated by

Stuart Copans, M.D.

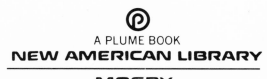

A PLUME BOOK
NEW AMERICAN LIBRARY

MOSBY

TIMES MIRROR
NEW YORK AND SCARBOROUGH, ONTARIO

Publisher: Thomas A. Manning
Assistant editor: Nancy L. Mullins
Manuscript editor: Judy Jamison
Production: Judy Bamert, Margaret B. Bridenbaugh

MOSBY MEDICAL LIBRARY

The ideas, procedures, and suggestions contained in this
book are not intended as a substitute for consulting with your physician.
All matters regarding your health require medical supervision.

This is a revised edition of a book previously published
by The C.V. Mosby Company entitled
Loosening the Grip: A Handbook of Alcohol Information.

NAL books are available at quantity discounts
when used to promote products or services. For information
please write to Premium Marketing Division,
The New American Library, Inc.,
1633 Broadway, New York, New York 10019.

PLUME TRADEMARK REG. U.S. PAT. OFF. AND FOREIGN COUNTRIES
REGISTERED TRADEMARK—MARCA REGISTRADA
HECHO EN FORGE VILLAGE, MASS., U.S.A.

SIGNET, SIGNET CLASSICS, MENTOR, PLUME, MERIDIAN and
NAL BOOKS are published by The New American Library, Inc.,
1633 Broadway, New York, New York 10019, in Canada, by
The New American Library of Canada, Limited,
81 Mack Avenue, Scarborough, Ontario M1L 1M8.

Library of Congress Cataloging in Publication Data

Kinney, Jean, 1943-
Understanding alcohol.

"A Plume book."
Rev. ed. of: Loosening the grip. 1978.
Bibliography: p.
Includes index.
1. Alcoholism—United States.   2. Alcoholics—United
States.   3. Alcohol—United States.   I. Leaton, Gwen,
1934-   .   II. Title.
HV5035.K56 1982   362.2'92   81-22557
ISBN 0-452-25338-1   AACR2

1   2   3   4   5   6   7   8   9   02/D/252

Printed in the United States of America

God of Compassion, if anyone has come to thine altar troubled in spirit, depressed and apprehensive, expecting to go away as he came, with the same haunting heaviness of heart; if anyone is deeply wounded of soul, hardly daring to hope that anything can afford him the relief he seeks, so surprised by the ill that life can do that he is half afraid to pray; O God, surprise him, we beseech thee, by the graciousness of thy help; and enable him to take from thy bounty as ungrudgingly as thou givest, that he may leave here his sorrow and take a song away.

AUTHOR UNKNOWN

Forewords

Alcohol has been called one of God's great gifts, and is used by most people with enjoyment and without problems. It has also been called "an invention of the devil" and the cause of most of the ills of mankind. In the battle between these two camps those people who have been unable to control their use of alcohol, and their families, have been the worst casualties—rejected by themselves, by the caring professions, and by most of the rest of us, as unworthy of consideration. They have been rejected by heavy drinkers as weaklings "who can't take it."

Until recently there has been almost no communication across the battlefield and little compassion for the casualties. Prejudice and ignorance have been perpetuated by the tunnel vision of the protagonists on both sides of the problem—both sides basing their opinions and prejudices on their limited experience; both sides convinced that they are right.

This book bridges the gap between ignorance, which has destroyed the lives and happiness of so many of our friends and neighbors, and understanding. One is impressed that the authors "have been there" and, with a minimum of professional jargon, are sharing their experience. They have looked at their experience free of preconceived notions and the cultural bias that most of us have.

Everyone in our society who would find some reliable answers to the problems of alcohol, and of alcoholic people and their families (and that should include all of us), will find their time well spent when they read *Understand-*

ing Alcohol. Although those who collaborated in the thought and creation of the book are medical people, including seven physicians, the book is readable and understandable by almost every one. It is needed, and I hope that it will be widely read to the end that our society may develop strategies and cultural norms that will reduce the tragedies associated with the unwise use and abuse of beverage alcohol.

John L Norris, M.D.
Medical Director (retired)
Eastman Kodak Company

In this present time the field of alcoholism is expanding beyond former boundaries until now it reaches into disciplines that just a couple of decades ago were far distant. Professionals, students, and interested laymen will find that this volume meets the need of the field for an organized and concise statement of the current state of the art. For indeed, before publication of *Loosening the Grip*, that most easily read book by the same authors which preceded this volume, there was no comprehensive treatise that gave all of us who are interested in alcoholism an integrated overview of the art, the science, and the spirituality of the field.

The authors are all eminent in their respective specialities, but since this can be said about most texts, the difference in this book is soon evident to the reader. The clear, and many times witty language and phrase, the respect for the gravity of the disease, the organization of the different aspects of this most complex illness, and the hope that is felt throughout as one reads from discipline to discipline, make this volume the currently definitive work in alcoholism.

It is obvious that the authors have a working knowledge, gained from much clinical practice. This book can be defined as a practical handbook as well as an integrated pool of alcoholism knowledge. It is particularly suited to the interested layman, and yet its sophistication should satisfy the professional.

Something rarely heard about a book that is both philosophical and technical, this book is delightful to read.

Joseph R. Cruse, M.D.
Medical Director,
Betty Ford Center at Eisenhower,
Rancho Mirage, California

James W. West, M.D.
Medical Coordinator,
Outpatient Alcohol Program,
Eisenhower Medical Center,
Rancho Mirage, California

Preface

Material on alcohol and alcoholism is mushrooming.
Books, articles, scientific reports, pamphlets. On present
use, past use, abuse. In teenagers, women, the labor force,
the elderly. When, where, why. . . .

Yet, while conducting an alcohol counselor training program at Dartmouth Medical School, we discovered that if
one didn't have all day to search library stacks, then it was
hard for those in the helping business to readily lay their
hands on the information that would be most useful. In
part to remedy that a text was written, the title, *Loosening
the Grip*. The goal was to pull together the basic information a counselor would use—synthesizing, organizing, and
sometimes "translating" the relevant information from
the fields of medicine, psychology, psychiatry, anthropol-
ogy, sociology, and counseling. It wasn't intended as the
last word, but we hoped it was a starting point.

While intended as a text, *Loosening the Grip* rather
quickly began to circulate among recovering alcoholics,
and their family and friends, who too were seeking author-
itative information on an illness that had so deeply touched
their lives. Or we heard of its being recommended to family
or close friends of an active alcoholic, those just recognizing and trying to make sense of the alcohol-induced chaos
in their lives. Thus, this edition, especially for the public,
was born and titled *Understanding Alcohol*. The bulk of
the basic content is identical to that found in the earlier
professional's edition, but with a focus on how it relates
personally to living with an alcohol problem, or just living

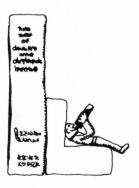

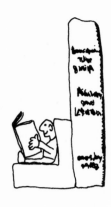

as we all do, in a world in which drinking is such a predominant feature.

It seems that an almost mandatory conclusion for book prefaces is an exhaustive listing of "all of those persons whose support and assistance. . . ." Trusting that our spouses, families, and professional colleagues know who they are, we wish to depart from that tradition. In fact, the most significant contribution to this work has been made by individuals whose names and identity are in many instances unknown to us—the alcohol counselors, those in the fellowship of AA, members of the clergy, school counselors, the medical profession, those whose efforts in their professional and private lives are what make loosening the grip on alcohol possible.

Jean Kinney
Gwen Leaton

Contents

Introduction

Remember . . .

Remember back to the time you wanted to learn how to ride a bicycle. . . . A *real* bicycle. A two-wheeler. (Close your eyes.)

Remember the street you lived on. . . . How about the big kids who had their own. . . . Can you feel how eager you were to join them? You could just picture yourself hopping on one of your own and winging off. . . . (Close your eyes and picture that scene.)

Continue in your imagination.

Suppose you had decided to seriously pursue your desire to ride a two-wheeler. Off to the town library, signing out a book on *Riding a Two-Wheeler in 20 Easy Steps.* Glossy pictures, diagrams, and sure enough, absolutely everything you'd need to know, to the smallest detail.

Step 1. Stand beside bicycle.

Step 2. Place hands on handlebars.

Step 3. With foot, push up kickstand.

Step 4. Walk briskly, pushing bicycle.

Step 5. Place left foot on left pedal (if standing on left side) and simultaneously swing right leg over bicycle and place on right pedal. (*Caution:* It is imperative to maintain forward motion during this step. Also critical to see that center of gravity of the body is properly positioned above bicycle.)

Step 6. Depress pedal in clockwise motion with ball of foot. And so forth. . . .

That isn't quite how it happened, is it? Had anyone ever suggested that was how you should go about it, there's no way you would not have spotted the ploy as the super con-job of the year.

So, how did you learn? By trying it! Getting your hands on a bike and simply climbing on! Unless you happened to

1

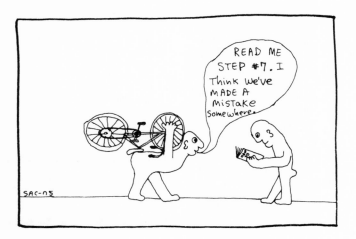

be the Joe Namath of the cycling set, you didn't smugly cruise down to the playground, either, on that first try. Wobbling along, training wheels, your mother or dad running beside holding the seat . . . spills, scuffs, tears, despair, forgetting how to brake in the crunch, more spills . . . and eventually it all clicked!

Living and working with alcoholics is pretty much like learning to ride a two-wheeler. It's a process. A series of trying things that occur over a period of time. Ideally *Riding a Two-Wheeler in 20 Easy Steps* has convinced you. That means learning by doing—feeling awkward, going shakily in the beginning, having someone close by for support and to provide advice. It will include some blows to your pride, moments of feeling silly or unknowledgeable.

How does this book fit in? It's not a do-it-yourself, step-by-step guide, that you can read, and go out to deal effectively with an alcohol problem, your own or others'. This book can be a guide. It can help you see things more clearly, what you can do, and those available to help you do it. To exhaust the bicycle comparison, in addition to your own willingness to get on and risk a brush burn or two, the other biggest thing in learning was likely the presence of someone else who ran along beside, whether it was dad, or mom, or older brother, or the "big kid" next door; but their giving encouragement, applauding your progress, *knowing* you could do it was vital. If you've an alcohol problem in your life, though the work is yours; there *are* people to help in just the same way.

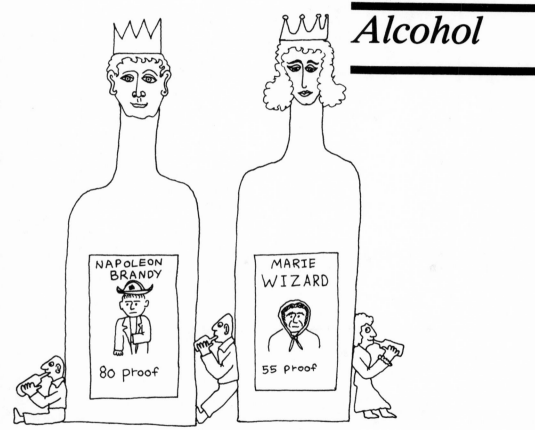

Alcohol

■ *Once upon a time . . .*

Imagine yourself in what is now Clairvoux, high in the Swiss hills. Stone pots dating from the Old Stone Age have been found that once contained a mild beer or wine. It probably was discovered very much like fire—nature plus curiosity. If any watery mixture of vegetable sugars or

*Ramses III distributed beer to
his subjects and then told
them the tingling they felt
radiated from him!*

*God made yeast, as well
as dough, and loves
fermentation just as dearly
as he loves vegetation.*

EMERSON

*Food without drink is like a
wound without a plaster.*

BRULL

starches is allowed to stand long enough in a warm place, alcohol will make itself. Say you're a caveman named Urg, coming back from a lengthier than usual flight from a dinosaur or some such thing. "Aha!" Some berries or barley left in a bowl in the sun. "Smells a bit funny, but so what! I'm thirsty and hungry and tired." Down it goes. Can you imagine what he thought as his first booze went down?

No one knows what kind of liquor was first, wine or beer or mead; but by the Neolithic Age, it was *everywhere*. Tales of the origin of liquor abound in the folklore. One legend relates that at the beginning of time the forces of good and evil contested with each other for domination of the earth. Eventually the forces for good won out. But a great many of these forces had been killed in the process, and wherever they fell, a vine sprouted from the ground. So it seems some considered wine to be a good force. Other myths depict the powers of alcohol as gifts from the gods. Some civilizations worshiped specific gods of wine: the Egyptians' god was Osiris; the Greeks', Dionysus; the Romans', Bacchus. Wine was used in early rituals as libations (poured out on the ground or altar or whatever). Priests often drank it as part of the rituals. The Bible, too, is full of references to sacrifices including wine.

Ritual uses broadened into convivial uses, and customs developed. Alcohol was a regular part of the meals, viewed as a staple in the diet, even before ovens were invented for baking bread. The Assyrians received a daily portion from their masters of a "gallon" of bread and a gallon of fermented brew (probably a barley beer). Bread and wine were offered by the Hebrews on their successful return from battle. In Greece and Rome wine was essential at

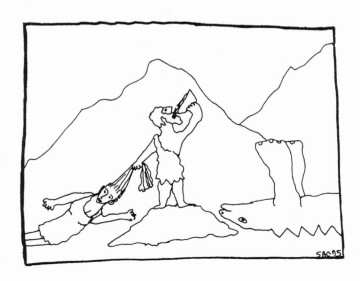

every kind of gathering. Alcohol was found to contribute to fun and games at a party; for example, the Roman orgies. Certainly its safety as opposed to water was a factor, but the effects surely had something to do with it. It's hard to imagine everyone drinking water at an orgy, or welcoming a victorious army with lemonade. By the Middle Ages alcohol use permeated everything, accompanying birth, marriage, death, the crowning of kings, diplomatic exchanges, signing treaties, and councils. The monasteries became the taverns and inns of the times, and travelers received the benefit of the grape.

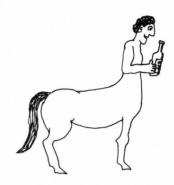

The ancients had figured that what was good in these instances might be good in others, and alcohol came into use as a medicine. It was an antiseptic and an anesthetic and was used in combinations to form salves and tonics. As a cure it ran the gamut from black jaundice to pain in the knee and hiccups. St. Paul advised Timothy, "No longer drink only water, but use a little wine for the sake of your stomach and your frequent ailments." Liquor was a recognized mood changer, nature's tranquilizer. The biblical King Lemuel's mother advises, "give wine to them that be of heavy hearts." The Bible also refers to wine as stimulating and cheering. "Praise to God, that he hath brought forth fruit out of the earth, and wine that maketh glad the heart of man."

■ *Fermentation and discovery of distillation*

Nature alone cannot produce stronger stuff than 14% alcohol. Fermentation is a combustive action of yeasts on plants: potatoes, fruit, grain, and so on. The sugar is exposed to wild yeasts in the air or commercial yeasts, which produce an enzyme, which in turn converts sugar into alcohol. Fermentive yeast cannot survive in solutions stronger than 14% alcohol. When that level is reached, the yeast, which is a living thing, ceases to produce and dies.

Now imagine the widespread joy when something stronger came along. In the tenth century an Arabian physician, Rhazes, discovered distilled spirits. Actually, he was looking for a way to release "the spirit of the wine." It was welcomed at the time as the "true water of life." European scientists rejoiced in their long-sought "philosopher's stone," or perfect element. A mystique developed, and alcohol was called "the fountain of youth," "eau-de-vie," "aqua vitae." *Usequebaugh* from the Gaelic *usige beath*, meaning breath of life, is the source of the word "whiskey." The word alcohol itself is derived from the Arabic *al kohl*. It originally referred to a fine powder of antimony used for staining the eyelids and gives rise to speculation on the ex-

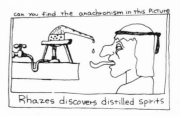

can you find the anachronism in this picture

Rhazes discovers distilled spirits

pression, "Here's mud in your eye!" The word evolved to describe any finely ground substance, then the essence of a thing, and eventually came to mean, "finely divided spirit," or the essential spirit of the wine. Nineteenth-century temperance advocates tried to prove that alcohol is derived from the Arabic *alghul*, meaning ghost or evil spirit.

Distilled liquor was not a popular drink until about the sixteenth century. Before that it was used as *the* basic medicine and cure for all human ailments. Distillation is a simple process that can produce an alcohol content of nearly 93% if it is refined sufficiently. Remember, nature stops at 14%. Start with a fermented brew. When it is boiled, the alcohol separates from the juice or whatever as steam. Alcohol boils at a lower temperature than the other liquid. The escaping steam is caught in a cooling tube and turns into a liquid again, leaving the juice or water behind. Voilà! Stronger stuff, about 50% alcohol!

Proof as a way of measuring the strength of a given liquor came from a practice used by the early settlers of this country to test their brews. They saturated gunpowder with alcohol and ignited it: too strong, it flared up; too weak, it sputtered. A strong blue flame was considered the sign of proper strength. Almost straight alcohol was diluted with water to gain the desired flame. Half and half was considered 100 proof. Thus, 86-proof bourbon is 43% alcohol. Since alcohol dilutes itself with water from the air, 200-proof, or 100%, alcohol is not possible. United States standards for spirits are between 195 and 198 proof.

▪ *Alcohol use in the New World*

Alcohol had come to America in company with the explorers and colonists. In 1620, the *Mayflower* crew decided to land at Plymouth because, it says in the ship's log, "We could not now take time for further search or consideration, our victuals having been much spent, especially our bere. . . ." The Spanish missionaries brought grapevines to the New World, and before the United States was yet a nation, there was winemaking in California. The Dutch opened the first distillery on Staten Island in 1640. In the Massachusetts Bay Colony brewing ranked next in importance after milling and baking. The Puritans did not disdain the use of alcohol as is sometimes supposed. A federal law passed in 1790 gave provisions for each soldier to receive a ration of one-fourth pint of brandy, rum, or whiskey. The colonists imported wine and malt beverages and planted vineyards, but it was Jamaican rum that became the answer to the thirst of the new nation. For its sake, New Englanders became the bankers of the slave

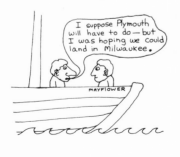

I suppose Plymouth will have to do — but I was hoping we could land in Milwaukee.

trade that supplied the molasses needed to produce it. Eventually whiskey, the backwoods substitute for rum introduced to America by Irish and Scots settlers in Kentucky, West Virginia, and Maryland, superseded rum in popularity. Sour-mash bourbon became the great American drink.

This is a very brief view of alcohol's history. The extent of its uses, the ways in which it has been viewed, and even the amount of writing about it that survives give witness to the value placed on this strange substance. It has been everywhere, connected to everything that is a part of everyday life. Growing the grapes or grains to produce it is even suspected as the reason for the development of agriculture. Whether making it, using it as a medicine, drinking it, or writing about it, people from early times have devoted a lot of time and energy to alcohol.

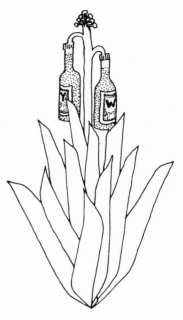

■ *Why bother?*

So alcohol happened, why didn't it go the way of the dinosaurs?

Think about the first time *you* ever tasted alcohol. Some people were exposed very early and do not remember the experience of having a little sherry in their bottle, or rubbed on their gums when they were teething. Some were allowed a taste of Dad's beer or the Christmas Day champagne at a tender age. Some sneaked sips at the first big wedding or party they were around. Some never even saw it until junior or senior high school. Still others were taught from infancy that it was evil and may not have touched it until college or the army took them away from home. And there are some, who for one reason or another, have never touched the stuff. If you are in the majority, however, you probably encountered it in a variation on one of the above themes.

Maybe you didn't like that first sip of Dad's beer or Aunt Tillie's sherry. Rather than admit it, you decided they must know what was good. So you took a sip every time it was offered. *"As you're fighting your way to the top, it helps to have a taste of what's up there."*

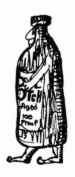

Or perhaps you were around for the preparations for a big do at your house. Ice, soda, and funny-colored stuff in big bottles were lined up with neat things like cherries, oranges, lemons, and sugar. The atmosphere was busy and exciting. When the guests began to arrive, the first thing they got was something from those bottles. Everyone seemed to talk and laugh quite a bit, and after awhile no one seemed to see you. Mom left her drink in the kitchen while she served some of those tasty cheese things she let you try earlier. One quick sip. *"To keep the party going, keep the best on hand."*

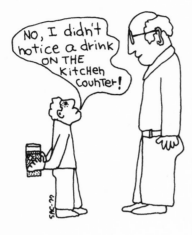

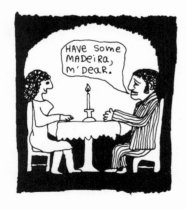

Perhaps people in your home drank on weekends, but not you. Mom and Dad said things like, "When you're of age" or "Wouldn't want to stunt your growth" or "This is a big people's drink." Anyway, you weren't getting any tastes. Somewhere along the school trail, you wound up at a party you'd expected to be like all the others you'd been to. Not this time. Someone brought some beer, and everyone else was having some. There might have been a brief flash of guilt when you thought of the folks, but who wants to stick out in a crowd? So you kept up with the gang. Soon you felt as grown-up as you'd ever be. *"On your night of nights, add that sophisticated touch."*

Or perhaps your folks never touched the stuff. They were really opposed to alcohol. They gave you lots of reasons: "It's evil," "People who drink get into terrible trouble," "Vile stuff, it just eats you up," or even, "God's against it." Well, you admired your folks, or were scared of them, or you really believed the part about God's stand. And, anyway, no one pushed you too much. Then came the army or college. It seemed as though everyone drank something, sometime, somewhere. They weren't dropping dead at the first sip, or getting into too much trouble that you could see. Even if there was a little trouble, someone said, "Oh, well, he/she was just drunk, sowing some wild oats." Lightning didn't strike. You didn't see the devil popping out of glasses. Just the opposite, most of your friends seemed to be having a lot of fun. *"When the gang gets together. . . ."* Bowling, fishing, sailing, hiking, beaching, everywhere.

It could be that you grew up with wine being served at meals. At some time you were initiated into the process as a matter of course. You never gave it a second thought.

You might have had a religious background that introduced you to wine as a part of your ritual acceptance into manhood or as a part of your particular church's worship.

With time, age, and social mobility, the reasons for continuing to drink become more complex. It's not unusual to drink a bit more than one can handle at some point. After one experience of being drunk, and/or sick, and/or hung over, some people decide never to touch the stuff again. But for most, something they are getting or think they are getting out of alcohol makes them try it again. Despite liquor's real effects on us, most of us search for an experience we have had with it, or want to have with it, or have been led to believe that we can have with its use. *"As an essential part of the Good Life,_____cannot be excelled."*

Theories to explain alcohol use

The theories advanced to explain the basic why behind drinking alcohol probably all contain some truth. *To escape anxiety*—''It calms me down, helps my nerves.'' ''It helps me unwind after a hard day.'' *The need for a feeling of power* over oneself or one's environment. Most people don't talk about the latter, but take a look at the heavy reliance of the liquor industry on he-man models, executive types, and beautiful women surrounded by adoring males. People in ads celebrate winning anything with a drink of some sort.

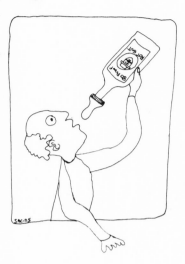

The anxiety thesis developed from Freud's work. He concluded that in times of anxiety and stress, people fall back on things that have worked for them in the past. In theory, the things you will choose to relieve anxiety are those you did when you last felt most secure. That neat, secure time might last have been at Mom's breast. It's been downhill ever since. In this case, use of the mouth (eating, smoking, drinking) would be chosen to ease stressful situations. This phenomenon is called *oral fixation*. Another version of the anxiety thesis comes from anthropological studies. It was observed that alcohol was used by primitive societies either ritually or socially to relieve the anxiety caused by an unstable environment. Drunken acts are acceptable and not punished. The greater the environmental stress, the heavier the drinking. Therefore, in this view, alcohol's anxiety-reducing property is the one universal key to why people drink alcohol. This theory has by and large been rejected as the sole reason for drinking.

Nonetheless, in our society today, feelings of uneasiness or pressure are often relieved by the business lunch, the cocktail party, etc. Seldon Bacon, head of the Rutgers School of Alcohol Studies, has explored this idea. He describes the original needs that alcohol might have served: satisfaction of hunger and thirst, medication or anesthetic, fostering of religious ecstasy. He maintains that modern, complex society has virtually eliminated these functions. All that is left is alcohol the depressant, the reliever of tension, inhibition, and guilt. Contemporary society, by cre-

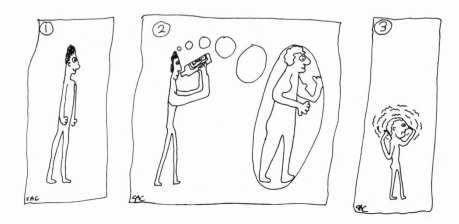

ating more and better tensions, has invented new needs that alcohol can meet.

The power theory was developed by researchers in the early 1970s, who explored folktales from both heavy- and light-drinking societies. They discovered that there was no greater concern with relief from tension or anxiety in heavy-drinking societies than in those that consumed less. To look at this further, they conducted a study with college men over a period of ten years. Without revealing the reasons for the study, they asked the students to write down their fantasies before, during, and after the consumption of liquor. The stories revealed that the students felt bigger, stronger, more influential, more aggressive, and more capable of great sexual conquest the more they drank. The conclusion was that people drink to experience a feeling of power. This power feeling was seen as having two different patterns, depending on the personality of the drinker. What was called *p-power* is a personal powerfulness, uninhibited and carried out at the expense of others; *s-power*, or social power, is a more altruistic powerfulness, power to help others. Social-power was found to predominate after two or three drinks; heavier drinking produced a predominance of p-power.

Another theory that has popped up from time to time is gaining in popularity. This thesis claims that every human being has some need to reach out toward some larger experience. People will try anything that suggests itself as a way to do that: alcohol, drugs, yoga, meditation, whatever. Some drugs are commonly known to "blow your mind" or are even designated as "mind-expanding drugs." Evidence cited for the seeking of altered states of consciousness begins with very young children who whirl, hyperventilate, and so on, to produce a change in their experience. When older, people learn that chemicals can produce different states. In pursuit of these states, alcohol is often used because it is the one intoxicant we make legally available. The drug scene is another answer to the same search. The drug scene also claims "better" highs. Purportedly this search arises from the "innate psychological drive arising out of the neurological structure of the human brain." In this view, we have put the cart before the horse in focusing attention on drugs, rather than on the states people seek from them. Thus, it is suggested society recognize the need itself and cope with it in a positive rather than a negative way.

The literature abounds with proponents of one or the other theory citing examples and experiments to prove their points. Indeed, there are instances when any theory fits like a glove. An inescapable fact is that from the very earliest recorded times, alcohol has been important to people.

*Absinthe makes the heart
grow fonder.*

ADDISON MIZNER

Myths are equally important to people. There are many who think alcohol makes them warm when they are cold (not so), sexier (in the courting, maybe; in the execution, not so), manlier, womanlier, cured of their ills (not usually), less scared of people (possibly), and better able to function (only if very little is taken). An exercise that asks many people what a drink does for them will expose a heavy reliance on myths for their "reasons."

Whatever the truth in the mixture of theory and myth, enough people in this country rely on the use of alcohol to accomplish *something* for them to support a $50 billion-a-year industry.

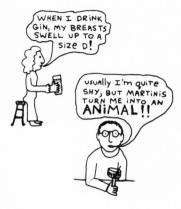

■ *Alcohol problems: the fly in the ointment*

Alcohol is many faceted. With its ritual, medicinal, dietary, and pleasurable uses, alcohol can leave in its wake confusion, pain, disorder, and tragedy. The use and abuse of alcohol has gone hand in hand in all cultures. With the notable exceptions of the Moslems and Buddhists, whose religions forbid drinking, temperance and abstinence have been the exception rather than the rule in most of the world.

Societies have come to grips with alcohol problems in a variety of ways. One of these regards drunkenness as a sin, a moral failing, and the drunk as a moral weakling of some kind. The Greek word for drunk, for example, means literally to "misbehave at the wine." An Egyptian writer admonished his friend with the slightly contemptuous "thou art like a little child." Noah, who undoubtedly had reason to seek relief in drunkenness after getting all those creatures safely through the flood, was not looked on kindly by his children as he lay in his drunken stupor. The complaints have continued through time. A Dutch physician of the sixteenth century criticized the heavy use of alcohol in Germany and Flanders by saying "that freelier than is profitable to health, they take it and drink it." Some of the most forceful sanctions have come from the temperance movements. An early temperance leader wrote that "alcohol is preeminently a destroyer in every department of life." As late as March 1974, the New Hampshire Christian Civic League devoted an entire issue of its monthly newspaper to a polemic against the idea that alcoholism is a disease. In their view the disease concept gives reprieve to the "odious alcohol sinner."

Others see the use of liquor as a legislative issue and believe the problem can be solved by laws. Total prohibition is one of the methods used by those who believe that legislation can sober people up. Most legal approaches through history have been piecemeal affairs invoked to deal with specific situations. Excessive drinking was so rampant in

Wine prepares the heart for love, unless you take too much.

OVID

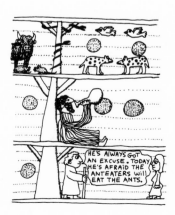

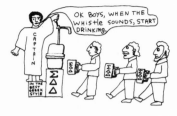

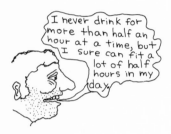

ancient Greece that "drinking captains" were appointed to supervise drinking. Elaborate rules were devised for drinking at parties. A perennial favorite has been control of supply. In A.D. 81, a Roman emperor ordered the destruction of half the British vineyards.

The sinful and legal views of drunkenness often go hand in hand. They have as a common denominator the idea that the drunk chooses to be drunk and is therefore either a sinner or a ne'er-do-well who can be handled by making drinking illegal. In 1606 intoxication was made a statutory offense in England by an "Act for Repressing the Odious and Loathsome Sin of Drunkenness." In the reign of Charles I, laws were passed to suppress liquor altogether. Settling a new world did not dispense with the problems of alcohol use. The traditional methods of dealing with these problems continued. From around 1600 to the 1800s attitudes toward alcohol were low-keyed. There were laws passed in various colonies and states to deal with liquor use, such as an early Connecticut law forbidding drinking for more than half an hour at a time. Another in Virginia in 1760 prohibited ministers from "drinking to excess and inciting riot." But there were no temperance societies, no large-scale prohibitions, no religious bodies fighting.

America's response to alcohol problems

Drinking in the colonies was largely a family affair and remained so until the beginning of the nineteenth century. With increasing immigration, industrialization, and greater social freedoms, drinking became less a family affair. The abuse of alcohol became more open and more de-

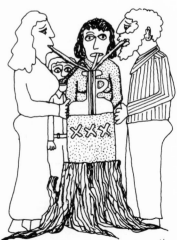

THE FAMily ThaT Imbibes together HAS GooD vibes Together.

structive. The opening of the West brought the saloon into prominence. The old and stable social and family patterns began to change. The frontier hero took to gulping his drinks with his foot on the bar rail. Attitudes began to intensify regarding the use of alcohol.

These developments hold the key to many modern attitudes toward alcohol, the stigma of alcoholism, the wet-dry controversy. Ways of looking at alcohol began to polarize America. The legal and moral approaches reached their apex in the United States with the growth of the temperance movement and the Prohibition Amendment in 1919.

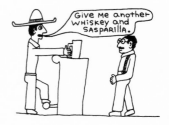

The temperance movement and Prohibition. The traditional American temperance movement did not begin as a prohibition movement. The temperance movement coincided with the rise of social consciousness, a belief in the efficacy of law to resolve human problems. It was part and parcel of the humanitarian movement, which included child labor and prison reform, women's rights, abolition, and social welfare and poverty legislation. It originally condemned only excessive drinking and the drinking of distilled liquor, *not all liquor or all drinking.* It was believed that the evils connected with the abuse of alcohol could be remedied through proper legislation. The aims of the original temperance movement were largely moral, uplifting, rehabilitative. Passions grow, however, and before long those who had condemned only the excess use of distilled liquor were condemning all liquor. Those genial, well-meaning doctors, businessmen, and farmers began to organize their social life around their crusade. Fraternal orders, such as the Independent Order of Good Templars of 1850, grew and proliferated. In a short span of time it had branches all over the United States, with churches, missions, and hospitals, all dedicated to the idea that society's evils were caused by liquor. This particular group influenced the growth of the Women's Christian Temperance Union and the Anti-Saloon League. By 1869 it had become The National Prohibition Party, which was the spearhead of political action. It advocated complete suppression of liquor by law.

People who had no experience at all of drinking got involved in the crusade. In 1874 Frances Willard founded the WCTU in Cleveland. Women became interested in the movement, which simultaneously advocated social reform,

All excess is ill, but drunkenness is of the worst sort.

WILLIAM PENN

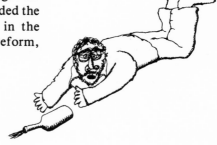

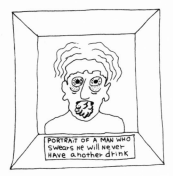

PORTRAIT OF A MAN WHO swears He will Never Have another drink

The front door of the Boston Licensing Board was ripped down by the crush to get beer licenses the day Prohibition ended.

prayer, prevention, education, and legislation in the field of alcohol misuse. Mass meetings were organized to which thousands came. Journals were published; children's programs taught fear and hatred of alcohol; libraries developed. The WCTU was responsible for the first laws requiring alcohol education in the schools, some of which remain on the books. All alcohol use—moderate, light, heavy, excessive—was condemned. All users were one and the same. Bacon, in describing the classic temperance movement, says there was "one word for the action—DRINK. One word for the category of people—DRINKER."

By 1895, many smaller local groups had joined the Anti-Saloon League, which had become the most influential of the temperance groups. It was nonpartisan politically and supported any candidate who was Prohibitionist. It pressured Congress and state legislatures and was backed by church groups in "action against the saloon." Political pressure mounted. The major thrust of all these activities was that the only real problem was alcohol, the only real solution, Prohibition. In 1919 Congress passed the Eighteenth Amendment, making it illegal to manufacture or sell alcoholic beverages. The Volstead Act had sixty provisions to implement Prohibition. The act was a messy and complicated affair. There was no precedent to force the public cooperation required to make the act work. From 1920 to 1933 Prohibition remained in effect. Prohibition shaped much of our economic, social, and underground life. The repeal under the Twenty-first Amendment in 1933 did not remedy the situation. Prohibition had failed. The real problems created by alcohol were obscured or ignored by the false wet-dry controversy. The quarrel raged between the manufacturers, retailers, and consumers on one side and the temperance people, many churches, and women on the other. Alcoholics and those with alcohol problems were ignored in the furor. When Prohibition was repealed the problem of abuse was still there, and the alcoholics were still there along with the stigma of alcoholism.

Another approach to alcohol problems is that of the "ostrich." The ostrich stance became popular after the failure of Prohibition and is still fashionable today. Problems are often handled with euphemisms, humor, ridicule, and delegation of responsibility, arising from conflicting values and beliefs. Our inconsistent attitudes toward alcohol are reinforced in subtle ways. For example, look at the hard-drinking movie heroes. There's the guy who drinks and drinks and then calls for more, never gets drunk, outdrinks the bad guys, kills off the rustlers, and gets the girl in the end. Then there's Humphrey Bogart, who is a drunken mess wallowing in the suffering of mankind until the pure and beautiful heroine appears, at which point he washes up, shaves, gets a new suit, and they live happily ever after.

Drunkenness versus alcoholism

It is important to see that alcoholism is not separate from alcohol. The alcoholic does not spring full-blown from some place in outer space. In general it is a problem that develops over time. Alcohol is available everywhere. A person really has to make a choice *not* to drink in our society. In some sets of circumstances one could drink for the better part of a day and never seem out of place at all. Some brunches have wine punch, Bloody Marys, or café brulet as their accompaniment. Sherry, beer, or a mixed drink is quite appropriate at lunchtime. Helping a friend with an afternoon painting project or even raking your own lawn is a reasonable time to have a beer. Then, after a long day comes the predinner cocktail, maybe some wine with the meal. Later, at cards with friends, drinks are offered. And surely, some romantic candlelight and a nightcap go hand in hand. For most people this combination of events would not be their daily or even weekend fare. The point is that none of the above would cause most people to raise an eyebrow. The accepted times of drinking can be all the time, anywhere. Given enough of the kind of days we described, the person who chooses to drink may develop problems. Alcohol is a drug and does have effects on the body.

Is alcoholism a purely modern phenomenon, a product of our times? There are no references to alcoholics as such in historical writing. The word itself is a modern one. But there are vague references, as far back in time as the third century, that distinguish between being merely intoxicated and being a drunkard. In a commentary on imperial law, a Roman jurist of that era suggests that inveterate drunkenness be considered a medical matter rather than a legal one. In the thirteenth century, James I of Aragon issued an edict providing for hospitalization of conspicuously active drunks. In 1655 a man named Younge, an English journalist, wrote a pamphlet in which he seemed to discern the difference between one who drinks and one who has a chronic condition related to alcohol. He says, "He that will be drawn to drink when he hath neither need of it nor mind to it is a drunkard."

History of alcohol treatment efforts

The first serious considerations of the problem of inebriety, as it was called, came in the eighteenth and nineteenth centuries. Two famous writings addressed the problem in what seemed to be a new light. Although their work on the physical aspects of alcohol became fodder for the temper-

When you ask one friend to dine,
Give him your best wine!
When you ask two,
The second best will do!

LONGFELLOW

*Wine is a bad thing.
It makes you quarrel with
    your neighbor,
It makes you shoot at your
    landlord,
It makes you—*miss *him.*

ance zealots, both Dr. Benjamin Rush and Dr. Thomas Trotter seriously considered the effects of alcohol in a scientific way. Rush, a signer of the Declaration of Independence and a surgeon general of the Army, wrote a lengthy treatise with an equally lengthy title, "An Inquiry into the Effects of Ardent Spirits on the Human Body and Mind, with an Account of the Means of Preventing and the Remedies of Curing Them." Rush's book is a compendium of the attitudes of the time, given weight by scholarly treatment. The more important of the two, and the first scientific formulation of drunkenness on record, is the classic work of Trotter, an Edinburgh physician. In 1804 he wrote "An Essay, Medical, Philosophical, and Chemical, on Drunkenness and Its Effects on the Human Body." He states: "In the writings of medicine, we find drunkenness only cursorily mentioned among the powers that injure health. . . . The priesthood hath poured forth its anathemas from the pulpit; and the moralist, no less severe, hath declaimed against it as a vice degrading to our nature." He then gets down to the nitty-gritty of the matter: "In medical language, I consider drunkenness, strictly speaking, to be a disease, produced by a remote cause, and giving birth to actions and movements in the living body that disorder the functions of health."

Trotter did not gain many adherents to his position, but small efforts were also being made in the United States at the time. Around the 1830s, in Massachusetts, Connecticut, and New York, small groups were forming to reform "intemperate persons" by hospitalizing them, instead of sending them to jail or the workhouse. The new groups, started by the medical superintendent of Worcester, Massachusetts, Dr. Samuel Woodward, and a Dr. Eli Todd, did not see inebriates in the same class with criminals, the indigent, or the insane. Between 1841 and 1874 eleven nonprofit hospitals and houses were set up. In 1876 the *Journal of Inebriety* started publication to advance their views and findings. These efforts were taking place against the background of the temperance movement. Naturally, there was tremendous popular opposition from both the church and the legislative halls. The *Journal* was not prestigious by the standards of the medical journals of that time, and before Prohibition the hospitals were closed and the *Journal* had folded.

There was also another group that briefly flourished. The Washington Temperance Society began in Chase's Tavern in Baltimore in 1840. Six drinking buddies were the founders, and they each agreed to bring a friend to the next meeting. In a few months parades and public meetings were being held to spread the message: "Drunkard! Come up here! You can reform. We don't slight the drunkard.

We love him!'' At the peak of its success in 1844, the membership consisted of 100,000 "reformed common drunkards" and 300,000 "common tipplers." A women's auxiliary group, the Martha Washington Society, was dedicated to feeding and clothing the poor. Based on the promise of religious salvation, the Washington Temperance Society was organized in much the same way as the ordinary temperance groups. There was this difference, however. It was founded on the basis of one drunkard helping another, of drunks telling their story in public. The society prospered all over the East Coast as far north as New Hampshire. A hospital, the Home for the Fallen, was established in Boston and still exists under a different name. There are many similarities between the Washington Society and Alcoholics Anonymous: alcoholics helping each other, regular meetings, sharing experiences, fellowship, reliance on a Higher Power, and total abstention from alcohol. The society was, however, caught up in the frenzies of the total temperance movement: the controversies, power struggles, religious fights, and ego trips of the leaders. By 1848, eight short years after its founding, it was absorbed into the total prohibition movement. The treatment of the alcoholic became unimportant in the heat of the argument.

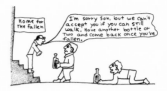

Recognition of the alcoholic as a sick person did not re-emerge until comparatively recently. The gathering of a group of scientists at Yale's Laboratory of Applied Psychology (later the Laboratory of Applied Biodynamics) and the Fellowship of Alcoholics Anonymous, both begun in the 1930s, were instrumental in bringing this about. It was also in the 1930s that a recovered Bostonian alcoholic, Richard Peabody, first began to apply psychological methods to the cure of alcoholics. He replaced the terms drunk and drunkenness with the more scientific and less judgmental alcoholic and alcoholism. At Yale, Yandell Henderson, Howard Haggard, Leon Greenberg, and later E. M. Jellinek founded the *Quarterly Journal of Studies on Alcohol* (since 1975 known as the *Journal of Studies on Alcohol*). Unlike the earlier *Journal of Inebriety*, the *QJSA* had a sound scientific footing and became the mouthpiece for alcohol information. Starting with Haggard's work on alcohol metabolism, these efforts marked the first attempt to put the study of alcohol and alcohol problems in a respectable up-to-date framework. Jellinek's masterwork, *The Disease Concept of Alcoholism*, was a product of the Yale experience. The Yale Center of Alcohol Studies and the Classified Abstract Archive of Alcohol Literature were established. The Yale Plan Clinic was also set up to diagnose and treat alcoholism. The Yale Summer School of Alcohol Studies, now the Rutgers School, educated professionals and laypeople from all walks of life.

Yale's prestigious influence had far-reaching effects. The National Council on Alcoholism, a volunteer organization, also grew out of the Yale School. It was founded in 1944 by the joint efforts of Jellinek and Marty Mann, a recovered alcoholic and the NCA's first president, to provide public information and education about alcohol.

On the other side of the coin, the Fellowship of Alcoholics Anonymous was having more success in treating alcoholics than any other group. AA grew, and in 1981 it estimated a membership of one million in both America and abroad. Its members became influential in removing the stigma that had been so long attached to the alcoholic. Lawyers, business people, teachers, people from every sector of society began to recover. They could be seen leading useful, normal lives without alcohol. (More will be said later on the origins and program of AA itself.) The successful recoveries of its members have unquestionably influenced the course of recent developments.

New attitudes

The new attitudes toward alcoholism have become the foundation for public policy. Since 1960 alcoholism has been gaining recognition by the federal government as a major public health problem. At the center of the federal efforts is the National Institute of Alcohol Abuse and Alcoholism, the NIAAA, established in 1971. The NIAAA sponsors research, training, public education, and treatment programs. The legislation creating NIAAA is a landmark in the history of society's responses to alcoholism. This bill, The Comprehensive Alcohol Abuse and Alcoholism Prevention, Treatment, and Rehabilitation Act of 1970, is also known as the Hughes Act. Its sponsor was former Senator Harold Hughes, himself a recovering alcoholic. It establishes what might be called a bill of rights for alcoholic individuals. It recognizes that they suffer from a "disease that requires treatment"; it provides protection against discrimination in hiring former alcoholic patients. In a similar vein, the Uniform Alcoholism and Intoxication Treatment Act dealing with public intoxication has been recommended for enactment by the states. This act mandates treatment rather than punishment. These acts incorporate the new attitudes emerging toward alcoholics and alcohol abuse: it is a problem; it is treatable.

On the heels of this, there has been a rapid increase during the 1970s in alcoholism treatment services, both public and private, both residential and outpatient. For example, each state has mandated alcohol (and drug abuse) services that focus on public information and education as well as treatment. Similarly, community mental health centers that receive federal support are required to provide alcohol services. Although not yet totally transformed, health insurance coverage more frequently is including rather than excluding alcoholism treatment for its subscribers.

With this increase in alcohol services, there has developed a new profession, the *alcohol counselor*, as the backbone for alcohol treatment. Education for all professionals involved with alcoholism has gained attention, with a proliferation of workshops, special conferences, and also courses to prepare counselors and other professionals. Marking the emergence of this new health care field, there have also been efforts to develop standards for the treatment personnel and alcohol treatment agencies. In many states, alcohol counselors' associations have been formed. In some instances these groups certify alcohol counselors; and in others, as the result of lobbying efforts, state licensure boards have been established. In sum, these efforts have resulted from and contributed to our society's response to alcohol problems as a major public health issue.

▪ *Alcohol costs—paying the piper*

In the United States, statistics on who drinks, what, where, and when have been kept since 1850. However, making comparisons between different historical periods is difficult. One reason is that statistics have only been gathered methodically and impartially since 1950. Another reason is that there have been changes in the way the basic information is organized and reported. A century ago, reports included numbers of "inebriates" or "drunkards." In the 1940s through the 1960s, "alcoholics" were often a designated subgroup. Then came the 1970s and another change. "Heavy drinkers" or "heavy drinkers with a high problem index" began to replace "alcoholics" as a category in reporting statistical information. Most recently "alcohol dependence syndrome" has emerged as another category. So the task of identifying changes in drinking practices is not an easy one.

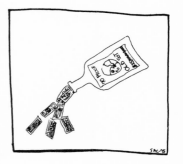

Who drinks what, when, and where

Nonetheless, among the maze of statistics available on how much Americans drink, where they drink it, and with what consequences, some are important to note. It is estimated that over three fourths, or 77%, of men and 60% of women drink alcohol. They comprise 68% of the adult population.

Per capita consumption has been on the rise. During the 1960s there was a 32% increase. In the early 1970s there was a leveling off, but per capita consumption is again on the upswing, having increased 5% between 1976 and 1978. In 1978 the statistically average American consumed the

There were roughly 100 beer cans per man, woman, and child manufactured in the United States in 1972.

equivalent of 2.82 gallons of ethanol. The "average" American drinks 2.6 gallons of liquor, 2.5 gallons of wine, and 26.6 gallons of beer. Since the alcohol content of each varies in terms of absolute alcohol, 39% of the alcohol comes from hard stuff, 12% from wine, and 49% from beer.

How does alcohol use in the United States compare to that of other countries? *The President's Task Force Report: Drunkenness for 1967* reported that the United States had the second highest rate of alcoholism in the world. France was then ranked first. (More recent figures are not available for comparison, because "alcoholics" have given way to "problem drinkers.") Among industrial countries, the United States then ranked eighth in per capita consumption for all categories of alcohol, but was second in distilled spirits. Ten years later (1976) the U.S. position had dropped from eighth to fifteenth out of a group of twenty-six industrial countries, in total alcohol consumption, although it fell to only third for distilled spirits. This change does not reflect a decline in U.S. drinking, but represents a more rapid increase in other countries.

A word of caution: all of the above figures describe the statistically average American, but it is important to realize that the "average" American is a myth. The typical American does not in fact drink his or her "statistical quota." First of all, recall that approximately one third do not use alcohol at all. And for the remaining two thirds there is wide variation in alcohol use. Seventy percent of the drinking population consumes only 20% of all the alcohol. The remaining 30% of the drinkers consume 80% of the alcohol. Most significantly it is one third of that 30% (or less than 7% of the total population) that consumes 50% of all alcohol.

Presently it is estimated that 7% of the total adult population of 145 million are problem drinkers. (This 7% figure is derived not from consumption figures but rather from the presence of problems attending to alcohol use. But the coincidence is striking!) There are also an estimated 3.3 million adolescents in the 14- to 17-year age range who have a serious drinking problem. The United States thus has an estimated 13.3 million persons with drinking problems. It is also estimated that for every person with an alcohol problem, four family members are directly affected. So approximately 53.3 million family members are touched by alcohol problems. A 1978 Gallup Poll found one person in four (24%) of those interviewed saying an alcohol problem had adversely affected his or her family life. This was twice the proportion that had reported alcohol as a cause of family problems just 4 years earlier. Note that these figures do not distinguish alcoholics from those who are nonalcoholic and abuse alcohol.

These nonalcoholic drinkers include the one-time drunken traffic offender who appears in court; the person who, when drunk for the one and only time in his life, puts his foot through a window and ends up in a hospital emergency room; and those who miss work after a particularly festive New Year's Eve. The alcohol abuser, though costly and troublesome, is not usually a habitual offender. The alcoholic tends to be.

In the alcoholic population itself only 5% are on skid row. At least 95% of problem drinkers are employed or employable; they make up 5% of the nation's work force and perhaps 10% of the executives. Most of them are living with their families. The vast majority live in respectable neighborhoods, are housewives, bankers, doctors, salespeople, farmers, teachers, clergy, and so forth. They try to raise decent children, go to football games, shop for their groceries, go to work, and rake the leaves. According to a 1974 survey, the highest percentage of problem drinkers live in the Northeast, Middle Atlantic, or Pacific Coast states. They are mostly males. However, the percentage of women problem drinkers is on the rise. This is frequently attributed to increased drinking among women and to less protection of the woman alcoholic. A high proportion of problem drinkers are unmarried or divorced, live in large cities, and are both the least and the most educated part of the population.

Economic costs

Although they are only a small portion of the drinking population, in combination both the alcohol abuser and the alcoholic cost the United States a huge amount of time and money each year. Following is a breakdown of the economic costs of alcohol misuse and alcoholism for 1975.

	Billions of dollars
Lost production	$19.64
Health and medical	12.74
Motor vehicle accidents	5.15
Violent crime	2.86
Social responses	1.94*
Fire losses	0.43
TOTAL	$42.75

*Includes the money spent on alcohol treatment, which comes to 2% of the total $42 + billion.

The other side of the cost coin is economic revenues. The total tax revenues on alcohol raised by federal and state authorities amounts to $10 billion. Interestingly, however, the federal tax rates on alcohol have not been raised since 1951. Alcohol, at least distilled spirits, is in fact a true bargain. With inflation, the consumer price index rose 42% during the 1970s, but liquor prices went up only 12%. The result was that the "average American" was able to drink more, for less money. Although per capita consumption went up, the proportion of income spent on alcohol declined, from about 5% of the family budget in the late 1960s to a little over 2% in 1977.

Personal costs

The personal cost of alcoholism is tremendous. An alcoholic's life expectancy is shortened by 10 to 12 years. Their mortality rate is two and a half times greater than that of nonalcoholics. In 1978, it was estimated alcohol-related deaths may run as high as 11% of all deaths each year. They have a higher rate of violent deaths. Alcohol use figures prominently in accidental death and violent death for alcoholics and nonalcoholics. Alcohol is the significant factor in approximately 50% of all motor vehicle fatalities. In fatal accidents involving pedestrians, as many as 40 to 50% of pedestrians and/or drivers had blood alcohol levels of 0.10%, the usual legal standard for intoxication. In fire-related deaths, alcohol is involved in up to 83% of all cases. Alcohol is believed to be involved in approximately 50% of home accidents, about 70% of all drownings, and 40% of all fatal industrial accidents. Alcohol plays a significant role in suicide. Studies indicate that in up to 65% of all suicide attempts, the individual had been drinking, and that 35 to 40% of all successful suicides are alcohol related. Half of all successful suicides are persons who were alcoholic.

Alcohol use is a significant factor in homicide and family violence. In as many as 50% of all homicides either the victim or the assailant, or both had been drinking. Similarly, drinking is seen as a precipitating factor in child abuse, spouse beatings, and other family disruptions. Although the data on family violence remain limited, the role of intoxication varies from 30% to over 70%, depending on the particular population studied.

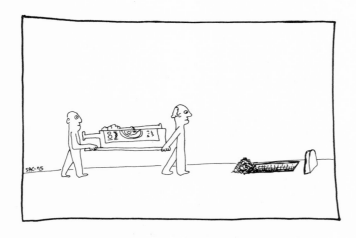

Crime and alcohol

Alcohol is also reflected in the crime statistics. As noted above, drinking is implicated in half of all homicides, and is believed to figure prominently in assaults and family violence. One half of all North American police officers killed while on duty in the mid-1970s were killed in the course of investigating family disputes. Alcohol is virtually a universal element in any family squabble reported to the police. In the early 1970s almost half of the yearly arrests were related to alcohol misuse. In many instances these were for public drunkenness and intoxication. However, with the decriminalization of public drunkenness in many states, this category of arrests has declined. At the same time there has been an increase in arrests for drunken driving. In sum, the most recent estimate of the total national bill for alcohol-related crimes and misdemeanors was $2.1 billion.

Health care and alcohol

Alcohol has an impact on the health care systems also. Studies have consistently shown that a minimum of 20% of all hospitalized persons have a significant alcohol problem whatever the presenting problem or admitting diagnosis is. The Veterans Administration estimates 50% of all VA hospital beds are filled by veterans with alcohol problems.

In terms of health care costs, alcohol figures prominently in our nation's annual medical bills. Medical costs of $12.8 billion annually for alcohol-related problems represent 12% of all adults' health expenditures. One large-scale study of patients' hospital costs found that a small proportion of patients, only 13%, had hospital bills equal to the remaining 87%. The only distinguishable characteristic of the "high-cost" group was not age, or sex, or economic status or ethnicity. It was that those persons were heavy drinkers and/or heavy smokers.

If one looks at the federal dollars spent on health research, alcohol is a health concern that is getting short shrift. In looking at morbidity figures, for every death attributable to cancer, $1,663 is being spent for research; for each alcohol death only $80 is expended for research. In terms of the number of persons afflicted, for each person with cancer, research expenditures amount to $209 per case. In comparison only $1 is spent on research for each case of alcoholism.

• • •

Television, radio, billboard, and magazine campaigns by the NIAAA, the National Council on Alcoholism, and other groups are designed to persuade Americans to examine the effects of drinking practices. A government survey

The habit of using ardent spirits, by men in office, has occasioned more injury to the public and more trouble to me than all other causes.

THOMAS JEFFERSON

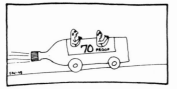

of American attitudes toward alcohol was done in 1973. It showed that 11% more persons questioned knew that alcohol is a drug in 1973 than in 1971, representing an 18% change; 13% more in 1973 than in 1971 felt that heavy drinking is a very serious problem in the country today, representing a 22% change. People are becoming aware of the toll that alcoholism and alcohol abuse can take in our public and private lives. What people will individually and collectively do with this knowledge is the question. Statistics in future years will reflect the answer.

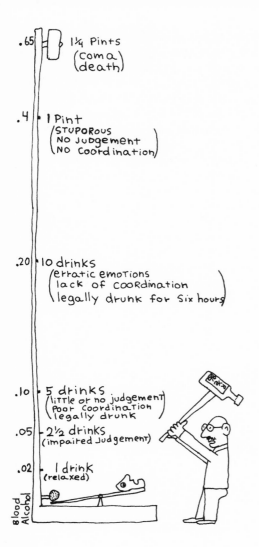

.65 — 1¼ Pints
(coma)
(death)

.4 — 1 Pint
(STUPOROUS
NO JUDGEMENT
NO coordination)

.20 — 10 drinks
(erratic emotions
lack of coordination
legally drunk for six hours)

.10 — 5 drinks
(little or no judgement)
(Poor coordination)
(legally drunk)

.05 — 2½ drinks
(impaired judgement)

.02 — 1 drink
(relaxed)

Blood Alcohol

Chapter 2

Alcohol and the body

Alcohol is a drug. When it is ingested, there are specific and predictable physiological effects on the body. Any body. Every body. Alcoholic and nonalcoholic. This is all too often overlooked. Instead, attention is paid to the physical impact of chronic use or what happens with excessive use. What gets lost are the normal, routine effects on *anyone* who uses alcohol. Let us examine what happens to alcohol in the body, how it is taken up, broken down, and thereby alters the normal functions of the body.

■ Digestion

The human body is well engineered to take the foods ingested and change them into substances the organism

<table>
<tr><td colspan="2" align="center">Calories</td></tr>
</table>

Beer, 12 oz. can	*173*
Martini, 3 oz. 3:1	*145*
olive, 1 large	*20*
Rum, 1 oz.	*73*
Sherry, sweet, 3 oz.	*150*
Fortified wines	*120–160*
Scotch, 1 oz.	*73*
cola, 8 oz.	*105*
pretzels, 5 small sticks	*20*

THE JOY OF COOKING

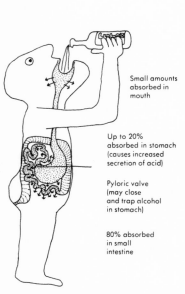

Small amounts absorbed in mouth

Up to 20% absorbed in stomach (causes increased secretion of acid)

Pyloric valve (may close and trap alcohol in stomach)

80% absorbed in small intestine

ABSORPTION OF ALCOHOL

needs to maintain life and to provide energy. Despite occasional upsets from too much spice or too much food, this process goes on without a hitch. The first part of this transformation is called digestion. A comparison might be made to the carpenter who dismantles an old building, salvages the materials, and later uses them in new construction. Digestion is the body's way of dismantling food to get the raw materials required by the body. Whether alcohol is properly termed a food was at one time a big point of controversy. Alcohol does have calories. One ounce of pure alcohol would contain 210 calories. To translate that into drinks, there are 75 calories in an ounce of whiskey or 150 calories in a 12-ounce can of beer. But alcohol's usefulness as a food is limited. Sometimes alcohol is described as providing "empty calories." It does not contain vitamins, minerals, or other essential substances. Also when alcohol is present, it interferes with the body's ability to use other sources of energy. As a food, alcohol is unique. It requires no digestion. Since alcohol is a liquid, no mechanical action by the teeth is required to break it down. And no digestive juices need be added to transform it into a form that can be absorbed by the bloodstream and transported to all parts of the body.

▪ *Absorption*

So what happens to alcohol in the body? Surprisingly, absorption of the alcohol begins almost immediately, with a very small amount being taken up into the bloodstream through the tiny capillaries in the mouth. But the majority goes the route of all food when swallowed: into the stomach. If other food is present in the stomach, the alcohol mixes with it. Here, too, some alcohol will seep into the bloodstream. Up to 20% can be absorbed directly from the stomach. The remainder passes into the small intestine to be absorbed.

The amount of food in the stomach when drinking takes place has important ramifications. Alcohol is an irritant. It increases the flow of hydrochloric acid, a digestive juice secreted by the stomach lining. Anyone who has an ulcer and takes a drink can readily confirm this. This phenomenon likewise explains the feeling of warmth in the tummy as the drink goes down. The presence of food acts to dilute the alcohol and therefore diminishes the irritant properties. The amount of food in the stomach is a big factor in determining the speed with which the alcohol is absorbed by the bloodstream. It is the rate of absorption that is largely responsible for the feelings of intoxication. In addition to the impact of food in the stomach, the rate of absorption will vary with the type of beverage. The higher the concentration of alcohol (up to 40%, or 80 proof), the more quickly it is absorbed. This partially explains why distilled spirits have more apparent "kick" than wine or beer. In addition, beer has some food substances that slow absorption. Carbon dioxide, which hastens the passage of alcohol from the stomach, has the effect of increasing the speed of absorption. Champagne, sparkling wines, or drinks mixed with carbonated soda give a sense of "bubbles in the head."

Meanwhile, on from the stomach to the pyloric valve. This valve controls the passage of the stomach's contents into the small intestine. It is sensitive to the presence of alcohol. With large concentrations of alcohol, it tends to get "stuck" in the closed position. When this pylorospasm happens, the alcohol trapped in the stomach may cause sufficient irritation and distress to induce vomiting. This phenomenon accounts for the nausea and vomiting that may accompany too much drinking. This "stuck" pylorus also may serve as a self-protective mechanism by preventing the passage into the small intestine of what might otherwise be life-threatening doses of alcohol.

■ *Blood alcohol concentration*

In considering the effects of alcohol, several questions come to mind. How much alcohol in how much person? How fast did the alcohol get there? And is the blood alcohol level rising or declining? Let's take each of these in turn. The concentration of alcohol in the blood is the first. One tablespoon of sugar mixed in a cup of water yields a much sweeter solution than a tablespoon diluted in a gallon of water. Similarly, a drink with one ounce of alcohol will give a higher blood alcohol level in a 100-pound woman than in a 200-pound man. In fact, it will be virtually twice as high. Her body contains less water than his.

The second factor is rate of absorption, which depends on the concentration of alcohol in the stomach and how rapidly it is ingested. So quickly drink a scotch on the rocks on an empty stomach, and you will probably be more giddy than if you drink more alcohol more slowly, say in the form of beer after a meal. Even with a given blood alcohol level, there is greater impairment the faster the level has been achieved. Impairment is based on both the amount absorbed and the rate of absorption. Finally, for any drinking occasion, there are different effects depending on whether the blood alcohol level is going up or coming down.

Once in the small intestine, the remainder of the alcohol (at least 80%) is very rapidly absorbed by the bloodstream. The bloodstream is the body's transportation system. It delivers nutrients the cells require for energy and picks up the wastes produced by cell metabolism. Thus alcohol diluted in the bloodstream is carried to all parts of the body.

Although *blood* alcohol levels are almost universally used as the measure of alcohol in the body, this isn't to imply that alcohol merely rides around in the bloodstream until the liver is able to break it down. Alcohol is highly soluble in water. It is able to pass through cell walls. Therefore it is distributed uniformly throughout the water content of all body tissues and cells. For a given blood alcohol level, the alcohol content in the tissues and cells varies in proportion to their amount of water. The alcohol content of liver tissue is 64% of that in the blood; of muscle, 84%; and that of the brain, 75%. It takes very little time for the tissues to absorb the alcohol circulating in the blood. For example, within 2 minutes, brain tissues reflect accurately the blood alcohol level.

Now that we have explained how alcohol is taken up by the body and distributed to the body tissues, what are the effects, and how is it broken down and removed?

■ *Breakdown and removal*

The removal of alcohol from the body begins as soon as the alcohol is absorbed by the bloodstream. Small amounts leave unmetabolized through sweat, urine, or the breath. At most, this accounts for only 5% of the alcohol consumed. The rest has to be changed chemically, metabolized. The first step in the metabolism of alcohol is its change to acetaldehyde. A liver enzyme, alcohol dehydrogenase, or ADH in chemical shorthand, accomplishes this. The acetaldehyde that is formed is acted on by yet another liver enzyme, acetaldehyde dehydrogenase. Very rapidly the acetaldehyde breaks down to form acetic acid. The acetic acid then leaves the liver and is dispersed throughout the body, where it is oxidized to carbon dioxide and water. In summary, the chain of events is:

alcohol—acetaldehyde*—acetic acid—carbon dioxide + water

As you can see, the liver holds the key position in this process. Almost any organ can break down the acetic acid. But only the liver can handle the first steps. The rate is set by

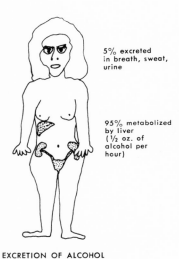

5% excreted
in breath, sweat,
urine

95% metabolized
by liver
(½ oz. of
alcohol per
hour)

EXCRETION OF ALCOHOL

---

*It is at this point that disulfiram (Antabuse), a drug used in alcoholism treatments, acts. Antabuse stops the breakdown of acetaldehyde by blocking acetaldehyde dehydrogenase. Thus, acetaldehyde starts to accumulate in the system. It is very toxic, and its effects are those associated with an Antabuse reaction. A better term would be an acetaldehyde reaction. The toxicity of acetaldehyde usually isn't a problem. It breaks down faster than it is formed. But Antabuse does not allow this to take place so rapidly. Thus the nausea, flushing, and heart palpitations. It has been observed that Orientals often have such symptoms when drinking. These are probably based on biochemical differences resulting from genetic differences. In effect, they have a built-in Antabuse-like response.

the availability of a key substance (nicotinamide adenine dinucleotide, or NAD^+) which is essential for the enzyme ADH to act. Generally the rate at which food is metabolized depends on the energy requirements of the body. Experience will confirm this, especially for anyone who has taken a stab at dieting. Chopping wood burns up more calories than watching the tube. Too much food, and a storehouse of fat begins to accumulate around the middle. By balancing calories taken in our meals with exercise, we can avoid accumulating a fat roll. Again, as a food, alcohol is unique. It is metabolized at a constant rate. The liver does not have a "piece rate" work-set when it comes to alcohol. The presence of large amounts does not prompt the liver to work faster. Despite alcohol's seeming potential as a fine source of calories, increased exercise (hence raising the body's need for calories) does not increase the speed of metabolism. This is probably not news to anyone who has tried to sober up a drunk. It's simply a matter of time. Exercise may only mean you have a wide-awake drunk, rather than a sleeping one, to contend with. The rate alcohol is metabolized by the liver may vary a little among people. It will also increase somewhat after an extended drinking career. Yet the average rate is around ½ ounce of *pure* alcohol per hour. That is roughly equivalent to one mixed drink of 86-proof whiskey or one 12-ounce can of beer. The unmetabolized alcohol remains circulating in the bloodstream, "waiting in line." The concentration of alcohol in the blood, and hence in the brain, is responsible for the intoxicating effects of alcohol.

■ *Alcohol's effects on the body*

What is the immediate effect of alcohol on the various body organs and functions?

Digestive system. As already noted, alcohol is an irritant. This explains the burning sensation as it goes down. Alcohol in the stomach promotes the flow of gastric juices. A glass of wine before dinner may thereby promote digestion by "priming" the stomach for food. But with intoxicating amounts, alcohol impedes or stops digestion.

Circulatory system. Alcohol has only minor effects on the circulatory system. Heartbeat and blood pressure are little affected. In moderate amounts, alcohol is a vasodilator of the surface blood vessels. These vessels expand near the skin surface. This accounts for the sensation of warmth and a flush to the skin that accompany drinking. Despite the feeling of warmth, body heat is being lost. Thus, whoever sends out the St. Bernard with a brandy cask to the aid of the snow-stranded traveler is misguided. Despite the illusion of warmth, a good belt of alcohol will further cool off the body.

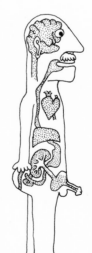

Interferes with brain activity, affecting first judgment, then muscular coordination, then sensory perception

Has few effects on heart or lungs except in high amounts, then may cause death

Interferes with liver's ability to maintain stable blood sugar

Leads to increased production of urine by kidneys

Irritates intestinal system; increases acid secretion by stomach

EFFECTS OF ALCOHOL

Kidneys. Anyone who has had a couple of drinks may well spend some time traipsing back and forth to the toilet. This increased urine output is not caused by alcohol's direct action on the kidneys and is not simply due to the amount of liquid consumed. This phenomenon is related to the effect of alcohol on the pituitary gland located at the base of the brain. The pituitary secretes a hormone regulating the amount of urine produced. As the pituitary is affected by alcohol, too little of the hormone is released, and the kidneys form a larger than normal amount of urine. This effect is most pronounced with a rising blood alcohol level, as the alcohol is still being absorbed.

Liver. The liver is very sensitive to the effects of alcohol (see Chap. 5 for more on the effects of alcohol on the liver). Thus in nonalcoholic volunteers it has been demonstrated that acute intake of even relatively small amounts of alcohol (1 to 2 ounces) can lead to accumulation of fat in liver cells.

The liver performs an incredible number of different functions. A very important one is its role in maintaining a proper blood sugar level. Sugar (the body's variety, called glucose) is the only source of energy that brain cells can use. Since the brain is the master control center of the body, an inadequate supply of food has far-reaching consequences. When alcohol is present in the system, the liver throws its whole attention, so to speak, to metabolizing it. There is a stored form of glucose in the liver (glycogen) that is usually readily available. But if glycogen is not present because of an inadequate diet or fasting for a day or two, the liver will normally go through a more complicated biochemical process to transform other nutrients such as protein into glucose. However, this complicated maneuver is blocked by the presence of alcohol. In these cases hypoglycemia can result. In a hypoglycemic state, there is a below-normal concentration of blood sugar. The brain is deprived of its proper nourishment. Symptoms include hunger, weakness, nervousness, sweating, headache, tremor. If the level is sufficiently depressed, coma can occur. Whereas, hypoglycemia may be more likely and more severe in individuals who already have liver damage from chronic alcoholism, it can occur in otherwise normal people with healthy livers who have been drinking heavily and have not been eating properly for as little as 48 to 72 hours.

In individuals with adequate diets, other metabolic effects of alcohol may cause abnormally high levels of blood glucose, called hyperglycemia, a state similar to that occurring in diabetics. In view of its potentially significant effects on blood sugar levels, the danger posed by alcohol for the diabetic patient is obvious.

The liver also plays an important role in the metabolism

of other drugs. The presence of alcohol can interfere with this and in part be responsible for some alcohol-drug interactions. As mentioned before, the liver enzyme ADH is essential to the metabolism of alcohol. Quantitatively it is the liver's major means of metabolizing alcohol. The liver, however, does have a "backup system." This secondary system is called MEOS (short for *m*icrosomal *e*thanol *o*xidizing *s*ystem) and it is located in certain structures within the cells, called microsomes. It is probably only after long-term heavy drinking that this secondary system begins to help out significantly in the metabolism of alcohol. But this system is mentioned here because it is a *major* system in metabolizing other drugs.

The MEOS activity is inhibited dramatically by the presence of alcohol. Therefore, other drugs are not broken down at the usual rate. If other drugs in the system have a depressant effect similar to alcohol's, this can be serious. The central nervous system (CNS) will be subjected to both simultaneously. However, problems can also result with other drugs. Say someone is taking a prescription drug at set intervals, such as Dilantin or Coumadin, and drinks. The presence of alcohol interferes with the metabolism of the medications. Therefore when the next scheduled dose is taken, substantial amounts of the earlier dose remain, and cumulative toxic or side effects may occur. With chronic long-term alcohol use the activity of MEOS is speeded up. In this instance the drugs are broken down faster, so that higher doses must be administered to achieve a given therapeutic effect. (See Table 1 in Chapter 5 for more alcohol-drug interactions.)

Central nervous system. The central nervous system, particularly the brain, is the organ most sensitive to the presence of alcohol. This sensitivity is what being high, drunk, or intoxicated is all about. The intensity of the effect is directly related to the concentration of alcohol in the blood. The drug alcohol is a CNS depressant. It interferes with or lowers the activity of the brain. Not all parts of the brain are uniformly affected. If they were, the same amount required to release inhibitions would also be lethal by simultaneously hitting the parts controlling breathing. Watch, or recall, someone becoming intoxicated and see the progression of effects. The following examples refer to CNS effects in men.

One drink. (The "drinks" here are a little under ½ ounce of pure alcohol, the equivalent of a 12-ounce beer or an ounce of 86-proof whiskey. Many generous hosts and hostesses mix drinks with more than 1 ounce of booze. So, as you read on, don't shrug off the "10-drink" section as an impossibility. Five generous ones could easily have as much alcohol!) With one drink, the drinker will be a bit more relaxed, possibly loosened up a little. Unless he chugged it rapidly, thus getting a rapid rise in blood alcohol, his behavior will be little changed. Being of average height, weighing 160 pounds, by the end of an hour his blood alcohol level will be 0.02. One hour later all traces of alcohol will be gone.

Two and a half drinks. With two and a half drinks in an hour's time, your party goer will have a 0.05 blood alcohol level. He's high. The "newer" parts of the brain, those controlling judgment, have been affected. That our friend has been drinking is apparent. He may be loud, boisterous, making passes; saying and doing things he might usually censor. These are the effects that cause people mistakenly to think of alcohol as a stimulant. The system isn't hyped up; the inhibitions have been suspended. At this time our friend is entering the danger zone for driving. With two and a half drinks in an hour, 2.5 hours will be required to metabolize the alcohol completely.

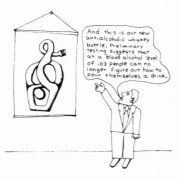

Five drinks. With five drinks in an hour, there is no question you've a drunk on your hands. The law would agree. A blood alcohol level of 0.10 is sufficient in most states to convict of driving while intoxicated. By this time judgment is nil. "Off coursh I can drive!" In addition to the parts of the brain controlling judgment, the centers controlling muscle coordination are depressed. There's a stagger to the walk and a slur to the speech. Even though the loss of dexterity and reaction time can be measured, the drinker, now with altered judgment, will claim he's never functioned better. Five hours will be required for all traces of alcohol to disappear from the system.

Ten drinks. This quantity of alcohol in the system yields a blood alcohol content of 0.20, and even more of the brain is affected besides the motor centers. Emotions are probably very erratic—from laughter to tears to rage. Even if your guest could remember he had a coat, he'd never be able to put it on. Ten hours will be required for all the alcohol to be metabolized. Six hours, and he'll still be legally drunk.

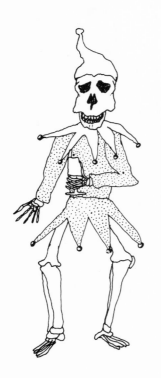

One pint of whiskey. With this amount of booze, the drinker is stuporous. Though not passed out, nothing the senses take in actually registers. Judgment is gone, coordination wiped out, and sensory perception almost gone. With the liver handling 1 ounce of alcohol per hour, it will be 16 hours, well into tomorrow, before all the alcohol is gone.

One and one-fourth pints of whiskey. At this point, the person is in a coma and dangerously close to death. The brain centers, which send out instructions to the heart and breathing apparatus, are partially anesthetized. At a blood alcohol level of 0.4 to 0.5, a person is in a coma; at 0.6 to 0.7, death occurs.

Substitute a 120-pound woman in these examples, and the weight differential would certainly speed up the process. With one drink in one hour, she would have a blood alcohol level of 0.03; two and a half drinks, she'd be up to 0.07. By five drinks, she'd have a 0.14 reading. Should she make it through a pint, she'd be in a coma with a level of 0.45. Tomorrow might not come as soon for her. Besides the differences in body weight, other factors can speed up or alter this process. Women and men differ in their relative amounts of body fat and water. Women have a higher proportion of fat and correspondingly lower amounts of water. Alcohol is not fat soluble. Therefore, a woman and a man of the same body weight, both drinking the same amounts of alcohol, will have different blood alcohol levels. Hers will be higher. She has less water than he has in which to dilute her alcohol.

There is another critical difference between men and women in regard to how they handle alcohol. A woman's menstrual cycle significantly influences her rate of absorption. This difference presumably relates to the changing balances of sex hormones and appears to be the result of several interacting factors. During the premenstrual phase of her cycle, a woman absorbs alcohol more rapidly. The absorption rate is significantly faster than in other phases of the menstrual cycle. So premenstrually a woman will get a higher blood alcohol level than she would get from drinking an equivalent amount at other times. In practical terms, a woman may find herself getting drunk faster right before her period. There is also evidence that women taking birth control pills also will absorb alcohol faster and thereby have higher blood alcohol levels.

Quite possibly other differences may exist between men and women in terms of alcohol's effects. Virtually all the physiological research has been conducted on men. The researchers have then blithely assumed the findings to be equally true for women. Though the basic differences between absorption rates of men and women were reported as early as 1932, they were forgotten and/or ignored until the mid-1970s. Believe it or not, the impact of the menstrual cycle was first reported in 1976! With this failure to examine the effects of the primary and obvious difference between males and females, who knows what more subtle areas have not been looked at. End of sermon!

Alcohol as anesthetic

Alcohol is an anesthetic, just as it shows in all the old western movies. By modern standards, it is not a very good one. The dose required to produce anesthesia is very close to the lethal amount. When the vital centers have been depressed by alcohol to produce unconsciousness, it only takes a wee bit more to put someone permanently to sleep. Sadly, a couple of times a year almost any newspaper obituary column documents a death from alcohol. Usually it involves chugging a fifth of liquor on a dare, or as a prank, which very quickly yields a lethal dose of alcohol.

Despite differences between people, each and every human body basically reacts in the same way to alcohol. This uniform, well-documented response is what enables the law to set a specific blood alcohol level for defining drunkenness. This can be easily measured by blood samples or the breathalyzer. Carbon dioxide in the blood diffuses across small capillaries in the lungs to be eliminated in the exhaled air. The amount or concentration of it in the exhaled air is directly proportional to the amount or concentration dissolved in the blood. Exactly the same thing happens with alcohol. The breathalyzer measures the concentration of alcohol in the exhaled air and from this, the exact concentration of alcohol in the blood can be determined.

▪ *Cumulative effects*

The immediate effects of the drug alcohol have been described. With continued drinking, changes take place. There are cumulative effects. Any drinker, not only the alcoholic, can testify to this. The first few times someone tries alcohol, with one drink they feel tipsy. With drinking experience, one drink no longer has that effect. In part this may reflect greater wisdom. The veteran drinker has learned "how to drink" to avoid feeling intoxicated, that is, by not chugging a drink or not drinking on an empty stomach. The other reason is that with repeated exposure, the CNS has adapted to the presence of alcohol. It can tolerate more alcohol and still maintain normal function. This is one of the properties that defines alcohol as an addictive drug. Over the long haul the body requires a larger dose to induce the effects earlier produced at lower levels. Not only does this adaptation occur over long spans of time, there are also rapid adaptive changes in the CNS every time someone drinks. A drinker is more out of commission when the blood alcohol level is climbing than when it is falling. If someone is given alcohol to drink and then performs certain tasks, there are predictable results. Impairment is greater on the ascending climb, or absorption phase. As the blood alcohol level drops in the elimination phase, the individual will be able to function better with the same blood alcohol content. It is as if one learns to function better, after "practice" with the presence of alcohol. Here, too, there are differences between men and women. Both have more impairment as alcohol levels rise. There are differences in the *kinds* of impairment. With intoxication, women appear to have greater impairment than men for tasks that require motor coordination. They are superior to men on tasks that require attention. Since driving requires both skills, neither appears the better bet on the highway.

▪ *Other alcohols*

In this discussion of alcohol, it is clear that we have been referring to "booze," "suds," "the sauce," "hooch," or any of the other colloquial terms for beverage alcohol. To be scientifically accurate, "our kind" of alcohol is called *ethanol, ethyl alcohol,* or *grain alcohol. Alcohol,* if one is precise, is a term used to refer to a family of substances. What all alcohols have in common is that each has a particular grouping of carbon, hydrogen, and oxygen atoms, linked up in the same way. They differ only in the number of carbons, and their associated hydrogens. Each alcohol is named according to the number of carbons aboard. Ethanol has two carbon atoms.

The other kinds of alcohol with which everyone is familiar are wood alcohol (methyl alcohol) with one carbon, and rubbing alcohol (isopropyl) with three carbons. With their different chemical makeup, they cause big problems if taken into the body. The difficulty lies in differences in rates of metabolism and the kinds of by-products formed. For example, it take nine times longer for methanol to be eliminated than ethanol. Although methanol itself is not especially toxic, when alcohol dehydrogenase acts on it, formaldehyde instead of acetaldehyde is formed. Formaldehyde is known to cause tissue damage, especially to the eyes. The formaldehyde then breaks down into formic acid, which is also not as innocent as the acetic acid produced by ethanol metabolism and can cause severe states of acidosis. Ingestion of methyl alcohol can lead to blindness and can be fatal; it requires prompt medical attention.

As an interesting aside, the treatment of acute methanol poisoning is one of the handful of places in clinical medicine where ethanol has a legitimate and important therapeutic role. In this situation giving ethanol will slow the rate of metabolism of methanol and reduce the level of toxic by-production. This happens because the ethanol successfully competes with methanol for ADH. This effect in conjunction with correction of acidosis may ameliorate or entirely eliminate serious complications.

Poisonings from nonbeverage alcohols don't just happen to alcoholics, who in desperation will drink anything. There's the toddler who gets into the medicine cabinet, or maybe the teenager or adult who doesn't know that all alcohols are not the same and have different effects.

At present, it is becoming common knowledge that anything taken into the body (or breathed in for that matter) has effects on the body. And all too often we are discovering these effects to be more harmful than had been previously thought. Chemical additives, fertilizers, and coloring agents are being found to be less benign than once supposed. Caution is urged in the use of all such agents, and the FDA has been outlawing some of them. Let us hope that this caution will begin to extend to the use of alcohol as well.

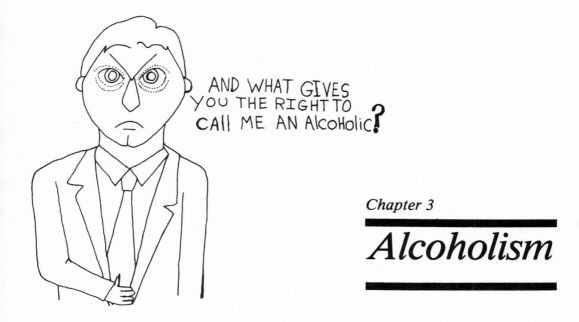

AND WHAT GIVES YOU THE RIGHT TO CALL ME AN AlCoHolic?

Chapter 3

Alcoholism

▪ *Definitions*

The social problems associated with the use and misuse of alcohol have been described. Even if there were no such phenomenon as alcoholism, the mere presence of alcohol would lead to the disruption of the social order and considerable costs to society. Yet all statistics on dented fenders caused by inebriated drivers, or dollars lost by industry, or even percentage of alcohol-related hospital admissions have a limited gut-level impact. Most of us would judge them to be unfortunate or nuisances, but they would not strike us as a national tragedy. Our major concern and compassion usually flows toward people, not things. Not unexpectedly, the problem of alcohol that captures our attention is the person for whom alcohol is no longer servant, but master. It is the 13 million plus alcoholics and the approximately 53 million family members who come immediately to mind when we consider the human dimensions of alcohol problems. The chances are very good that this concern is particularized, with the faces of people we know or have known coming to mind.

What is alcoholism? Who is the alcoholic? A number of definitions are available from a variety of sources. The word alcoholic itself can provide some clues. The suffix *-ic* has a special meaning, according to *Webster's New Collegiate Dictionary*.

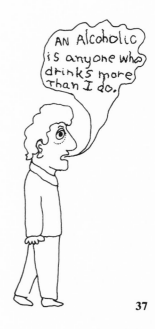

AN AlCoHolic is anyone who drinks more than I do.

37

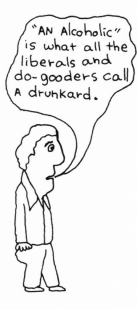

-ic n suffix: One having the character or nature of: one belonging to or associated with: one exhibiting or affected by.

Attaching *ic* to alcohol, this word means a person whom those around him link with alcohol. O.K., that's a start. Clearly not all drinkers are linked with alcohol, just as all baseball players are not linked with the Boston Red Sox. Why the link or association? The basis is probably frequency of use, pattern of use, quantity used, or frequency of signs that indicate the person has been tippling. "Belonging to" has several connotations, including an individual's being possessed by or under the control of. The Chinese have a saying that goes: "The man takes a drink, the drink takes a drink, and then the drink takes the man." This final step closely approximates what the word alcohol*ic* means. And the progression itself provides a good picture of the progression of alcohol*ism*.

It is worth noting that the discussion or debate on who is alcoholic and what is alcoholism is quite recent. This doesn't mean society has never noticed the alcoholic before. Certainly, persons in trouble with alcohol have been recognized for centuries. But their existence was accepted as a fact, without question. To the extent there was debate, it centered on why, and how the alcoholic should be handled. Essentially two basic approaches prevailed. One was that "obviously" the alcoholic was morally inferior. The evidence cited was the vast majority of people who drank moderately, without presenting problems for themselves or the community. The other view has been that "obviously" the alcoholic was possessed, since no one in his right mind would drink like that of his own volition.

With increasing scientific study and knowledge of "the drink taking the man" phenomenon, the more complicated the task of definition has become. Though the awareness prevails that these persons are distinctly different from the many who drink moderately, the other clear discovery is that all alcoholics are *not* alike. Not all develop DTs when withdrawn from alcohol. There are big differences in the quantity of alcohol consumed or the number of years drinking before family problems arise. Many alcoholics develop cirrhosis, but more do not. The more time spent on study, the less is known with certainty. In some instances, what was previously seen as a single problem, alcoholism, is now discussed as alcoholisms.

Now that you have been forewarned that there is no easy single, agreed-upon definition, and that the situation is becoming more complicated, we list a sample of the common formulations:

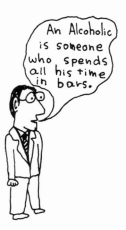

E. M. Jellinek (1946), a pioneer of modern alcohol studies. "Any use of alcoholic beverages that causes any damage to the individual or to society or both."

Marty Mann (1950s), a founding member of the National Council on Alcoholism. "An alcoholic is a very sick person, victim of an insidious, progressive disease, which all too often ends fatally. An alcoholic can be recognized, diagnosed, and treated successfully."

Mark Keller (1960), former editor of *Journal of Alcohol Studies.* Alcoholism is "a chronic disease manifested by repeated implicative drinking so as to cause injury to the drinker's health or to his social or economic functioning."

Alcoholics Anonymous. AA has no official definition, but the concept of Dr. William Silkworth, one of AA's friends, is sometimes cited by AA members: an obsession of the mind and an allergy of the body. The obsession or compulsion guarantees that the sufferer will drink against his own will and interest. The allergy guarantees that the sufferer will either die or go insane. An operative definition in use in AA is that "an alcoholic is a person who cannot *predict* with accuracy what will happen when he takes a drink."

World Health Organization (WHO) (1951). The Alcoholism Subcommittee defined alcoholism as "any form of drinking which in extent goes beyond the traditional and customary 'dietary' use, or the ordinary compliance with the social drinking customs of the community concerned, irrespective of etiological factors leading to such behavior, and irrespective also of the extent to which such etiological factors are dependent upon heredity, constitution, or acquired physiopathological and metabolic influences."

American Psychiatric Association (APA) (1968). According to the Committee on Nomenclature and Statistics, "alcoholism: this category is for patients whose alcohol intake is great enough to damage their physical health, or their personal or social functioning, or when it has become a prerequisite to normal functioning." Three types of alcoholism were further identified.

Episodic excessive drinking. If alcoholism is present and the individual becomes intoxicated as frequently as four times a year, the condition should be classified here. Intoxication is defined as a state in which the individual's coordination or speech is definitely impaired or his behavior is clearly altered.

Habitual excessive drinking. This diagnosis is given to persons who are alcoholic and who either become intoxicated more than twelve times a year or are recognizably under the influence of alcohol more than once a week, even though not intoxicated.

Alcohol addiction. This condition should be diagnosed when there is direct or strong presumptive evidence that the patient is dependent on alcohol. If available, the best directive evidence of such dependence is the appearance of withdrawal symptoms. The inability of the patient to go one day without drinking is presumptive evidence. When heavy drinking continues for 3 months or more it is reasonable to presume that addiction to alcohol has been established.

American Medical Association (1977). "Alcoholism is an illness characterized by significant impairment that is directly associated with persistent and excessive use of alcohol. Impairment may involve physiological, psychological or social dysfunction." (From *Manual on Alcoholism* edited by the AMA Panel on Alcoholism.)

Interestingly, the definitional situation is further simplified or confused—depending on your perspective—by actions taken by both the WHO (1977) and the APA (1980). Neither group is disputing the existence of the phenomenon of "alcoholism." However, in large measure because of the multiple definitions that do abound, both groups have for medical-scientific purposes substituted "alcohol-dependence syndrome." This new terminology also is seen as introducing more consistency with other syndromes related to substance use. Thus, the current APA *Diagnostic and Statistical Manual* distinguishes two types of alcohol-dependence syndrome: alcohol abuse and alcohol dependency. Both include impairment in social or occupational functioning. The essential distinguishing feature is the presence of tolerance or withdrawal in the latter.

As if this were not confusing enough, in addition there are all the definitions casually used by each of us and our neighbors. Here we find considerable variation, from "alcoholism is an illness," to "it's the number one drug problem," to "when someone's drunk all the time."

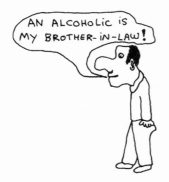

Although not necessarily conflicting, each of the expert definitions has a different focus or emphasis. Several concentrate on the unfortunate consequences associated with alcohol use. Others zero in on hallmark signs or symptoms, especially loss of control or frequency of intoxication. This is true of both expert and lay definitions. Note that generally laypeople seem to have more permissive criteria! One other distinction between the available definitions is that some are descriptive and others attempt to handle the origins of the problem.

Criteria for choosing a definition

Before supplying another definition, or examining those just listed, a little digression is in order. That is, how does one know the "true" definition or select the best one? There are guidelines used by physical scientists worth examining. When faced with a choice between two possible explanations, they judge on the basis of two criteria. The first is called the Law of Parsimony. This means that the better explanation is the one that adequately explains the data with the fewest number of factors. An example will help to illustrate this.

A worker in a mental health clinic has a client who is feeling down, isn't getting along at work, finds his wife is bitching at him, and his liver is acting up. One explanation is that by chance, his job is oppressive, his boss is obnoxious, by nature his wife has a nasty temperament, and furthermore, fate has conspired to give him a cirrhotic liver. Thus his feeling blue is a natural response to an unfortunate set of circumstances. An alternative explanation is that he is an alcoholic. The simplest explanation that fits the facts is the best.

The second criterion the scientist uses when selecting among competing theories is heuristic value. This means taking into account the theory or explanation's usefulness as a guide to action. A car mechanic has an understanding of what makes an automobile tick. When it goes on the blink, he therefore has some sense of how to go about correcting the situation. The same holds here. Any definition of what alcoholism *is* should provide some clues about what *should be done*.

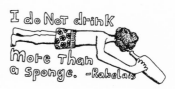

Applying these criteria to the many definitions available, which makes the most sense? This is going to depend on what someone is trying to do. Probably what most people are trying to determine is whether the drinking of a particular person is normal or not, or whether there are grounds for concern. So the definition used should help answer that question. Presumably, it should be faithful to the facts. Also, it should be applicable to persons in the early as well as the later stages of the disease. This is the major failing of most lay definitions. They are so specific and geared to the later stages that approximately 95%, or most alcoholics, cannot qualify.

A definition that seems to fit most of our purposes is a short one, closely following Jellinek or Keller. "Alcoholism is a disease in which the person's use of alcohol *continues* despite problems it causes in any area of life." Every definition has plusses and minuses. The utility of this one is its simplicity and its ability to cover people at various stages. The reference to disease suggests the potential for treatment and asserts the sufferer is entitled (as are all sick people) to care, not punishment or ostracism. Its weakness is the failure to address the issue of causes. Since the causes of alcoholism are not neat and clear-cut as yet, ignoring that point may not be a bad idea.

The remainder of the chapter will be devoted to examining alcoholism as a disease, and then examining two major pieces of work that have led to our present understanding of what alcoholism is, its complexity, and how to recognize it. First of these is the work of E. M. Jellinek, who has been termed the father of alcohol studies in the United States and the world. Second is the guidelines established by a committee of the National Council on Alcoholism for diagnosing alcoholism, published in 1972.

■ *A disease?*

Anyone who is sufficiently interested in alcoholism to have gotten this far is probably well accustomed to hearing alcoholism referred to as an illness, disease, or sickness.

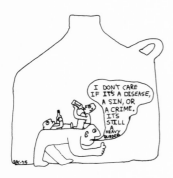

This has not always been the case. As discussed earlier, alcoholism has not always been distinguished from drunkenness. Or it has been seen as a lot of drunkenness and categorized as a sin or character defect. The work of E. M. Jellinek has largely been responsible for the shift to an illness model. In essence, through his research and writings, he said, "Hey, world, you guys mislabeled this thing. You put it in the sin bin, and it really belongs in the disease pile." How we label something is very important. It provides clues on how to feel and think, what to expect, and how to act. Whether a particular bulb is tagged as either a tulip or an onion is going to make a big difference (especially from the bulb's point of view). Depending on which I think it is, I'll either chop and sauté or plant and water. Very different behaviors are associated with each. An error may lead to strange-flavored spaghetti sauce and a less colorful flower bed next spring.

Implications of disease classification

Placing alcoholism in the category of disease has had a dramatic impact. Sick people are generally awarded sympathy. The accepted notion is that sick people do not choose to be sick, being sick is not pleasant, and care should be provided to restore health. During the period of sickness, people will not be expected to fill their usual roles or meet their responsibilities. A special designation is given to people in this situation: patient. Furthermore, sick persons are not to be criticized for manifesting the symptoms of their illness. To tell a flu victim to stop "fevering" would be seen as pointless and unkind. With alcoholism an illness, the alcoholic is thought of as a sufferer and victim. Much of the bizarre behavior displayed is recognized as unwillful and a symptom of illness. No longer the object of scorn, the alcoholic is now seen to require care. The logical place to send the alcoholic is no longer jail, but a hospital or rehabilitation center. There has been a gradual shifting in public attitudes since the 1940s. In a recent nationwide poll, over 80% of the respondents said they believed alcoholism to be an illness. Although Jellinek's efforts may have triggered this shift, a number of other events added impetus. The National Council on Alcoholism put its efforts into lobbying and public education. The American Medical Association and American Hospital Association published various committee reports. State agencies developed programs for treating alcoholics. Probably the biggest push came from the presence of recovering alcoholics, especially through the work of AA. Virtually everyone today has personal knowledge of an apparently hopeless alcoholic who has gone off the sauce and seems a new, different person.

The formulation of alcoholism as a disease has opened up possibilities for treatment that were nonexistent. It has brought into the helping area the resources of medicine, nursing, social work, and others, who before had no mandate to help alcoholics. Also it is gradually removing the stigma associated with alcoholism. This improves the likelihood that individuals and families will seek help rather than cover up. Finally, the resources of the federal government have been focused on alcoholism as a major public health problem. A host of treatment and educational programs have been brought into being.

The early sales pitch for selling alcoholism as a disease was probably the slogan: ''Alcoholism is an illness, just like any other.'' With a little imagination, you can picture folks going around the radio talk show circuit flashing this phrase. Now that the notion has gained acceptance, the time may be approaching for a new, or refined, formulation. For there have been some disadvantages or limitations to the disease concept.

Refinement of disease classification

There have been some who have been critical of the disease concept. Among the objections are that it possibly has put too much emphasis on the physician as the major helper. The doctor certainly has a role to play in diagnosis and physical treatment. But medical training has not necessarily prepared physicians to do counseling. Even if it has, a physician's time might be used more efficiently in other areas and counseling left to others. Yet the disease concept may imply the doctor alone is qualified to provide or direct treatment. Criticism is frequently leveled at doctors for being uninterested or unconcerned with the problems of alcoholism. Possibly the misuse of the disease concept may also foster unrealistic expectations and place undue burdens on them.

In a similar vein, the disease concept may create the false idea that alcoholism can be treated with a pill and that the alcoholic does not have to do anything. This notion is a mistake and an oversimplification of what the art of medicine is. This age has been an age of wonder drugs—penicillin, polio vaccines, measles vaccines, and so on. Were a cancer vaccine to be developed, all would be delighted, but few shocked. Television commercials constantly push ''wonder drugs'' for instant relief of headaches, insomnia, muscle pains, the blahs. We expect quick results. The side of the picture we neglect, since it isn't so spectacular, is the field of rehabilitative medicine. For instance, with physical therapy, accident victims learn to walk again. In these cases, patients are required to take active part in their recovery. To be successfully treated, an alcoholic must also take an active part.

The most important distinction usually *not* made is between acute and chronic disease. Acute disease means you get sick, get treated, become better, and that's the end of it. Chronic diseases are different: once you have it, you have it. Chronic diseases may be amenable to treatment and arrested. A person might be able to get along as well as before. But there is always a possibility of relapse. Treatment is intended to help you live around the illness, in spite of it. Diabetes falls into this category as do some forms of bronchitis, arthritis, and alcoholism.

In this book considerable emphasis will be placed on alcoholism as a chronic disease. There are several general points to be made at the outset. Medically speaking, one does not talk of curing chronic illness. By definition, given the current state of knowledge, chronic diseases are incurable. The medical approach to chronic illness is summed up by the term "management." Management may include specific medical treatments, but always there's more to it. Take the example of diabetes: insulin may be prescribed, but that isn't all that is done. A nutritionist will work with the diabetic around diet, the patient will be taught to check his or her urine, and in light of the diabetic's susceptibility to other health problems, some modifications of daily routine may be introduced. The person with a chronic illness is not the passive recipient of a physician's doctoring. The chronically ill person becomes an active collaborator with the physician, and assumes considerable responsibility for caring for and managing his or her own illness. Characteristically the management of chronic disease involves treatment of acute flare-ups; emotional support (after all no one likes having a chronic illness); education, so the individual can be informed about the illness and assist in self-care; and rehabilitative measures, to make the life changes necessary to live with the limitations imposed by the illness.

The other noteworthy characteristic of chronic illnesses is that they tend to develop slowly. Quite conceivably with acute illness such as flu, one can go to bed feeling quite well and wake up the next morning sick. It literally happened overnight. However, one does not become diabetic, arthritic, or alcoholic overnight. The disease state develops slowly and there will be warning signs and symptoms prior to the point at which it is unequivocably present. For alcoholism, we have E. M. Jellinek to thank for sketching out this progression.

Another major criticism of the disease concept is that it can be used by alcoholics as a cop-out. "Don't look at me, I'm not responsible. I'm sick. Poor me (sigh, sigh)." Expect a drinking alcoholic to try shooting holes into any definition. Those who criticize the disease concept on this basis are possibly those who have been victims of the alcoholic's con game. Our sympathy goes out to them. Alcoholics do have a knack for immobilizing those around them, so that their drinking can continue undisturbed. A one-liner that seems to handle the situation fairly well comes from a billboard on the Boston skyline. "There's nothing wrong with being an alcoholic, if you're doing something about it."

▪ *Phases à la Jellinek*

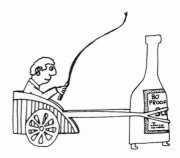

How did Jellinek arrive at his disease formulation of alcoholism? A biostatistician by training, he was logically fascinated by statistics, the pictures they portray, and the questions they raise. Much of his work has been descriptive, defining the turf of alcoholism. Who, when, where. One of his first studies, published in 1952, charted the signs and symptoms associated with alcohol addiction. This work was based on a survey of over 2,000 members of Alcoholics Anonymous. Although differences certainly existed between persons, the similarities were more remarkable. There was a definite pattern to the appearance of the symptoms. There was also a progression of the disease in terms of increasing dysfunction. The symptoms and signs tended to go together in clusters. Thus Jellinek developed the idea of four different phases of alcohol addiction: the prealcoholic, prodromal, crucial, and chronic phases. These have been widely used in alcohol treatment circles. The four phases are often portrayed graphically on a chart.

In the *prealcoholic phase*, the individual's use of alcohol is socially motivated. However, the prospective alcoholic soon experiences psychological relief in the drinking situation. Possibly this person's tensions are greater than other persons', or possibly he or she has no other way of handling tensions. It does not matter. Either way, he or she learns to seek out occasions where drinking will occur. At some point the connection becomes conscious. Drinking then becomes the standard means of handling stress. But the drinking behavior will not look different to the outsider. This phase can extend from several months to 2 years or more. An increase in tolerance gradually develops.

Suddenly the prealcoholic will enter the *prodromal phase*. (Prodromal means warning or signaling disease.) According to Jellinek, the behavior that heralds the change is the occurrence of "alcoholic palimpsests"—or blackouts. Blackouts are amnesia-like periods during drinking. The person seems to be functioning normally but later has no memory of what happened. Other behaviors emerge that give evidence that alcohol is no longer "just" a beverage, but a "need." Among these are sneaking extra

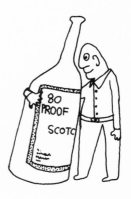

drinks before or during parties, gulping the first drink or two, and guilt about the drinking behavior. Here consumption is heavy, yet not necessarily conspicuous. To look "okay" requires conscious effort by the drinker. This period can last from 6 months to 4 or 5 years, depending on the drinker's circumstances.

The third phase is the *crucial phase.* The key symptom that ushers in this phase is loss of control. Now taking a drink sets up a chain reaction. The drinker can no longer control the amount consumed once he or she takes a drink. However, whether or not to take a drink is still under the person's control. So it is possible to go on the wagon for a time. With loss of control, the drinker loses his or her cover-up. His or her drinking is now clearly different. This requires explanation, so rationalizations begin. Simultaneously, the alcoholic attempts a sequence of strategies to regain control. The thinking goes, "If I just _____, then it will be okay." Common maneuvers attempted are periods of abstinence, changing drinking patterns, geographical escapes, changing jobs. These are doomed to failure. The alcoholic responds to these failures, becoming alternately resentful, remorseful, and aggressive. Life has become alcohol centered. Family life and friendships deteriorate. The first alcohol-related hospitalization is likely. Morning drinking may begin to creep in, foreshadowing the next stage.

The final stage in the process is the *chronic phase.* In the preceding crucial phase, the drinker may have been somewhat successful in maintaining a job and social footing. Now, as drinking begins earlier in the day, intoxication is an almost daily, day-long phenomenon. Benders are more frequent. The drinker may also go to dives and drink with persons previously below his or her social class. Not unexpectedly alcoholics find themselves on the fringes of society. When ethanol is unavailable, they'll drink poisonous substitutes. During this phase, marked physical changes occur. Tolerance for alcohol drops sharply. No longer able to hold his liquor, the alcoholic is stuporous after a few drinks. Tremors develop. Many simple tasks are impossible in the sober state. The alcoholic is beset by indefinable fears. Finally, the rationalization system fails. The long-used excuses are revealed as just that, excuses. The alcoholic is spontaneously open to treatment. Often, drinking

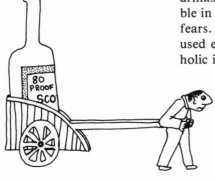

is likely to continue because the alcoholic can imagine no way out of his or her dilemma. Jellinek did emphasize that alcoholics are not destined to go through all four stages before treatment can be successful.

■ *Species*

The pattern on the preceding pages describes the stages of alcohol addiction. Jellinek continued his studies on alcoholics, focusing on alcohol problems in other countries. The differences he found could not be accounted for simply by the phases of alcohol addiction. These differences seemed more of kind than degree of addiction. This led to his formulation of species, or categories, of alcoholism. Each of these types he named with a Greek letter.

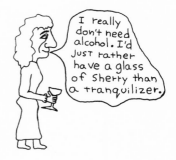

Alpha alcoholism. A purely psychological dependence on alcohol. There is neither loss of control nor an inability to abstain. What is evident is the reliance on alcohol to weather any, or all, discomforts or problems in life. This use may lead to interpersonal, family, or work problems. A progression is not inevitable. Jellinek notes that other writers may term this species *problem drinking.*

Beta alcoholism. Present when the various physical problems resulting from alcohol use develop, such as cirrhosis or gastritis, but the individual is not psychologically or physically dependent. This species is likely to occur in persons from cultures where there is widespread heavy drinking and inadequate diet.

Gamma alcoholism. Marked by a change in tolerance, physiological changes leading to withdrawal symptoms, and a loss of control. In this species there is a progression from psychological to physical dependence. It is the most devastating species in terms of physical health and social disruption. This is the species Jellinek originally studied. It progresses in four phases: prealcoholic, prodromal, crucial, and chronic. The gamma alcoholic appears to be the most prominent type in the United States. This species is the most common among the members of AA.

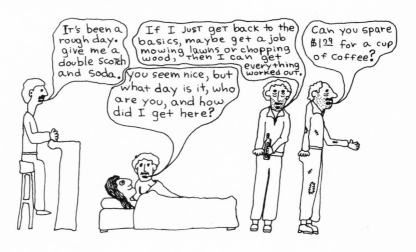

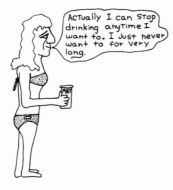

Characteristics of this species alone are often seen as synonymous with alcoholism.

Delta alcoholism. Very similar to the gamma variety. There is psychological and physical dependence, but there is no loss of control. On any particular occasion the drinker can control intake but cannot go on the wagon for even a day without suffering withdrawal.

Epsilon alcoholism. Not studied in depth, but appeared to be significantly different from the others. Jellinek called this *periodic alcoholism*, marked by binge drinking. Though not elaborating, he felt this was a species by itself, not to be confused with slips by gamma alcoholics.

Having described these various species, Jellinek concluded that possibly not all species are properly categorized as a disease. Maybe alpha and epsilon varieties are symptoms of other disorders. There was in his mind no question that gamma and delta, each involving physiological changes and progression, are diseases. By more adequately classifying and categorizing the phenomena of alcoholism, he brought scientific order to a field that before had been dominated by beliefs. That was no modest contribution.

■ *Guides for diagnosis*

The next major step taken was in 1972 with a paper entitled "Criteria for the Diagnosis of Alcoholism," published in two major medical journals. This article was prepared by a special committee of the National Council on Alcoholism. Their task was to establish guidelines to be used in diagnosing alcoholism. Physicians are thereby provided a firm set of standards to use in making a diagnosis.

The committee collected all the signs and symptoms of alcohol use that can be discovered through a physical examination, medical history, social history, laboratory tests, and clinical observations. They then organized these signs and symptoms into two categories, or tracks, of data. The first track is the physiological and clinical data. Included there are the things a physician can discover through a physical examination, laboratory tests, or medical history. The second track is termed the behavioral, psychological, and attitudinal; it includes what the patient or the family report about the client's life situation, or a social history, or what the doctor may directly observe about the patient's involvement with alcohol. Finally, each of the potential signposts is weighted as to whether it "definitely," "probably," or "possibly" indicates alcoholism.

For example, items that are deemed to be *definitely* indicative of alcoholism include:

• Physiological dependence, evidenced by withdrawal syndromes when alcohol use is interrupted or decreased

- Evidence of tolerance, by blood alcohol level of 0.15 without gross evidence of intoxication, or consumption of the equivalent of a fifth of whiskey for more than one day by a 180-pound man
- Continued drinking, despite strong medical indications known to patient, such as liver or gastrointestinal problems
- Drinking despite serious social problems
- Blood alcohol level of 0.3 or more at any time
- Blood alcohol level of 0.1 in routine examination

Among those seen as *probably* indicative of alcoholism are:

- Major alcohol-related illness in a person who drinks regularly such as:
     fatty liver
     alcoholic hepatitis
     cirrhosis
     pancreatitis
     chronic gastritis
- Odor of alcohol on breath at time of medical appointment
- Patient's complaint of loss of control
- Repeated attempts at abstinence
- Unexplained changes in family, social, or business relationships
- Spouse's complaints about drinking

There are many similarities between the symptoms of alcohol addiction developed by Jellinek and the criteria published in 1972. However, Jellinek composes his list based on the self-reports of recovered alcoholics. So the signs are from their subjective point of view. A good number of the symptoms Jellinek included involve deception and the alcoholic's attempts to appear normal. This provides little assistance to the physician or helper interviewing a drinking alcoholic. What further complicates diagnosis based on the Jellinek items is that many of the behaviors included are not the kind of thing a physician can easily detect. What the criteria have accomplished is to pinpoint *objective* measures for the physician.

In the criteria, alcoholism is further described as a chronic progressive disease. Although incurable, it is very treatable. Since it is a chronic disease, this means the diagnosis once made can *never* be dropped. An individual successfully involved in a treatment program would have the diagnosis amended to "alcoholism: arrested" or "alcoholism: in remission." Suggested criteria are provided for determining when this change in diagnosis is appropriate. The panel recommends that factors other than the length of sobriety be taken into account. Among the factors they list as signs of recovery are full, active participation in AA, active use of other treatments, use of Antabuse-like preparations, no substitution of other drugs, and resumption of work. The paper is primarily interested in diagnosis, not treatment. Yet implicit in the standards suggested for diagnosing ''alcoholism: arrested'' is a view that alcoholism requires a variety of treatment and rehabilitative efforts.

In his book *The Disease Concept of Alcoholism*, Jellinek humorously notes that a disease is ''simply anything the medical profession agrees to call a disease.'' Therefore, alcoholism is officially a disease. And, with the addition of the criteria, we finally have some clear direction for determining who's got it.

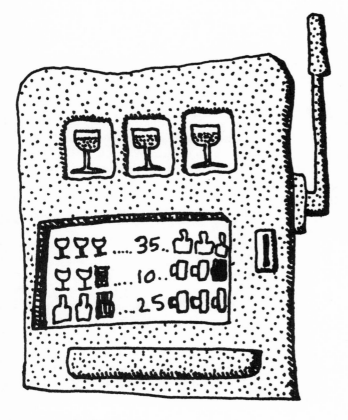

Chapter 4

Etiology of alcoholism

■ *Why alcohol?*

What are the causes of alcoholism? As more knowledge is gained, the answers become more complex. It might be useful to make a comparison to the common cold. Once you have "it," there isn't much question. The sneezing, the runny nose, the stuffed-up feeling the cold tablet manufacturers describe so well leave little doubt. But why you? Because "it" was going around. Your resistance was down. Others in the family have "it." You became chilled when caught in the rain. You forgot your vitamin C. Everyone has a pet theory and usually chalks it up to a number of factors working in combination against one. There does seem to be some chance factor involved. There are times we do *not* catch colds that are going around. Explaining the phenomenon cannot be done with great precision. It's more a matter of figuring out the odds and proba-

51

bilities, as the possible contributing factors are considered. The folks in the public health field have developed a systematic way of tackling this problem of disease, causes, and risks of contracting one. First, they look at the agent, the thing that causes the disease. Next they take a look at the host, the person who has the illness, to find characteristics that may have made him or her a likely target. Finally, the environment is examined, the setting in which the agent and host come together. A thorough look at these three areas ensures that no major influences will be overlooked.

■ *Public health model*

Alcoholism certainly qualifies as a public health problem. It is the third leading cause of death in the United States. It affects one out of every twelve adults. If alcoholism were an infectious disease such as polio, it would constitute an epidemic. People would be clamoring for a place in line to get vaccine. The response to alcoholism is pale in comparison.

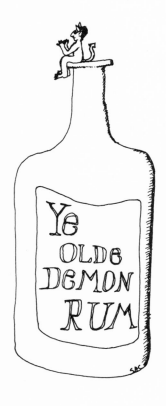

From the public health viewpoint, the first item to be examined as a possible cause of alcoholism is the agent. For alcoholism, the agent is the substance, alcohol. This is such an obvious fact that it might seem silly to dwell on it. No one can be alcoholic without being exposed to alcohol. The substance must be used before the possibility of alcoholism exists. Alcohol is an addictive substance. With sufficient quantities over a long period, the organism will undergo physiological changes. When this has occurred and the substance is withdrawn, there is a physiological response, withdrawal. For alcohol there is a well-defined set of symptoms that may accompany cessation of alcohol use in an addicted person. An individual can be addicted to alcohol. To use this fact alone to explain alcoholism represents untidy thinking. That alcohol is addicting does not explain why anyone would drink enough to reach the point of addiction. Temperance literature tries to paint a picture of an evil demon in the bottle. Take a sip, and he's got you. This may appear humorous to those comfortable with drinking alcoholic beverages. It is obvious that drinking need not inevitably lead to a life of drunkenness. Let's look at the action of the drug itself. What invites its use and makes it a candidate for use sufficient to cause addiction?

The agent—alcohol

We humans take any number of substances into our bodies—from meats to sweets, as solids or liquids. Although everyone overeats occasionally, abusing these substances is extremely unlikely. The notion of being addicted to cornflakes sounds ridiculous to our ear. Part of the humor of the Frito Bandito on the tube is that you *know* you can't be addicted to the product. So the notion is amusing, not terrifying. There is simply nothing that cornflakes or Hershey bars or soda pop can do for us *so* good, that we're likely to *need* a Hershey fix every few hours for example. Alcohol does do that something. It's a depressant drug. One of its first effects is on the central nervous system, the "higher" centers related to judgment, inhibition, and the like. What is more important is what this feels like, how it is experienced. With mild intoxication comes relaxation, a more carefree feeling. It is generally experienced as a plus, a high. Preexisting tensions are relieved. A good mood can be accentuated. Alcohol is experienced as a mood changer, in a good direction. This capacity of alcohol is one factor to remember in trying to understand use sufficient for addiction.

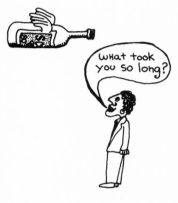

A common expression is "I sure could use a drink *now*." It may be said after a hard day at work, after a round of good physical exercise, or after a period of chaos and emotional stress, when the wobbly knees are setting in. This expression certainly includes the recognition that alcohol can be a mood changer. Equally as important is the word *now*. There is a recognition that the effects are immediate. Not only does alcohol make a difference, it does so very rapidly. If alcohol had a delayed reaction time, say 3 days, or 3 weeks, or even 3 hours, it wouldn't be a useful method for changing one's mood. Most people's lives are sufficiently unpredictable, so that drinking now for what may happen later would seem silly. So the speed of the mood change is another characteristic of the drug alcohol that enhances its likelihood of abuse.

Alcohol has another characteristic common to all depressant drugs. With mild inebriation, behavior is less inhibited, there are feelings of relaxation. However, at the same time there is a gradual increase of psychomotor activity. The drinker is unaware of this while feeling the initial glow. As the warm glow subsides, the increased psychomotor activity will become apparent. He may feel wound up, edgy, very similar to the feelings caused by too much coffee, especially in combination with cigarettes. The increase in psychomotor activity builds up gradually and extends beyond the feeling of well-being. Since it is delayed and its onset masked, the drinker is not very likely to recognize it as a product of the alcohol use. Instead, he thinks the edginess is his "normal" self. In fact, it is more probable that the drinker is feeling less serene or calm than when he began. What would be the rational thing to do? Have another drink! It is quite possible that many people, including nonalcoholics, have a second or third to get rid of

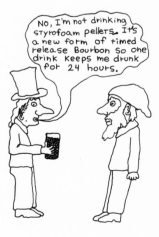

the very feelings created by earlier drinks. There is one nasty catch to this approach. The agitation phase, which accompanies alcohol consumption, extends considerably beyond the relaxed initial experience. A second drink will only temporarily cover the edginess of the first drink. The second drink, with its own edge coming on behind, will combine with the edge left over from the first. Were this to continue, a point would be reached when the accumulated tensions and increased psychomotor activity could no longer be masked by adding more alcohol. Normally, people are wholly unaware of this phenomenon because it is interrupted after two or three drinks. They've set their limit. They have dinner and go on to other activities. They go to bed.

These particular characteristics of alcohol do not alone account for the phenomena of alcoholism, but they are certainly responsible for the *possibility* of alcoholism. As other factors are examined, we can see how an interaction may work.

The host—genetic factors

The belief that alcoholism runs in families has long been a part of the folk wisdom. In your childhood, possibly, a great-aunt explained away the town drunk with "He's his father's son." No further comment was necessary. The obvious truth was so clear: that many of life's misfortunes are the result of "bad" genes. Just such an inadequate understanding of genetics, supported by warped theological views, led to statutes that authorized the sterilization of the feebleminded, hopelessly insane, and chronically drunk.

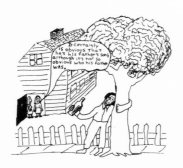

In the face of new knowledge, such an approach has fallen into disrepute. It is now clear that heredity isn't as simple as it seemed. Each individual, at the point of conception, receives a unique set of genetic material. This material is like a set of internal "instructions" that guide the individual's growth. In some respects, the genetic endowment simply sets down limits, or predispositions. The final outcome will depend on the life situation and environment in which the person finds (or places) himself or herself. Thus, there are some people who tend to be slim, and some who tend to put on weight easily. Such a *tendency* is probably genetic. But whether we are fat, thin, or just right depends on us.

Nature versus nurture. What are the facts about heredity in alcoholism? Actually, alcoholism does run in families. The child of an alcoholic parent *is* more likely to become alcoholic. One study tracing family trees found that 50% of the descendents of alcoholics were also alcoholics. Though that figure is a bit higher than other similar studies, it is simply a more dramatic example of the typical finding.

Drunkards beget drunkards.

PLUTARCH

That something's running in families is not proof that it is inherited. After all, speaking French runs in families—in France. Recognizing the role of psychological factors influencing behavior, separating nature from nurture becomes a complex, but necessary, job. Certainly an alcoholic parent must have an impact on a growing child. It's not unreasonable to expect that inherent in the family lies the soil of addiction. But again, simply because this sounds reasonable does not make it true.

The most current hypothesis is that heredity does play a role in the development of alcoholism in some persons. Which persons, and by what mechanisms, has not been established. Considerable research is being done in this particular area of alcoholism, and much has been learned since the early 1970s when the first papers were published.

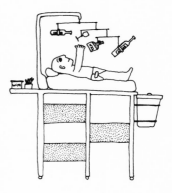

If heredity is a factor, there must be some basic biochemical differences between those who are alcoholism prone and those who are not. The observations of people working in the area of alcohol rehabilitation and treatment would tend to support a constitutional vulnerability. Certain individuals develop alcoholism very early in their life, and it progresses very rapidly in the absence of any unique, identifiable, psychological stress. At AA meetings the remark may be heard, "I was an alcoholic from my first drink." Usually this means that for seemingly idiosyncratic reasons the speaker never drank "normally" as did his peers, but used, and was affected by, alcohol differently.

Twin and adoption studies. Scientific investigational methods using an experimental model are not possible in the task of separating nature and nurture. Human research requires locating persons with particular life experiences or characteristics and then comparing them to people with other backgrounds. Twin studies and adoption studies are the two classical methods for doing this. Dr. Donald Goodwin is an alcoholism researcher who has worked extensively on the topic of alcoholism and heredity. Many of his (and others') studies have used data from Scandinavia, because these countries keep very complete records of marriages, births and so on, making tracing families easier. One early study was based on a large sample of twins. In each set, *one* twin was alcoholic. The researchers determined if the twins were identical or fraternal. They then interviewed the twin of the known alcoholic. The prediction: if alcoholism has a hereditary base, the other twin of identical sets would then be more likely to be alcoholic also than if that twin was fraternal. This assumption was made because identical twins share the same genetic material. That proved to be the case. However, the hereditary endowment does *not* act to dictate entirely the development

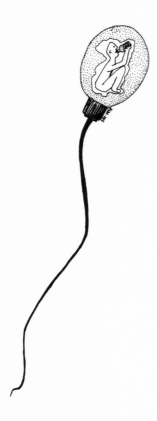

of alcoholism because not all the identical twins were both alcoholic. It was further discovered that there exists an apparent predisposition toward having, or being spared, the social deterioration associated with alcoholism. If both twins were alcoholic, the best predictor of the other twin's life situation was *not* how much, or how long he had been drinking. The life situation of the first twin was more reliable. So there appears to be both a hereditary predisposition to alcoholism and also to the social problems associated with it.

An adoption study conducted by Goodwin using Danish subjects further supports the influence of heredity. He traced children born of alcoholic parents. These children had been adopted by age 6 weeks. He then compared them to adopted children of nonalcoholic biological parents. The adoptive families of both groups were essentially the same. He discovered that those whose natural parents were alcoholic were in adulthood themselves more likely to be alcoholics. Thus, the alcoholism cannot be attributed simply to the home environment. In passing, Goodwin recalls Jellinek's speculation that cases of "early onset" alcoholism may have a heredity base. The average age of the individuals in Goodwin's study was 30 years. If the children of nonalcoholic parents were to be studied again in 15 or 20 years, possibly new cases of alcoholism would become apparent. Such a finding would lend support to Jellinek's hypothesis.

Genetic marker studies. Finally, another group of studies are given the shorthand title of "genetic marker" studies. In such investigations, attempts are made to link alcoholism to any traits that are known to be inherited. This would establish a genetic base for alcoholism. Some of the possibilities that have been studied include blood types. It's known that blood type is inherited and the genes controlling this may also be responsible for other characteristics. Other leads that have been followed include other blood substances; ability to taste or not taste phenylthiocarbamide; and blue-yellow color blindness. Nothing definite has resulted, although research continues.

Animal studies. Another avenue of investigation involves animal studies. These studies cannot be directly generalized to humans. However, work with chimps, baboons, or rats can shed light on the promising areas for human investigation and provide clues. Some of the more curious studies involve rats. Different strains of rats were given a choice of water or water spiked with alcohol of differing concentrations. Inevitably, they sampled each and usually opted for plain water. If the only liquid available had alcohol added, they'd drink it. Several strains of rats were important exceptions. They preferred alcohol and water solutions of around 5%. These "drinking rats" could be inbred and produce offspring who preferred even higher alcohol concentrations. The tentative conclusion is that biochemically they are different from their water-drinking counterparts. Interestingly, even "drinking rats" very rarely choose to drink to intoxication. Though a taste for alcohol may exist, they don't go on to become alcoholic. Dogs are apparently different. They will drink to intoxication more frequently. They'll even indulge in several days of "heavy" drinking, but they stop spontaneously. Despite the fact that the dogs seem to experience what the experimenters interpret as a hangover or mild withdrawal, the animals abstain. Unless the dogs were binge drinkers, it would appear that alcoholism is a human problem.

Studies of nonalcoholic blood relatives. Any genetic difference between those biologically alcoholism prone and those who are not will, as noted, be manifested in some biochemical differences. One of the not unreasonable hypotheses would be that there is a difference in the way the body handles alcohol. The differences could conceivably be differences of metabolism, or differences in response to chronic exposure to ethanol, or possibly a unique response to a single dose—for example, those at high risk having greater pleasure and those at low risk more discomfort. These studies are just now being conducted. The results are very preliminary, but there does seem to be a difference in metabolism. In one study, a group of presently nonalcoholic young men with an alcoholic father or brother showed greater acetaldehyde levels during alcohol metabolism than another similar group who did *not* have an alcoholic family member. Another preliminary study, looking at how alcohol's effects are experienced using young men who exhibit no symptoms of alcoholism, reports that those having an alcoholic family member describe a lesser response to a single dose of alcohol than those with no alcoholic blood relative. To translate this, those with a family history of alcoholism didn't feel as "high" as did those without alcoholism in the family. It would be premature to even speculate on what this might mean. More work needs to be carried out. But what is clear is that a promising area of research has been opened up.

The host—psychological factors

Psychological theories attempt to explain alcoholism by looking at the personalities of the people who become alcoholic. The question to be answered: "Is there anything in the person's character, or personality makeup, that makes him likely to become an alcoholic?" Many people drink, but in proportion, few become alcoholic. Alcoholism is a deviant behavior. It is not the normal, average state of affairs. What are the conditions within an individual that render him or her a likely target, or host, for this abnormal situation?

Historically the first modern efforts to understand the causes of alcoholism focused exclusively on psychological factors. These early efforts assumed that physiological factors or environmental factors were irrelevant. To put this into historical context, be aware that the genetic influence was then unknown. Furthermore, to look at behavior "psychologically" was to be quite up to date in the late 1930s and 1940s. Though the attempt to explain the origins of alcoholism solely on the basis of psychological or personality factors has been discredited, these earlier approaches to alcoholism, even if not scientifically acceptable now, still color popular thinking. The almost instinctive response of all of us to understanding an alcoholic's drinking is to look for psychological motives.

Our present almost unthinking acceptance of psychological factors as the significant determinants of behavior represents a revolution in approaching human behavior that began less than a century ago. The credit for this revolution goes to Dr. Sigmund Freud. A testimony to his influence is our common daily use of words such as "unconscious," "neurotic," "repressed," "anxious," "Freudian slip," to describe behavior. Although Freud might not consider our usage proper, nonetheless these words have been added to our vocabularies.

Psychological needs. It is now generally recognized that our behavior is at least partially determined by factors of which we are unaware. What are these factors? Our grade school geography classes usually focused on food, clothing, and shelter as the three basic human needs. But there are emotional needs, just as real and important, if people are to survive healthy and happy. What do we need in this realm? Baruch, in her book *New Ways of Discipline: You and Your Child Today*, puts it this way:

> What are the emotional foods that every human being must have regardless of age? What are the basic emotional requirements that must come to every small infant, to every growing child, to every adult?
>
> In the first place, there must be affection and a lot of it. Real down-to-earth, sincere loving. The kind that carries the conviction through body warmth, through touch, through the good mellow ring of the voice, through the fond look that says as clearly as words, "I love you because you are you."
>
> Closely allied with being loved should come the sure knowledge of belonging, of being wanted, the glow of knowing oneself to be a part of some bigger whole. *Our town, our school, our work, our family*—all bring the sound of togetherness, of being united with others, not isolated or alone.

Every human being needs also to have the nourishment of pleasure that comes through the senses. Color, balanced form and beauty to meet the eye, harmonious sounds to meet the ear. The hearty enjoyment of touch and taste and smell. And finally, the realization that the pleasurable sensations of sex can be right and fine and a part of the spirit as well as the body.

Everyone must feel that he is capable of achievement. He needs to develop the ultimate conviction, strong within him, that he can do things, that he is adequate to meet life's demands. He needs also the satisfaction of knowing that he can gain from others recognition for what he does.

And most important, each and every one of us must have acceptance and understanding. We need desperately to be able to share our thoughts and feelings with some other person, or several, who really understand. . . . We yearn for the deep relief of knowing that we can be ourselves with honest freedom, secure in the knowledge that says, "This person is with me. He accepts how I feel!"*

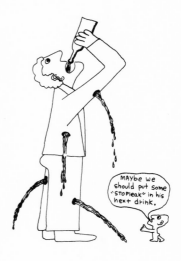

If these needs are not satisfactorily met, the adult is not whole. A useful notion to assess what has happened is to think of the unmet needs as "holes." Everybody has some "holes." They can vary in number, size, and pattern. What is true for all is that "holes" are experienced as painful. Attempts are made to cover up, patch over, or camouflage our holes. Thus we feel more whole, less vulnerable, and more presentable.

Psychological approaches to alcoholism. The various psychological approaches that have emerged essentially are all attempting to categorize the nature of the "holes," their origins, and the devices used to cover them up.

PSYCHOANALYTIC THEORIES. The first family of personality theories is the psychoanalytic, based on the work of Freud. Freud himself never devoted attention to alcoholism. However, his followers did apply aspects of his theory to this disease. It is impossible to present briefly the whole of Freud's work. He recognized that psychological development is related to physical growth. He identified stages of development, each with its particular, peculiar hurdles that a child must overcome on the way to being a healthy adult. Tripping over one of the hurdles, he felt, led to difficulties in adulthood. Some of the events of childhood are especially painful, difficult, and anxiety producing. The situation may persist unrelieved by the environment. This makes the child feel incompetent, resulting in a hole. He would seek his own ways to patch over the holes he feels. However, the existence of the hole shapes future behavior. It may grow larger, requiring more patchwork. The hole

*From Baruch, Dorothy. *New ways of discipline: you and your child today.* New York: McGraw-Hill Book Co., 1949. Used with permission of McGraw-Hill Book Co.

may render the child more vulnerable to future stress and lead to new ones.

The concept of *oral fixation* has been used in applying psychoanalytic theory to alcoholism. This means the holes began way back in earliest childhood. Observe infants and see how very pleasurable and satisfying nursing and sucking are. Almost any "dis-ease" or discomfort can be soothed this way. An individual whose most secure life experiences are associated with this period will tend to resort to similar behaviors in times of stress. These people will also, as adults, tend to have the psychological characteristics of that life period. The major psychological characteristics of the oral period are the infant's egocentricity and inability to delay having his needs met. He's hungry when he's hungry, be it a convenient time from mother's viewpoint or not. And he's oblivious to other persons except as they fit into his world. Thus the alcoholic, according to this theory, is likely to be an individual who never fully matured beyond infancy. He is stuck with childlike views of the world and childlike ways of dealing with it. He is easily frustrated, impatient, demanding, wants what he wants when he wants it. . . . He has little trust that people can help him meet his needs. He is anxious and feels very vulnerable to the world. Nursing a drink seems an appropriate way of handling his discomforts. Alcohol is doubly attractive, since it works quickly: bottled magic.

Another psychoanalytic concept applied to male alcoholics is that of *latent homosexuality*. Its origins are seen to be rooted in the *oedipal period*, which corresponds to the preschool, kindergarten age. According to Freud, an inevitable part of every little boy's growing up is a fantasy love affair with his mother. There is an accompanying desire to get Dad out of the picture. Given the reality of Dad's size, he has a clear advantage in the situation. The little boy eventually gives up and settles on being *like* Dad, rather than taking his place. Through this identification process, the little boy assumes a male role. There are several possible hitches that can occur. Maybe the father is absent, or the father is not a very attractive model. In such instances, the child will not grow to manhood with a sense of himself as a healthy, whole male. As an adult he may turn to alcohol to instill a sense of masculinity. Or he may like drinking because it provides a socially acceptable format for male companionship.

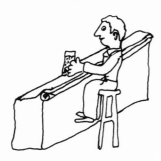

FEELINGS OF DEPENDENCY. Other personality theorists have focused on different characteristics. Adler latched onto the feelings of dependency. He saw the roots of alcoholism being planted in the first 5 years of life. He thought firstborn children were most likely to become either alcoholic or suicidal. In this view the dynamics of both are essentially the same. The firstborn is displaced or dethroned by the next child. He or she loses a position of being pampered by both parents and feels less important. If the parents are unable to provide reassurance, he or she has increased feelings of inferiority and pessimism. The feelings of inferiority or the longing for a sense of power require strong proofs of superiority for satisfaction. When new problems arise, arousing anxiety, the person seeks a sense of *feeling* superior rather than really overcoming difficulties. Theoretically, then, drinking as a solution is, to the alcoholic, intelligent. Alcohol does temporarily reduce the awareness of anxiety and gives relief from the inferiority feelings. Without the relief of alcohol, the inferiority feelings and anxiety could build up and lead to the ultimate escape of suicide.

THE ALCOHOLIC PERSONALITY. Another psychological approach to alcoholism attempts to define the "alcoholic personality." The hope was to identify common characteristics by looking at groups of alcoholics. So far these attempts have met with little success, and the search has largely been abandoned. Since active alcoholics were studied, what appeared to be the "alcoholic personality" was in fact a set of symptoms for alcoholism. Thus the behavior being studied was either drugged or behavior essential to continue the drugged state. Although an alcoholic personality exists, it is seemingly unrelated to the prealcoholic personality.

In 1960, William and Joan McCord published their *Origins of Alcoholism*. Their studies used quite extensive data. The data had been collected on 255 boys throughout their childhood. What they found negated many of the psychoanalytic theories. In brief, oral tendencies, latent homosexuality, and strong maternal encouragement of dependency were not, in fact, predictors of alcoholism. From their analysis, a consistent, statistically significant picture emerged. The typical alcoholic, as a child, underwent a variety of experiences that heightened inner stress. This stress produced the paradoxical effect of intensifying both his need for love and his strong desire to repress this need. The conflict produced a distorted self-image. McCord and McCord examined "the personality of alcoholics, both in childhood and in adulthood. In childhood, the alcoholics appeared to be highly masculine, extroverted, aggressive, 'lone-wolfish'—all manifestations . . . of their denial of the need to be loved. An analysis of the personality of adult alcoholics leads to the conclusion that the disorder itself produces some rather striking behavioral changes." Their contribution was significant. They highlighted the complexity of the social and psychological interactions.

• • •

In the past decade, there has been an emergence of what has been called the *human potential*, or *growth movement*. In essence it has been devoted, not to "curing" mental illness, but to applying the expertise of psychology and psychiatry to assisting "normal" people to function better (whatever that means to them). Tied in with this has been the emergence of new psychological or personality theories. The primary question has become, "What is going on now, and how can the individual/client/patient change?" The previously important question, "Why, or how, did the sickness or screwed-up-ness originate?" is less important. Transactional analysis, popularly known as TA, and reality therapy are two of these recent arrivals. Both have made a big splash in lay circles as well as in the professional community. Both have been used to address the problem of alcoholism.

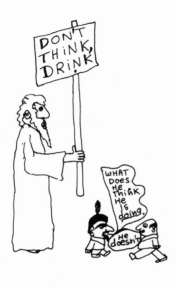

TRANSACTIONAL ANALYSIS (TA). *Games Alcoholics Play* by Claude Steiner has applied TA to alcoholism and the alcoholic. According to this thesis, the origins of alcoholism lie in the alcoholic's childhood conditions and his responses to them. The child finds himself in a predicament with his parents. When he behaves in a way that feels good or makes sense to him, he runs into problems. He discovers the real him isn't O.K. To overcome this and become O.K., he adopts a life-style or script for himself. In the script, he attempts to respond so as to counterbalance the message that said, "You're not O.K." For the alcoholic, the dominant script theme, according to Steiner, is "Don't think." This originates in a home where there are clear disparities between what is going on and what the parents say is happening. An observant child picks this up. If he points it out, he gets a "You just do what I say," or "You just mind your own business," or "Don't get sassy." To survive, he needs to find mechanisms for tuning out, turning off. As an adult, being an alcoholic is a fine way to continue the "Don't think" script.

REALITY THERAPY. William Glasser developed reality therapy. He believes that besides the obvious and inborn biological needs, all humans have two basic needs: to love and be loved, and to feel that we are worthwhile to ourselves and others. Failure to fill these needs leads to pain. A possible solution is the route to addiction; use of some substance or behavior that, while it continues, completely removes the pain.

• • •

Learning theories. The other major class of psychological theories used to explain alcoholism has come from a different branch of psychology. These are the learning theories, which look at behavior quite differently. They see behavior as a result of learning motivated by an individual's attempt to minimize unpleasantness and maximize pleasure. What is pleasant is a very individual thing. A child might misbehave and be "punished," but the punishment, for him, might be a reward and more pleasant than being ignored.

In applying learning theories to alcoholism, the idea is that alcoholic drinking has a reward system. Either alcohol, or its effects, are sufficiently reinforcing to cause continuation of drinking by the individual. Behavior most easily learned is that with immediate, positive results. The warm glow and well-being associated with the first sips are more reinforcing than the negative morning-after hangover. This theory would hold that anyone could become alcoholic if the drinking were sufficiently reinforced. Vernon Johnson, founder of a highly successful treatment program and author of a book, *I'll Quit Tomorrow*, gives great emphasis to the importance of learning in explaining drinking. He notes that users of alcohol learn from their first drink that alcohol is exceedingly trustworthy (it works every time) and that it does good things. This learning is highly successful, sufficient to set up a lifetime relationship with alcohol. The relationship may alter gradually over time, finally becoming a destructive one. But the original positive reinforcement keeps the person seeking the "good old days" and minimizing the destructive elements. Looked at in this light, alcoholics are not so far distant from people who remain in what are now unsatisfactory marriages, jobs, or living situations out of habit or some hope that the original zest will return.

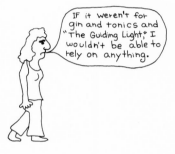

In summary, many of the aforementioned theories were formulated in the "salad days" of psychology and alcohol studies. No knowledgeable individual is likely nowadays to rely on any one of them as a single definitive explanation of a person's actions.

Current thinking. Psychology is the study of behavior. Within the field of psychology, it is currently recognized that a number of different influences need to be considered in explaining behavior. This general approach is now being applied to alcoholism as a behavior. For lack of a better phrase, this may be termed the "slot-machine theory." To be alcoholic requires getting three cherries. An individual may be born with a physiological cherry. The environment and culture he is raised in may provide a second, or sociological, cherry. And his personality makeup, with its unique set of holes, may be the third cherry. Or it may be some variation: say two-thirds psychological and one-third sociological. But one lone cherry is not an accurate predictor of who becomes alcoholic.

At this point, a comment on the relationship between alcoholism and mental illness is in order. By way of preface it must be noted that the modern approach to mental illness is identical to the one being presented for alcoholism. Psychiatrists and psychologists too are looking at biological predispositions to mental illness. It would probably be fair to say that increasingly behavior is being seen as a result of the interaction of biological and psychological factors, in the context of an individual's environment. Hence the old body *or* mind approach is here too out of date. In terms of the relationship between alcoholism and mental illness, alcoholics do not have a substantially greater incidence of mental illness than the general population. To put it crassly, being "crazy" doesn't cause alcoholism; nor on the other hand, is being alcoholic a protection against mental illness occurring. However, persons with mental illness may tend to use alcohol as a self-medication, and if the mental illness goes undiagnosed, they may inadvertently—so to speak—become alcoholic. In one area there does appear to be some relationship between mental illness (namely depression) and alcoholism, particularly in women. Because a biological predisposition to depression is strongly suspected, it is not inconceivable that the same, or similar, mechanism may be related to both these illnesses.

There is one approach that has not received the attention we believe it deserves. It fits neatly into neither the sociological or psychological approaches to the etiology of alcoholism. It was advanced in a provocative paper by the late Gregory Bateson, a maverick anthropologist-sociologist. One of his many concerns was how people process information, drawing upon their culture and their own style of thinking. An essay published in 1972, "The Cybernetics of 'Self': A Theory of Alcoholism," offers some intriguing ideas on why alcoholism may be reaching epidemic proportions in Western cultures. It certainly provides an interesting hypothesis on why abandoning alcohol is so difficult for the alcoholic.

Bateson points out that Western and Eastern cultures differ significantly in the way they view the world. Western societies focus on the individual. The tendency of Eastern cultures is to consider the individual in terms of the group or in terms of his relationships. To point out this difference, consider how you might respond to the question, "Who is that?" The "Western" way to answer is to respond with the person's name, "That's Joe Schmoe." The "Eastern" response might be, "That's my neighbor's oldest son." This latter answer highlights the relationship of several persons.

One of the results of Westerners' zeroing in on the individual is an inflation of the sense of "I." We think of ourselves as wholly separable and independent. Also we may not recognize the relationships of ourselves to other persons and things and the effects of our interactions. According to Bateson, this can lead to problems. One example he cites is the relationship of humans to the physical environment. If nothing else, the ecology movement has taught us the old rallying cry of "man against nature" doesn't make sense. Humans can't beat nature. We only win, that is survive, if we allow nature to win some rounds too. To put it differently, now we are starting to see humans as a part of nature.

How does this fit in with alcohol? The same kind of thinking is evident. The individual who drinks expects, and is expected, to be the master of alcohol. If problems develop, you can count on hearing "control your drinking," "use willpower." The person is supposed to fight the booze and win. Now there's a challenge. Who can stand losing to a "thing?" So the person tries different tactics to gain the upper hand. Even if he quits drinking for awhile, the competition is on: me versus it. To prove that he is in charge, sooner or later, he will have "just one." If disaster doesn't strike then, the challenge continues to "just one more." Sooner, or later. . . .

Bateson asserts that successful recovery requires a change of world views by the person in trouble with alcohol. The Western tendency to see the self (the I) as separate and distinct from, and often in combat with, alcohol (or anything else) has to be abandoned. The alcoholic has to learn the paradox of winning through losing, the limitations of the I and its interdependence with the rest of the world. He continues with examples of the numerous ways in which Alcoholics Anonymous fosters just this change of orientation.

The environment—sociological factors

Genetic and psychological approaches taken alone or together fall short of fully explaining the phenomenon of alcoholism. This is because they concentrate on why isolated individuals are, or become, alcoholic. Looking at the larger picture shows something else at work. The particular society or culture in which someone lives makes a big difference. All groups or cultures do not have similar difficulty with alcohol. Statistically, the odds on becoming alcoholic vary significantly from country to country. Through studies in epidemiology it is known that the Irish, French, Chileans and Americans have a high incidence of alcoholism. The Italians, Jews, Chinese, and Portuguese have substantially lower rates. The difference seems to lie with the country's habits and customs. Indeed, whether someone drinks at all depends as much on culture as it does on individual characteristics.

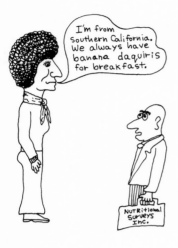

Culture includes the unwritten rules and beliefs by which a group of people live. Social customs set the ground rules for behavior. The rules are learned from earliest childhood and are followed later, often without a thought. Many times it is such social customs that account for the things we do "just because." The specific expectations for behavior differ from nation to nation, and between separate groups within a nation. Differences can be tied to religion, sex, age, or social class. The ground rules apply to drinking habits as much as to other customs. Cultures vary in attitudes toward alcohol use just as they differ in the sports they like or what they eat for breakfast.

Cultural orientation's effects on alcoholism rates. Several distinctive drinking patterns and attitudes toward alcohol's use have been identified. Which orientation predominates in a culture or a cultural subgroup is influential in determining that group's rate of alcoholism. One such attitude toward drinking is *total abstinence*, as with the Moslems or Mormons. With drinking forbidden, the chances of alcoholism are mighty slim. Expectedly, the group as a whole has a very low rate of alcoholism. An interesting twist we'll get to later, relates to what happens when members leave the group. Another cultural attitude toward alcohol promotes *ritual use.* The drinking is primarily connected to religious practice, ceremonies, and special occasions. Any heavy drinking in other contexts would be frowned upon. When drinking is tied to social occasions, with the emphasis on social solidarity and camaraderie, this is termed *convivial use.* Finally, there is *utilitarian use.* The society "allows" people to drink for their own personal reasons, to meet their own needs, for example, to relax, to forget, or to chase a hangover. Rates of alcoholism are highest where utilitarian use is dominant.

Differences among nations are growing less noticeable with television, jet planes, increased travel, and so forth. Italy has adopted the cocktail party; America is on France's wine kick. Nonetheless, a look at some of the differences between the *traditional* French and Italian drinking habits shows cultural attitudes toward the use of alcohol can influence the rate of alcoholism. Both France and Italy are wine-producing countries, France first in the world, Italy second; both earn a substantial part of their revenue from the production and distribution of wine. Yet the incidence of alcohol addiction in Italy in 1952 was less than one-fifth that of France.

In France there are no controls on excess drinking. Indeed, there is no such thing as excessive drinking. Wine is publicly advertised as good for the health, creating gaiety, optimism, and self-assurance. It is seen as a useful or indispensable part of daily life. Drinking in France, as in Ireland, is a matter of social obligation; a refusal to drink is

met with ridicule, suspicion, and contempt. It is not uncommon for a Frenchman to have a little wine with breakfast, to drink small amounts all morning, to have half a
bottle with lunch, to sip all afternoon, to have another half
bottle with dinner, and to nip until bedtime, consuming 2
liters or more a day. Frenchmen do get drunk. On this
schedule, drunkenness does not always show up in drunken
behavior. The body, however, is never entirely free of alcohol. Even people who have never shown open drunkenness
have withdrawal symptoms and even delirium tremens
when they abstain. The "habit," and the social atmosphere
that permits it, are obviously facilitating factors in the high
rate of alcoholism in France.

Italy, on the other hand, which has the second highest
wine consumption in the world, consumes only half of
what is consumed in France. Italy has a low rate of alcoholism on a world scale. The average Italian doesn't drink
all day, but only with his noon and evening meals. One
liter a day is the accepted amount, and anything over that
is considered excessive. There is no social pressure for
drinking as in France. As Jellinek said, "In France, drinking is a must. In Italy it is a matter of choice." Drunkenness, even mild intoxication, is considered a terrible thing,
unacceptable even on holidays or festive occasions. A guy
with a reputation for boozing would have a hard time getting along in Italy. He would have trouble finding a wife.
Both she and her parents would hesitate to consent to a
marriage with such a man. His social life would be hindered,
his business put in jeopardy, he would be cut off from the
social interaction necessary for advancement.

Jews have a low rate of alcoholism. Jewish drinking patterns are similar to the Italians', and there is the additional
restraint of religion. The Irish are more like the French and
have a high incidence of alcoholism for many of the same
reasons. The Irish have many ambivalent feelings toward
alcohol and drunkenness, which can produce tension and
uneasiness. Drinking among the Irish (and other groups
with high rates) is largely convivial on the surface; yet

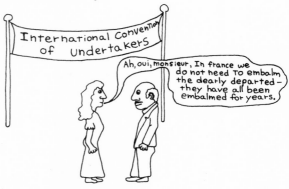

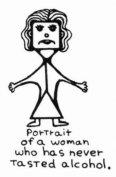

Portrait
of a woman
who has never
Tasted alcohol.

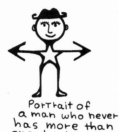

Portrait of
a man who never
has more than
one drink.

purely utilitarian drinking—often lonely, quick, and sneaky —is a tolerated pattern.

What, then, are the specific factors that account for the differences? These are obviously not based on abstinence. Among the Italians and Jews, many use alcohol abundantly and yet they have a low incidence of alcoholism. In cultures with low rates of alcoholism, children are gradually introduced to alcohol in diluted small amounts, on special occasions, within a strong, well-integrated family group. Parents who drink a small or moderate amount with meals, who are consistent in their behavior and their attitudes set a healthy example. There is strong disapproval of intoxication. It is neither socially acceptable, stylish, funny, nor tolerated. A positive acceptance of moderate, nondisruptive drinking and a well-established consensus on when, where, and how to drink create freedom from anxiety. Drinking is not viewed as a sign of manhood and virility, and abstinence is socially acceptable. It is no more rude to say no to liquor than to coffee. Liquor is viewed as an ordinary thing. No moral importance is attached to drinking or not drinking; it is neither a virtue nor a sin. In addition, alcohol is not seen as the primary focus for an activity; it accompanies rather than dominates or controls.

High rates of alcoholism tend to be associated with the reverse of the above patterns. Wherever there is little agreement on *how* to drink and *how not to* drink, alcoholism rates go up. In the absence of clear, widely agreed-upon rules, whether one is behaving or misbehaving is uncertain. Ambivalence, confusion, and guilt can easily be associated with drinking. Those feelings further compound the problem. Persons who move from one culture to another are especially vulnerable. Their guidelines may be conflicting, and they are caught without standards to follow. Thus persons who belong to groups that promote abstinence similarly run a very high risk of alcoholism if they do drink.

The focus has been on the unwritten rules that govern drinking behavior and influence the rates of alcoholism. How about the rules incorporated into law, that govern use and availability? What impact do they have on the rates of alcoholism? Though their impact is less than the factors just discussed, which permeate all of daily life, they do make a difference. Think back to the nation's experience of Prohibition, which can only be described as a fiasco. Few would maintain Prohibition was successful in significantly curtailing consumption or reducing alcoholism. What is clear is that laws if they are to work must, to a large degree, reflect how people want people to behave.

Change our culture, change our drinking behavior? Short of Prohibition, there are still significant ways society can influence the use of alcohol. Among these are cost of alcoholic beverages, regulations on advertising, and when and where alcohol may be sold. Evidence from other countries would suggest that the rate of alcoholism is related to per capita consumption. So banning advertising, increasing taxes, and so on, to thereby reduce sales might achieve a lower rate of alcoholism. Discussion is hot and heavy on these issues. Many states are now busy either raising or lowering the legal drinking age as a way to handle alcohol problems. Several years ago the governor of Alaska, in what he acknowledged was a drastic and probably unpopular move, proposed a legislative package to "combat the grim statistics" of alcohol abuse in the state: among the proposals were allowing bush villages to establish possession limits on alcohol, adopt unlimited sales taxes on alcohol, and impose a 2-week lag time between purchase and pickup.

It must be noted here that in the United States, the laws in reference to alcohol use are set by the states for the most part. The blood alcohol level used to define legal intoxication is not even universally the same in the United States. States may vary on when, where, and what a citizen may drink within their borders. And some states even vary from county to county (Texas for example). These laws go from dry to beer only to anything at all but only in private clubs, to sitting down but not walking with drink in hand, ad infinitum.

As a society we are attempting to "have our booze and drink it too." We want alcohol without the associated problems. Since that is not possible, the question is what compromises are we willing to make. The Uniform Code, mentioned in Chapter 1, which promotes treatment, not punishment, of alcohol abusers is a step in the right direction. But what other inconveniences and costs is society willing to assume? Will we accept a ban on package sales after 10 P.M. on the assumption that folks who want to buy alcohol at that hour don't need it? Will we allocate a reasonable share of the alcohol tax dollar to help the inevitable percentage who get into trouble with the drug?

America in the 1980s has not achieved a consensus on how, when, and where to drink. Convivial and utilitarian drinking have largely replaced ritual use of alcohol. In some quarters, it is manly and sophisticated to drink. In others, drinking is felt to be unnecessary, if not outright decadent. The attitudes toward alcohol embodied in our liquor laws testify to this contradiction. The law implies minors should not drink, yet on the magical twenty-first (maybe eighteenth) birthday, they are treated as if they suddenly knew how to handle alcohol appropriately.

With alcohol everywhere, until agreement emerges on appropriate and inappropriate use, American society will continue to be a fertile breeding ground for alcoholism.

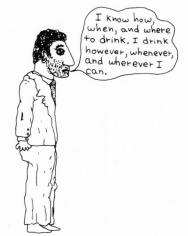

Chapter 5

Medical complications

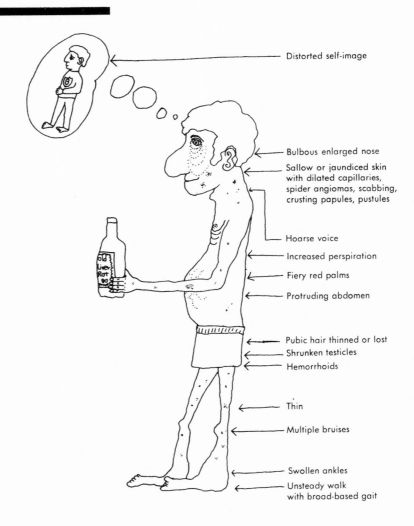

Distorted self-image

Bulbous enlarged nose

Sallow or jaundiced skin
with dilated capillaries,
spider angiomas, scabbing,
crusting papules, pustules

Hoarse voice

Increased perspiration

Fiery red palms

Protruding abdomen

Pubic hair thinned or lost

Shrunken testicles

Hemorrhoids

Thin

Multiple bruises

Swollen ankles

Unsteady walk
with broad-based gait

Alcoholism is one of the most common chronic diseases in all of medicine, occurring at a rate of 7% in the population at large. Untreated, its natural history is a predictable, gradually progressive downhill course. The early symptoms and manifestations of the primary disease alcoholism are for the most part behavioral and nonphysical. Later in its course it causes a wide variety of secondary pathological changes and medical complications, in a multitude of different organ systems. These are associated with a host of different physical signs and symptoms.

It is important to emphasize the distinction between the primary disease alcoholism and its late secondary medical complications. Alcoholism the disease is one of the most highly treatable of chronic illnesses and if recognized and treated early—that is, *before* major medical complications have occurred—may be entirely arrested. Treated patients can function quite normally, their only long-term disability being that they cannot use alcohol. Its complications, on the other hand, may be irreversible and may, if the underlying alcoholism is not treated, have a fatal outcome.

Other chapters in this book focus on the primary disease alcoholism, particularly as it appears at an early and highly treatable stage. This chapter focuses on the late secondary medical complications of alcoholism. Many physicians in the past have tended to view these as the major reason for their involvement with alcoholics and alcoholism. If physicians recognized and treated the primary disease alcoholism early enough there would be virtually no late secondary medical complications. Unfortunately, this does not happen often enough; thus the frequent occurrence of a broad spectrum of serious medical complications.

An acquaintance with all of the secondary medical complications of chronic alcoholism is equivalent to familiarity with an exceedingly broad cross section of medical disease, since nearly every organ system is affected. In this section we will touch briefly, in a systems-oriented fashion, on most of the major alcohol-related problems. First, however, let us examine a composite picture of a person afflicted with the visible stigmata of chronic alcoholism.

■ *The visible signs and stigmata of chronic alcoholism*

Statistically, the typical alcoholic is male; thus we will say he. However, women alcoholics can and do show virtually all the same signs of chronic alcohol use, except those involving the reproductive organs. Bearing in mind that any given alcoholic may have many or only a few of these visible manifestations, let us examine a hypothetical chronic drinker who has them all.

There are more old drunkards than old physicians.

RABELAIS

He is a typically thin, but occasionally somewhat bloated appearing, middle-aged individual. Hyperpigmented, sallow, or jaundiced skin accentuates his wasted, chronically fatigued, and weakened overall appearance. He walks haltingly and unsteadily with a broad-based gait (ataxia); multiple bruises are evident. He perspires heavily. His voice is hoarse and croaking, punctuated by occasional hiccups, and he carries an odor of alcohol.

The abdomen protrudes and closer examination of it may reveal the *caput medusae* (a prominent superficial abdominal vein pattern). There is marked ankle swelling, and he has hemorrhoids. His breasts may be enlarged, his testicles shrunken, and his chest, axillary, and/or pubic hair entirely lost or thinned. Inspection of the skin reveals dilated capillaries, acne-like lesions, and maybe a bulbous enlarged nose. There is scabbing and crusting secondary to generalized itching. He has spider angiomas on the upper half of the body. These are small red skin lesions that blanch with light pressure applied to their centers and spread into a spidery pattern with release of pressure. His palms are fiery red (liver palms), and he may have "paper money" skin, so called because tiny capillaries are distinctly visible much like the tiny red-colored filaments in a new dollar bill. In colder climates, there is evidence of repeated frostbite. The fingernails are likely to be affected. They may have either transverse white-colored bands (Muehrcke's lines) or transverse furrows, or may be totally opaque without half-moons showing at the base of the nail. He may well have difficulty fully extending the third, fourth, and fifth fingers due to a flexion deformity called Dupuytren's contracture. A swelling of the parotid glands in the cheeks, giving him the appearance of having the mumps, is known as "chipmunk facies." Finally, a close look at the whites of the eyes reveals small blood vessels with a corkscrew shape.

Now, with this as an externally visible picture, let us look inside the body at the underlying diseased organ systems and see how they may account for it.

■ Gastrointestinal system

Alcohol affects the gastrointestinal system in a variety of ways. This is the route by which alcohol enters the body and is absorbed. It is where the first steps of metabolism take place. Moderate amounts of alcohol can disturb and alter the normal functioning of this system. And chronic use of alcohol can raise havoc. Alcohol can have both direct and indirect effects. Direct effects are any changes that occur in response to the presence of alcohol. Indirect effects would be whatever occurs next, as a consequence of the initial, direct impact.

Many a man keeps on drinking till he hasn't a coat to either his back or his stomach.

GEORGE D. PRENTICE

Irritation, bleeding, and malabsorption

Chronic use of alcohol, as does any alcohol use, stimulates the stomach lining's secretion of hydrochloric acid and irritates the gut's lining. It also inhibits the muscular contractions called peristalsis that pass food along the intestines. In combination, these effects can lead to a generalized irritation of the mucous membrane lining the gut, especially in the stomach. Chronic heavy drinkers may also complain of frequent belching, loss of appetite, alternating diarrhea and constipation, morning nausea, and vomiting.

Irritation, rather than being found throughout the gastrointestinal system, is more often localized to particular portions. If the esophagus is irritated, esophagitis results. This is experienced as midchest pain and pain on swallowing. Acute and chronic stomach irritation by alcohol involving inflammation, abdominal pain, and maybe even bleeding, results in gastritis. Chronic alcohol use, if not indeed causing ulcers, can certainly aggravate ulcers of the stomach or duodenum (the first section of the small intestine). Bleeding can occur at any of the irritated sites. This represents a potentially serious medical problem. Bleeding along the gastrointestinal system can either be slow or massive. Either way, it is serious. Frequently, for reasons to be discussed later on, the alcoholic's blood clots less rapidly. So the body's built-in defenses to reduce bleeding are weakened. Surgery may be required to stop it in some cases.

In addition to the causes of gastrointestinal bleeding just mentioned, there are several other causes. The irritation of the stomach lining, not unexpectedly, upsets the stomach. With that can come prolonged violent nausea, vomiting, and retching. This may be so severe as to cause mechanical tears in the esophageal lining and bring on massive bleeding. Another cause of massive, and often fatal upper gastrointestinal bleeding is ruptured dilated veins along the esophagus (esophageal varices). The distention and dilation of these veins occurs as a result of chronic liver disease and cirrhosis, as we shall see shortly.

Chronic irritation of the esophagus by a combination of long-standing heavy alcohol consumption and cigarette smoking significantly increases the risk of developing cancer there. Chronic excessive use of alcohol can lead to abnormal absorption of a variety of foodstuffs, vitamins, and other nutrients as a result of its effects on the small intestinal function.

Although there are no specific diseases of the large intestine caused by alcohol abuse, diarrhea frequently occurs. Hemorrhoids, also a by-product of liver disease and cirrhosis, are common in chronic alcoholics.

Pancreatitis

Alcohol is frequently the culprit causing acute inflammation of the pancreas, known as acute pancreatitis. The pancreas is a gland tucked away behind the stomach and small intestine. It makes digestive juices, which are needed to break down starches, fats, and proteins. These juices are secreted into the duodenum through the pancreatic duct, in response to alcohol as well as other foodstuffs. They are alkaline and thus are important in neutralizing the acid contents of the stomach, thereby helping to protect the intestinal lining. The pancreas also houses the islets of Langerhans, which secrete the hormone insulin, needed to regulate sugar levels in the blood.

Currently there are two major theories as to how alcohol causes acute pancreatitis. The first suggests that the pancreatic duct, opening into the duodenum, can become swollen if the small intestine is irritated by alcohol. As it swells, digestive juices cannot pass through it freely; they become obstructed or "stopped up." The pancreas then becomes inflamed as the digestive juices that cannot escape, in effect, auto-digest it. The second theory holds that some of the excess fats in the bloodstream mobilized by excessive drinking are deposited in the pancreas and digested by pancreatic enzymes whose usual task is breaking down dietary fats. The products of this process, free fatty acids, cause cell injury in the pancreas and result in further release of fat-digesting enzymes, thereby perpetuating a vicious cycle.

A drunkard is like a whiskey bottle, all neck and belly and no head.

AUSTIN O'MALLEY

The symptoms of acute pancreatitis include nausea, vomiting, occasional diarrhea, and severe upper abdominal pain radiating straight through to the back. Chronic inflammation of the pancreas can lead to calcification, visible on abdominal x-ray films. This is a relapsing illness almost always associated with long-standing alcohol abuse. Diabetes can result from the decreased capacity of the pancreas to produce and release insulin as a result of chronic cell damage.

Liver disease

The liver is a most fascinating organ. You recall that it is the liver enzyme, alcohol dehydrogenase, that begins the breakdown process of alcohol. The liver is also responsible for a host of other tasks. It breaks down wastes and toxic substances. It manufactures essential blood components, including clotting factors. It stores certain vitamins, such as B_{12}, which is essential for red blood cells. It helps regulate the blood sugar level, a very critical task, since that is the only food the brain can use. Liver disease occurs because the presence of alcohol disturbs the metabolic machinery of the liver. Metabolizing alcohol is always a very high-priority liver function. Therefore, whenever alcohol is present, the liver is "distracted" from other normal and necessary functions. For the alcoholic, this can be a goodly part of the time.

As you may know, liver disease is one of the physical illnesses most commonly associated with alcoholism. There are three major forms of liver disease associated with alcohol abuse. The first is acute *fatty liver*. This condition may develop in anyone who has been drinking heavily. Fatty liver gets its name from the deposits of fat that build up in normal liver cells. This occurs because of a decrease in breakdown of fatty acids and an increase in the synthesis of fats by the liver as a result of the "distracting" metabolic effects of alcohol (see Chapter 2). Acute fatty liver occurs whenever 30 to 50% or more of the dietary calories are in the form of alcohol. This is true even if the diet is otherwise adequate. Acute fatty liver is a reversible condition if alcohol use is stopped.

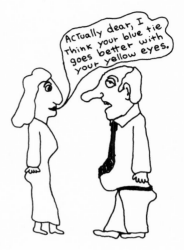

Alcoholic hepatitis is a more serious form of liver disease. It often follows a severe or prolonged bout of heavy drinking. Although more commonly seen in alcoholics, like acute fatty liver, this condition may occur in nonalcoholics as well. There is actual inflammation of the liver and variable damage to liver cells. Liver metabolism is frequently seriously disturbed. Jaundice is a usual sign of hepatitis. Jaundice refers to the yellowish cast of the skin and the whites of the eyes. The yellow color comes from the pigment found in bile, a digestive juice made by the liver. The bile is being handled improperly and is therefore circulating in the bloodstream in excessive amounts. Other symptoms of alcoholic hepatitis may include weakness, easy fatigability, loss of appetite, occasional nausea and vomiting, low-grade fever, mild weight loss, increasing ascites, dark urine, and light stools. Whereas in some patients it is completely reversible with abstinence from alcohol, in others it may be fatal or go on to become a smoldering chronic disease. Among patients who stop drinking, only one in five will go on to develop *alcoholic cirrhosis*; whereas from 50 to 80% of those who continue to drink will develop it. Alcoholic hepatitis is in many cases clearly a forerunner of alcoholic cirrhosis, but it is thought that alcoholic cirrhosis can also appear without the prior occurrence of alcoholic hepatitis.

Cirrhosis of the liver is a condition in which there is widespread destruction of liver cells and replacement by nonfunctioning scar tissue. In fact, the word cirrhosis simply means scarring. There are many different types and causes of cirrhosis, but long-term heavy alcohol use is the cause of the vast majority of cases. It is estimated that about one in ten long-term heavy drinkers will eventually develop alcoholic cirrhosis. Given the nature of the disease, it is accompanied by very serious and often relatively irreversible metabolic and physiological abnormalities. That is very bad news. In fact, more than half of the patients who continued to drink after the diagnosis of alcoholic cirrhosis has been made were dead within 5 years. In alcoholic cirrhosis the liver is simply unable to perform its work properly.

Toxic substances, normally removed by the liver, circulate in the bloodstream, creating problems elsewhere in the body. This is particularly true of the brain, as we shall see below. The liver normally handles the majority of the blood from the gut or intestinal tract as it returns to the heart. The cirrhotic liver, now a mass of scar tissue, is unable to handle the usual blood flow. The blood, unable to move through the portal vein (the route from the blood vessels around the intestines to the liver), is forced to seek alternative return routes to the heart. This leads to pressure and "backup" in these alternative vessels. It is this pressure that causes the veins in the esophagus to become distended, producing esophageal varices and inviting hemorrhaging. The same pressure accounts for hemorrhoids. Another phenomenon associated with cirrhosis is ascites. Here the liver, again because of back pressure, "weeps" tissue fluid directly into the abdominal cavity. This fluid would normally be taken up and transported back to the heart by the hepatic veins and lymphatics. Large amounts of liquid can collect and distend the abdomen, and a woman, for example, can look very pregnant. If you were to gently tap the side of a person with ascites, you would see a wavelike motion in response, as fluid sloshes around. Another result of alcoholic liver disease is diminished ability of the liver to store glycogen, the body's storage form of sugar, and produce glucose from other nutrient such as proteins. This can lead to low blood sugar levels (see also Chapter 2). This is an important fact when it comes to treating an alcoholic diabetic because insulin also lowers the blood sugar. Another situation in which this is important is in treating apparent coma in any alcoholic. Insufficient amounts of blood sugar may cause coma, essentially because the brain is without enough of a fuel supply to function. Intravenous glucose may be necessary to prevent irreversible brain damage.

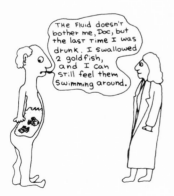

On the other hand, alcohol and alcoholic liver damage may lead to states of diabetes-like, higher than normal blood glucose levels. This occurs in large part because of the effects of alcohol and alcoholic liver disease on certain other glucose-regulating hormones in the body besides insulin.

Hepatic coma (due to severe hepatic encephalopathy) can be one result of cirrhosis. In this case, the damage comes from toxins circulating in the bloodstream. In essence, the brain is "poisoned" by these wastes and its ability to function seriously impaired, leading to coma. Cancer of the liver is another complication of long-standing cirrhosis. Another source of bad news is that, of people who get cirrhosis, as many as 50% will also have pancreatitis. So these persons have two serious medical conditions. Still other complications may include gastrointestinal bleeding, salt and water retention, and renal failure.

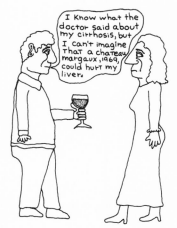

The main elements of treatment for cirrhosis are abstinence from alcohol, multivitamins, a nutritionally balanced, adequate diet, and bed rest. Even with such treatment, the prognosis of cirrhosis is not good and many of the complications just described may occur.

The different forms of alcohol-related liver disease result from specific changes in liver cells. Unfortunately, there is no neat and consistent relationship between a specific liver abnormality and the particular constellation of symptoms that develop. Although laboratory tests indicate liver damage, they cannot pinpoint the kind of alcohol-related liver disease. Therefore, some authorities believe a liver biopsy, which involves direct examination of a liver tissue sample, is essential to properly evaluate the situation.

Until fairly recently, it was believed that liver damage common to alcoholism was *not* a direct effect of the alcohol. Rather, it was believed the damage was caused by poor nutrition. It has since been learned that alcohol itself plays a major direct role. Liver damage can occur even in the presence of adequate nutrition when excessive amounts of alcohol are consumed.

■ *Hematological system*

The blood, known as the hematological system, is the body's major transportation network. The blood carries oxygen to the tissues. It takes up waste products of cell metabolism and carts them off to the lungs and kidneys for removal. It carries nutrients, minerals, and hormones to the cells. The blood also protects the body through the anti-infection agent it carries. Although the blood looks like a liquid, it contains formed elements (solid components). These formed elements include red blood cells, white blood cells, and platelets. They are all suspended in the serum, the fluid or liquid part of the blood. Each of the formed elements of the blood is profoundly affected by alcohol abuse.Whenever there is a disturbance of these essential blood ingredients, problems arise.

Red cells

Let us begin with the red blood cells. The most common problem here is anemia, too few red blood cells. Anemia is a general term like fever. It simply means insufficient function or amounts. Logically, one can imagine this result coming about in a number of ways. Too few can be manufactured if there is a shortage of nutrients to produce them. If they are produced, they can be defective. They can be lost (e.g., through bleeding), or they can actually be destroyed. In fact, alcohol contributes to anemia in each of these ways.

How does alcohol abuse relate to the first situation, inadequate production? The most likely culprit here is inadequate nutrition. Red blood cells cannot be manufactured if the bone marrow does not have the necessary ingredients. Iron is a key ingredient. Alcohol is thought to inhibit the bone marrow's ability to use iron in making hemoglobin, the oxygen-carrying part of the blood. Even if there is enough iron in the system, it "just passes on by." On the other hand, because of a poor diet, not uncommon in the alcoholic, the iron intake may be insufficient. There may also be chronic gastrointestinal bleeding as a result of chronic alcohol abuse. If so, the iron in the red blood cells is lost and not available for recycling. This type of anemia is called *iron-deficiency anemia*. Another variety is *sideroblastic anemia*. It, too, is related to nutritional deficiencies, too little vitamin B_6, pyridoxine. This vitamin is also needed by the bone marrow cells to produce hemoglobin.

These first two varieties account for the inadequate production of red blood cells. Another variety, *megaloblastic anemia*, is also related to nutritional deficiencies. There is too little folate. This happens because it is not in the diet, and/or the small intestine is unable to absorb it properly because of other effects of chronic alcohol abuse. What results then is defective red blood cell production. Without these vitamins, red blood cells cannot mature. They are released from the bone marrow in primitive, less functional forms that are larger than normal.

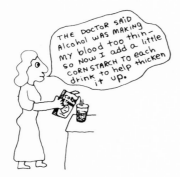

Chronic loss of blood from the gut—gastrointestinal bleeding—can result in anemia. Here the bone marrow simply cannot make enough new cells to keep up with those that are lost. The body normally destroys and recycles old red blood cells, through a process called *hemolysis*. Abnormal forms of hemolysis may occur. One abnormal cause of hemolysis is hypersplenism, which results from chronic liver disease. The spleen, enlarged and not working properly, destroys perfectly good red blood cells as well as the old worn-out ones. Toxic factors in the serum of the blood are also thought to be responsible for three other varieties of hemolysis. *Stomatocytosis* is a transient anemia related to binge drinking and unrelated to severe alcoholic liver disease. *Spur cell anemia* is associated with severe, often end-stage, chronic alcoholic liver disease. The name comes from the shape of the red cell, which, when seen under the microscope, has jagged protrusions. *Zieve's syndrome* is the co-occurrence of jaundice, transient hemolytic anemia, and elevated cholesterol levels, as well as acute fatty liver disease, without enlargement of the spleen in an alcoholic patient.

In France, and maybe elsewhere, other changes in red blood cells have been reported in persons who drink at least 2 to 3 quarts of wine each day. These are changes typically seen with lead poisoning. (Lead, even in low concentrations, can mean trouble.) Excessive intake of wine in France is thought to be a significant source of dietary lead. In the United States, there are periodically reports of lead poisoning connected with alcohol use. However, the circumstances are different; the beverage has not been wine, but moonshine! In these cases, old car radiators were used in the distilling process.

White cells

On to the effects of alcohol on white blood cells. These cells are one of the body's main defenses against infection. The chronic use of alcohol affects white cells. This contributes to the increased susceptibility to and frequency of severe infections, especially respiratory tract infections in alcoholics. Alcohol has a direct toxic effect on the white blood cell reserves (bone marrow granulocytes), which produces a relative lack of white cells to fight infection. Chemotaxis, or white cell mobilization, is diminished by alcohol. In other words, although the white cells' ability actually to take in and kill the bacteria is not affected, they have difficulty reaching the site of infection in adequate numbers. Alcohol also interferes with white cell adherence to bacteria, which is one of the body's defensive inflammatory reactions. The ability of serum (the unformed elements of the blood) to kill gram-negative bacteria is also impaired by alcohol. This may be related to the diseased liver's lowered ability to produce complement, an important agent in the body's inflammatory response. Many immune and defensive responses depend on its presence.

Platelets

Alcoholics are frequently subject to bleeding disorders. They bruise easily. Bleeding can occur in the gastrointestinal tract, the nose, and the gums. This is largely explained by the effect of alcohol in decreasing the number of platelets. Platelets are a major component of the body's clotting system and act like a patch on a leak. Alcohol has a direct toxic effect on bone marrow production of platelets. One out of every four alcoholic patients will have abnormally low platelet counts. It can also cause hypersplenism, which destroys platelets as well as red blood cells. When the

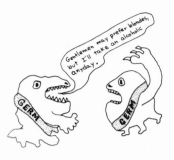

liver's metabolic processes are disrupted by the effects of chronic alcohol use, there is a decrease in the production of some of the necessary serum clotting factors. One thing to bear in mind is that there are thirteen to fifteen different substances needed to make a clot. Of these, five are liver produced; ergo, liver disease may lead to bleeding problems in alcoholics.

Another area of current research is examining other ways the immune system may be altered by alcohol. Actually, there are two different immune systems. One is associated with circulating antibodies, called *immunoglobulins*, in the blood system. The other is associated with antibodies attached to individual cells. Changes in both systems induced by alcohol may in part account for the increased susceptibility to infection seen in cases of severe alcoholism. Recent research has suggested that alcohol-induced changes in some white cells together with changes in the cell-based immune system may lead to an increased production of certain types of fibrous tissues. It is just such fibrous tissues that are characteristic of cirrhosis. A current $64 question is whether the scar tissue of cirrhosis can at least in part be attributed to white cell changes and alterations in the cells immune response that are induced by chronic alcohol use. Even though the hematological complications of chronic heavy alcohol use are many and potentially quite serious, they are in general totally reversible following abstinence. The speed with which they reverse themselves can be enhanced in many instances by administering the deficient substances, such as folate, pyridoxine and iron, in addition to a fully adequate diet.

▪ *Cardiovascular system*

Long-term heavy alcohol use is thought to be directly responsible for a specific but not too common form of heart disease, *alcoholic cardiomyopathy.* This is a severe condition with low-output heart failure, shortness of breath with the least exertion, and dramatic enlargement of the heart, occurring most commonly in middle-aged males. It often responds well to discontinuation of alcohol plus long-term bed rest. Another form of heart disease with high-output congestive heart failure known as *beriberi heart disease* may be seen in alcoholism. This is caused by impaired dietary intake and thiamine (vitamin B_1) deficiency and may respond dramatically to replacement of thiamine in the diet.

As an aside, a rather unusual and specific type of severe cardiac disease was noted to occur a few years ago among drinkers of a particular type of Canadian beer. It was found to be due not to alcohol per se, but rather to the noxious effects of small amounts of cobalt, which had been added to the beer to maintain its "head." These cases occurred in the mid to late 1960s with a mortality rate of 50% to 60%. Fortunately, the cause has been eliminated, and this will hopefully no longer happen.

A variety of *abnormalities in cardiac rhythm* have been associated with alcohol. In fact, nearly the entire spectrum of such abnormalities may be caused by acute and chronic alcohol intake. The upper chambers (atria) of the heart are like the primers to the lower (ventricular) part that acts as the pump. Thus ventricular irregularities tend to be more serious. Atrial fibrillation and atrial flutter occur in the upper heart muscles and produce an ineffective atrial beat. These conditions are frequently associated with acute and chronic heavy drinking. Paroxysmal atrial tachycardia is another alcohol-induced irregular rhythm in the upper part of the heart producing a different and more rapid than usual beat. Alcohol also causes an increase in the frequency of premature ventricular contractions. These are irregular or in-between contractions of the lower part of the heart. They can be a very dangerous condition, and if the irregular contractions occur in a particular pattern, which may be induced by alcohol, they can cause sudden death. A fourth effect is sinus tachycardia with palpitations, which is thought to occur because of the effects of alcohol and its metabolite, acetaldehyde, in releasing norepinephrine. The sinus node is the normal pacemaker of the heart, and its rate of firing can be greatly increased by the amount of circulating epinephrine and norepinephrine.

Recently there have been reports of a new alcohol-induced, arrhythmia-related syndrome. It goes by the name *holiday heart.* As you might expect with that name, arrhythmias occur after heavy alcohol intake, around holidays and on Mondays after weekend binges. The syndrome includes palpitations and arrhythmias, but no evidence of cardiomyopathy or congestive heart failure. The signs and symptoms clear completely after a few days of abstinence.

Alcohol, even in moderate amounts, exacerbates certain preexisting abnormalities of blood fats, especially *Type IV hyperlipoproteinemia.* This is an elevated fat level of a particular kind that has been suggested to increase the rate of development of arteriosclerosis, or hardening of the arteries. The coronary arteries become increasingly occluded or blocked, hence making premature heart attacks more likely. Even a small amount of alcohol can badly affect this disorder.

Alcohol is well known to cause dilation of peripheral superficial blood vessels and capillaries. It does not have the same effect on the coronary blood vessels. Therefore, despite its use in this condition in the past, it is not currently thought to be helpful in treating angina.

Somewhat surprisingly perhaps, on the other hand, some recent experimental evidence suggests that moderate amounts of alcohol (two or fewer drinks per day) may provide a protective effect against the occurrence of heart attacks in people without blood fat abnormalities. Such reports suggest that one cocktail a day has roughly the same effect on serum cholesterol as the average lipid-lowering diet. It causes increased levels of high-density lipoprotein (HDL) cholesterol and decreased levels of low-density lipoprotein (LDL) cholesterol. High and low levels of these substances, respectively, are associated with lower risks of heart attacks. So moderate daily use of alcohol may be desirable from your heart's point of view.

In work recently reported, a definite link was shown between heavy drinking and *hypertension.* Heavy drinkers had both elevated systolic and diastolic blood pressures. This was true even when weight, age, serum cholesterol, and smoking were controlled for. Although this relationship seems well established, the role alcohol plays in the development of atherosclerosis is much less clear.

*Wine is at the head of all
medicines.*

TALMUD; BABA BATHRA, 58b

▪ Genitourinary system

Urinary tract

The kidneys, almost uniquely, are not directly affected by alcohol. What happens in the kidneys is the result of disordered function elsewhere in the body. For example, alcohol promotes the production of urine through its ability to inhibit the production and output of antidiuretic hormone (ADH) by the hypothalamic region of the brain. The blood goes to the kidney for filtering, and water and wastes are separated from it and excreted through the bladder. Normally, in this process, ADH allows water to be reabsorbed by the kidney to meet the body's needs. When the hormone levels are suppressed, the kidney's capacity to reabsorb water is diminished. It is therefore excreted from the body. Alcohol only inhibits this hormone's production when the blood alcohol level is rising. This is so with as little as 2 ounces of pure alcohol. When the blood alcohol level is steady, or falling, there is no such effect. In fact, the opposite may be true. There may be a retention of fluids by the body.

Alcohol can lead to acute urinary retention and recurrence and exacerbation of urinary tract infections and/or prostatitis. This is due to its ability to cause spasm and congestion in diseased prostate glands as well as in the area of previously existing urethral strictures.

A nearly uniformly fatal, but fortunately uncommon,

consequence of chronic alcohol abuse is the so-called *hepatorenal syndrome*. This is thought to be caused by a toxic serum factor, or factors, secondary to severe liver disease. These factors cause shifts in kidney blood flow and diminish effective perfusion (filtering through) of the kidney. Unless the underlying liver disease is somehow reversed, irreversible kidney failure can occur. Interestingly, there is nothing intrinsically wrong with the kidneys themselves. They can be transplanted into a patient without underlying liver disease and perform normally.

Reproductive system

Chronic heavy alcohol use affects the reproductive system. In women there may be skipped menstrual periods; in men, diminished libido and on occasion, even sterility. In addition to its many other functions, the liver plays an important role in the balance of sex hormones. So when the liver is impaired, an imbalance of sex hormones results. Both male and female sex hormones are present in both sexes, only in different proportions. The increased levels of female hormones in alcoholic men can also lead to "feminization" of features. Breasts can enlarge, testicles shrink, and a loss or thinning of body hair can occur. Sex hormone changes in males also result from alcohol's direct action on the testes, which decreases the production of testosterone, a male sex hormone. Testosterone levels may be lowered as well by alcohol's direct inhibiting effect on various brain centers, such as the hypothalamus and pituitary gland, which produce luteinizing hormone (LH), which in turn prompts the release of testosterone. This is currently under investigation. These latter hormonal effects are the direct results of alcohol. They are independent of any liver or nutritional problems. The situation in women in terms of sex hormone changes is not as completely understood in part because the female reproductive system, located within the body, is less accessible for research. Also, the use of alcohol by women as a distinct area of inquiry is a very recent development.

Finally, although sexual interests and pursuits may be heightened by alcohol's release of inhibitions, ability to perform sexually can be impaired. For example, in men there may be either relative or absolute impotency.

■ *Alcohol and pregnancy*

Fetal alcohol syndrome

Since 1971, there has been considerable attention directed toward the effects of chronic alcohol use during pregnancy. At that time, a researcher reported his observations of infants born to alcoholic mothers. The constellation of features observed has since been termed the fetal alcohol syndrome. Alcohol can pass through the placenta to the developing fetus and interfere with prenatal development. At birth, infants with fetal alcohol syndrome are smaller, both in weight and length. The head is small, probably due to a decrease in brain growth. These infants also have a "dysmorphic facial appearance"—that is, they are strange looking, just appear "different," although the difference is not easily described. At birth the infants are jittery and tremulous. Whether this jitteriness is the result of nervous system impairment from the long-term exposure to alcohol and/or miniwithdrawal is unclear. There have been reports of newborn infants having the scent of alcohol on their breath. Cardiac problems and retardation are also associated with the fetal alcohol syndrome. This syndrome is now being seen as the third leading cause of mental retardation. (See Chapter 7 for further discussion of the effects of maternal alcoholism on children.)

Fetal alcohol effects

It is now well established that a mother *does not* have to be an alcoholic to expose her unborn baby to the risks of alcohol during pregnancy. Nor do alcohol's effects on the fetus have to occur as the full-blown fetal alcohol syndrome; they can occur with variable degrees of severity, and when less severe are referred to as fetal alcohol effects.

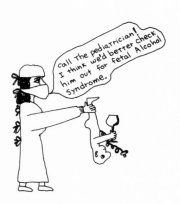

Perhaps even more worrisome than the fetal alcohol syndrome are recent reports on the effects of drinking in excess of two drinks (one ounce of pure alcohol) on the unborn baby. As little as two drinks a day may lead to increased risk of abnormalities. This two-drink figure is *not* a numerical average. It refers to the amount of alcohol consumed on any one day. As the amount of alcohol consumed on any given day rises, the risk also increases:

Less than two drinks	Very little risk
Two to four drinks	10% risk of abnormalities
Ten drinks	50% risk of abnormalities
Over ten drinks	75% risk of abnormalities

Based on this information, in the summer of 1977 the National Institute on Alcohol Abuse and Alcoholism issued a health warning, advising expectant mothers not to have more than two drinks a day.

How alcohol interferes with normal prenatal growth is not fully understood. Nor is it known if there are critical periods during pregnancy when alcohol is especially hazardous. Research with animals suggests that alcohol crosses the placenta freely and diffuses throughout fetal tissues in much the same fashion as in adults and that the alcohol level of some of the fetal tissues may be higher than that of the mother. If this is the case the reason has not been clearly identified. One would predict that the alcohol, since it can pass freely through the placenta to the fetus, should be able to exit just as easily. Therefore both mother and fetus would be expected to have equivalent blood alcohol levels.

However, case reports of women who drank alcohol during delivery, and in whom blood alcohol level studies were done, indicate that the newborn baby's blood and tissue alcohol levels do not drop as fast as the mother's. The reason presumably is that the infant has an immature liver. Newborns do not have the fully developed enzyme systems (alcohol dehydrogenase) necessary to metabolize and eliminate alcohol as rapidly as their mothers do. Thus for a given maternal blood alcohol concentration, the fetus may have a somewhat higher blood and tissue alcohol concentration for a longer period of time than might have been expected.

▪ Respiratory system

Alcohol affects the respiration rate. Low to moderate doses of alcohol increase the respiration rate, presumably by direct action on the medullary respiration center in the brain. In larger, anesthetic, and/or toxic doses the respiration rate is decreased, and this latter effect may contribute to respiratory insufficiency in persons with chronic pulmonary disease.

Whereas in the past it was thought that alcohol largely spared the lungs as far as the direct harmful effects were concerned, recently such effects have been increasingly recognized and investigated. These include interference with a variety of important defensive cellular functions—both mechanical and metabolic—an important contribution to chronic airflow obstruction, and a possible role in producing bronchospasm in some individuals. There are also a variety of noxious effects that occur in an indirect fashion. The combination of stuporousness, or unconsciousness, and vomiting from alcohol abuse can lead to aspiration of mouth and nose secretions or gastric contents. On the one hand, the mouth and nose contents can lead to bacterial aspiration pneumonias and anaerobic pulmonary infections with lung abscesses. On the other, aspiration of gastric contents can lead to chemical pneumonias with secondary bacterial infection. With the alcoholic's diminished defenses against infection, pulmonary infections, especially with pneumococci and gram-negative bacteria, seem to occur more frequently than in nonalcoholics. Also, with decreases in defenses the incidence of reactivated tuberculosis is increased in alcoholics. Thus, any alcoholic with a newly positive skin test for tuberculosis should be considered for treatment to prevent possible reactivation of the dormant tuberculosis bacteria.

▪ *Endocrine system*

The endocrine system is composed of the glands of the body and their secretions, the hormones. Hormones can be thought of as chemical messengers, released by the glands into the bloodstream. They are vital in regulating countless body processes. There is a very complex and involved interaction between hormonal activity and body functioning.

Alcohol can affect the endocrine system in three major ways. Although there are many glands, the pituitary gland, located in the brain, can be thought of as the "master gland." Many of its hormonal secretions are involved in regulating other glands. So one way that alcohol can affect the endocrine system is by altering the function of the pituitary. If this happens, then other glands are unable to function properly because they are not receiving the proper hormonal instructions. Alcohol can also affect other glands directly. Despite their receiving the correct instructions from the pituitary, alcohol can impede their ability to respond. Finally, interference with the endocrine system can develop as a result of liver damage. One of the functions of the liver is to break down and metabolize hormones, thereby removing them from the system. With liver disease, this capacity is diminished and hormonal imbalances can result.

Several hormonal changes have already been mentioned. The level of testosterone, the male sex hormone, is lowered by alcohol, possibly in several ways. The first is the direct inhibiting action of alcohol on the testes. Next there is inhibition of the portion of the pituitary gland that secretes luteinizing hormone (LH), the hormone that stimulates the testes' secretion of testosterone. Another factor is that the peripheral clearance of testosterone may be increased in the alcoholic. Finally, malnutrition, which frequently occurs in alcoholics may inhibit the hypothalamic-pituitary-testicular axis at all levels.

Serious liver disease reduces the liver's ability to break down another of the pituitary's hormones, melanocyte-stimulating hormone (MSH). This may result in increased levels of MSH, which leads to the "dirty tan" skin color.

The adrenal glands are also affected by alcohol. The adrenals produce several hormones and thus serve multiple functions. One function known to us all comes from the release of epinephrine (adrenaline) when we are frightened or fearful. The effects of this charge of epinephrine, rapid heartbeat and sweating, comprise "the fight-or-flight response." Heavy intake or withdrawal of alcohol prompts increased discharge of catecholamines by the adrenals. This may be partly responsible for the rapid heartbeat and hyper-tension during withdrawal. Another adrenal hormone, aldo-sterone, which plays a major role in regulating the body's salt and water levels, is increased with both heavy use and withdrawal. This often leads to significant and potentially serious salt and water imbalances visible clinically as swell-ing or edema. Increased aldosterone levels are also frequent-ly seen in cirrhosis with ascites. These are thought to be in part the cause of the peripheral edema that is often seen with this condition. In response to alcohol's action on the pitu-itary, the adrenals secrete excess cortisol, causing a condi-tion like Cushing's disease, except that it clears rapidly with abstinence from alcohol.

Animal research is raising several interesting questions about alcohol's effects on the endocrine system. In animals, heavy drinking increases the levels of norepinephrine in the heart. So the question is asked whether this may contribute to the development of alcoholic cardiomyopathy.

Another area of research is whether alcohol's effect on the endocrine system can contribute to the development of several kinds of cancer. Heavy drinkers have a higher in-cidence of skin, thyroid, and breast cancer. Recall that the pituitary gland is the master control gland. It influences the activity of various other gland tissues through the hor-mones it releases. Alcohol inhibits the breakdown of pitu-itary MSH. It also stimulates the release of hormones that promote thyroid activity and milk production by the breast. These three hormones have one thing in common: they af-fect their target tissues, the skin, thyroid gland, and breast, by causing these tissues to increase their metabolic activity. Aha, so the pieces may be falling into place. Cancer, simply put, occurs when there is uncontrolled or abnormal cellu-lar metabolic activity and growth. Is it possible that alco-hol's presence over long periods of time produces so many hormonal messages to the skin, thyroid, and breast tissues that in certain patients in some as yet undetermined fash-ion, tumors may be produced? Maybe.

▪ Skin

Chronic alcohol use affects the skin in a variety of ways both directly and indirectly. Its most pronounced direct ef-fect is dilatation of the vessels of the skin, but a variety of pathological effects on other systems are mirrored indirect-ly by the condition of the skin. For example, a chronic flushed appearance, itching, jaundice, thinning of the skin, changes in hair distribution, and the presence of spider angiomas, all reflect significant liver dysfunction, whereas bruising, paleness, and skin infections may reflect major abnormalities in the hematological system.

Heavy and chronic alcohol use, among other causes, will

precipitate or aggravate a condition called rosacea in predisposed persons. This condition includes flushing and inflammation especially of the nose and middle portion of the face. Particularly striking is the excessive growth of the subcutaneous tissue of the nose, a condition called rhinophyma or "rum nose."

Another skin condition associated with chronic alcoholism and alcoholic liver disease is porphyria cutanea tarda, which includes increased pigmentation, hair growth, and blistering in sun-exposed areas.

It has been thought by some that there may be a causal link between major primary skin diseases such as psoriasis, eczema, and scleroderma and alcoholism. Others feel that it is more likely that these conditions are simply much harder to manage and therefore seem to be more severe in alcoholics because of the multitude of other medical problems, nutritional inadequacy, and poor treatment compliance often seen in them.

■ *Musculoskeletal system*

Chronic alcohol abuse affects the skeletal system in four major ways. It causes osteoporosis, a thinning or demineralization of the bones, especially in the elderly. This condition, which can lead to a 25% decrease in bone mass, in turn frequently leads to fractures of the hip (especially the neck of the femur), the wrist, the upper arm bone or humerus, or the vertebral bodies in the spinal column. Rib fractures are also quite common in chronic alcoholism, but are more likely attributable to an increased frequency of falls and trauma than to osteoporosis per se. The possible causes of osteoporosis in alcoholics are many and include alcohol-induced loss of calcium and/or magnesium through the kidneys, decreased absorption of calcium and/or vitamin D by the small intestine as a result of the effects of chronic alcohol abuse, and the demineralizing effects of adrenal corticosteroid hormones, the release of which is stimulated by alcohol.

Aseptic necrosis, or bone death (especially of the head of the femur), due to blockage of adequate blood supply to that region, is another condition especially frequent in alcoholic men. In fact, as many as 50% of patients with this condition (of whom two thirds are men) will have a history of heavy alcohol use. Deformity of the hip joint often results from this condition and can lead to severe arthritis, which can be disabling and may require total hip joint replacement. The cause is postulated to be fat emboli, which are quite common in alcoholism and are probably due to alcohol-induced abnormalities in the liver's metabolism of fats (see Chapter 2). These emboli probably lodge in the small arterial vessels supplying the femoral head and cut off necessary nutrition and oxygenation to that area.

Degenerative arthritis (also known as osteoarthritis) of a variety of other joints besides the hips, also occurs more frequently in the setting of chronic heavy alcohol abuse. This is probably due to the higher frequency of falls, injuries, and fractures in alcoholics.

Septic arthritis or infection in the joint space is also seen more frequently in those who use alcohol heavily over long periods than in others. This is probably a result of at least two factors. First, osteoarthritis, which causes a roughened joint surface where blood-borne infectious agents may be more likely to settle, is more frequent in alcoholics. Second, the bodily defenses against such pathogenic agents are in general diminished in alcoholics.

■ *Nervous system*

The central nervous system (CNS) of all the major organ systems, is perhaps most widely and profoundly impacted by the effects of both acute and chronic alcohol use. The major acute effect of alcohol on the CNS is that of a depressant. The common misconception that alcohol is a stimulant comes from the fact that the depressant action disinhibits many higher cortical functions. Parts of the brain are released from their usual inhibitory restraints, thus behaviors that would not ordinarily occur may be seen. Acute alcohol intoxication, in fact, induces a mild delirium. Thinking becomes fuzzy, and orientation, recent memory, and other higher mental functions may be altered. An EEG done when someone is high would show a slowing of normal brain waves, associated with this mild state of delirium. These acute effects are, of course, completely reversible.

Physical dependence

Chronic alcohol use can lead to physical dependence and addiction. This state is marked by the development of tolerance and withdrawal symptoms. What is tolerance? This refers to changes that occur as a result of repeated exposure to alcohol. There are changes in how the body handles the alcohol (metabolic tolerance) and changes in alcohol's impact on the nervous system (functional or behavioral tolerance). There are both an increased rate of metabolism of alcohol and a decrease in impairment for a particular blood alcohol level. The nontolerant individual will have a relatively constant and predictable amount of impairment for a given dose of alcohol. As tolerance develops, the person requires increasing amounts of alcohol to get the effects previously achieved at lower doses. Tolerance represents the nervous system's ability to adapt and function more or less normally despite the presence of alcohol. This adaptation occurs rapidly. For example, if the blood alcohol levels are raised slowly, virtually no signs of intoxication may be seen. The reason(s) are unclear. The best guess is that there are subtle shifts or adjustments in nerve metabolism. Furthermore, if the dose of alcohol leading initially to high blood alcohol levels is held constant, nonetheless the blood alcohol level may decrease somewhat and clinical evidence of intoxication may decrease. The basis for this metabolic tolerance has not been established. Chronic heavy drinkers well along in their drinking careers often experience a sharp drop in tolerance. Rather than being able to drink more, with only a drink or two they become intoxicated. This phenomenon is referred to as *reversed tolerance.* The reason for this drop in tolerance is thought to be related, in part, to the decreased ability to metabolize alcohol.

Withdrawal

In chronic alcohol users, the most dramatic effects on the nervous system are those associated with an *acute lack* of alcohol. An individual who has regularly abused alcohol —that is, developed tolerance—will have withdrawal symptoms whenever there is a relative absence of alcohol. (Alcohol does not have to be entirely discontinued for withdrawal symptoms to occur. All that has to happen is for chronically elevated blood alcohol levels to decrease significantly through decreased intake.) These symptoms can include intention tremors (the shakes when he tries to do something), which are rapid and coarse, involving the head, tongue, and limbs. Most likely these will be worse in the morning, assuming that the last drink was the night before and the blood alcohol level has dropped since then. Another manifestation of alcohol withdrawal in the early stages is the all too familiar "hangover headache." This is most likely related to vascular change and actually has nothing to do with the brain. The brain itself has no pain receptors. So any headache pain must be from the nerves of the surrounding lining, skin, vessels, or muscles.

If the chronic alcohol drinker does not take more alcohol, he is likely to develop other symptoms of withdrawal. The withdrawal syndrome is the nervous system's response to the lack of alcohol. It is thought to represent the overactivity of certain brain regions no longer suppressed by high levels of alcohol in the bloodstream and brain. The severity of the symptoms of withdrawal can vary widely, depending on the length of time of heavy drinking and the amount of alcohol consumed, plus individual differences in people. Symptoms of withdrawal can include tremulousness, agitation, seizures, and hallucinations. This will be discussed later in detail.

Pathological intoxication

Aside from withdrawal symptoms, there are other important nervous system disorders related to alcohol use. A relatively unusual manifestation is a somewhat controversial condition called *pathological intoxication.* Some susceptible persons, for reasons unknown, have a dramatic change of personality when they drink even small amounts of alcohol. It is a transient psychotic state, with a very rapid onset. The individual becomes confused and disoriented, may have visual hallucinations and be very aggressive, anxious, impulsive, and enraged, and may carry out senseless, violent acts. This can last for only a few minutes or several hours. Then the person lapses into a profound sleep and has amnesia for the episode. Were he to be interviewed later, he might be very docile, not at all the madman he was during the episode. Most likely he'd report: "I don't know what happened, I just went bananas." Whether or not pathological intoxication is related neurologically to other organic impulse intermittent explosive disorder syndromes or perhaps even to certain types of epilepsy is unclear.

Organic brain disorders

Chronic alcohol use can also lead to varying degrees of dementia and organic brain disease. The particular type of brain disease, its name and associated impairment, is determined by the portion of the brain that is involved. *Wernicke's syndrome* and *Korsakoff's psychosis* are two such syndromes closely tied to alcoholism. Sometimes they are discussed as two separate disorders. Other times people lump them together as Wernicke-Korsakoff's syndrome. Both are caused by nutritional deficiencies—especially thiamine, a B vitamin—in combination with whatever toxic effects alcohol has on nerve tissue. The difference, pathologically, is that Wernicke's syndrome involves injury to the midbrain, cerebellum, and areas near the third and fourth ventricle of the brain; Korsakoff's psychosis results from damage to the diencephalon and hippocampal formation, areas important to memory function, and is often associated with evidence of damage to peripheral nerve tissue as well. Prognostically, Wernicke's syndrome has a brighter picture, often when recognized and treated early, responding very rapidly to thiamine therapy. Korsakoff's psychosis is much less likely to improve. Someone with Korsakoff's psychosis will probably require chronic nursing home care.

Clinically, a person with Wernicke's syndrome is apt to

be confused, delirious, and apprehensive. There is a characteristic dysfunction called *nystagmus* and/or paralysis of the eye muscles that control eye movements. Nystagmus is often one of the first symptoms to appear. Also, the development of ataxia—that is, difficulty in walking due to peripheral and/or cerebellar nerve damage—is likely.

Korsakoff's psychosis presents a somewhat different picture. There is severe memory loss and confabulation. Confabulation—that is, making up tales, talking fluently with no regard whatever to facts—is the hallmark sign. It occurs for the most part in an individual who is otherwise alert and responsive and able to attend to and comprehend the written as well as spoken word. In other words, the memory dysfunction is greatly out of proportion to other cognitive dysfunctions. Because of the severe damage to areas of the brain crucial to memory, the person simply cannot process and store information. Thus in order to fill in the memory gaps, he makes up stories; he confabulates. These are not deliberate lies. Trickery would require more memory and intent than someone with Korsakoff's psychosis could muster. For example, were you to ask someone with this disorder if he had met you before, his response might be a long, involved story about the last time you had been together. It would be pure fantasy. This is the phenomenon of confabulation. Memory for things that happened recently as well as long ago is variably but often severely impaired. Both retrograde amnesia and an inability to learn new information occur. Things simply are not stored for recall, and the person cannot remember things even 5 minutes later. With Korsakoff's psychosis, ataxia is also possible. There is a characteristic awkward walk, with the feet spread apart to assist in walking. Korsakoff's and Wernicke's diseases can both have a sudden, rapid onset in patients who have drunk heavily for long periods of time. However, it is not infrequently the case that Korsakoff's psychosis follows a bout of the DTs. Cerebral atrophy, diffuse loss of brain tissue, often can occur in chronically alcoholic persons in their fifties and sixties, and is associated clinically with what in the past was known as the "alcoholic deteriorated state" or alcoholic dementia. A variety of factors most likely combine to cause this condition.

Treatment of these diseases includes administration of thiamine and discontinuation of alcohol. This is more successful in reversing the signs and symptoms of Wernicke's syndrome. Only about 20% of persons with Korsakoff's psychosis recover completely. The recovery process is slow. It may take from 6 months to a year. The mortality rate of the combined disorder is around 15%. The dementia due to chronic alcoholism is irreversible.

Alcoholic cerebellar degeneration is a late complication of chronic alcohol use. It is more likely to occur in men, usually only after 10 to 20 years of heavy drinking. In such cases patients gradually develop a slow, broad-based, lurching gait, as if they were about to fall over. This results from the fact that the cerebellum, the area of the brain that is damaged, is what coordinates complex motor activity. There is *no* cognitive or mental dysfunction, since the portions of the brain governing such activities are not affected.

Another brain syndrome associated with alcoholism is *chronic hepatocerebral disease.* This is a complication of long-standing liver disease, when the brain is adversely affected by toxins circulating in the bloodstream. The brain becomes scarred (astrocytic). There is a corresponding loss of function, with dementia, ataxia, impairment of speech (dysarthria), and sometimes bizarre movements. Brain tissue cannot be repaired. Any such loss is permanent. Such patients require chronic care facilities.

Two final organic brain diseases, which are quite obscure but potentially serious, are also related to alcohol abuse and nutritional deficiencies. *Central pontine myelinosis* involves a part of the brain stem known as the pons. This disease can vary in intensity from being inapparent to rapidly causing death over a 2- to 3-week period. The pons controls respiration. As it degenerates, coma and finally death occur from respiratory paralysis. Second, *Marchiafava-Bignami disease*, also exceedingly uncommon, involves the nerve tracts connecting the frontal areas on the two sides of the brain. Their degeneration leads to diminished language and motor skills, gait disorders, incontinence, seizures, dementia, and hallucinations.

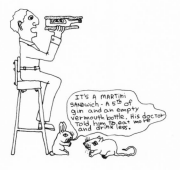

A term one is likely to hear in discussion of alcoholism and the effects of alcohol on the nervous system is "wet brain." A physician would most likely look blank if you were to use this term in a discussion. There is *no* specific medical condition that goes by this name. Probably it developed colloquially among nonmedical alcohol workers to encompass nonreversible organic brain syndromes other than Korsakoff's psychosis. The confabulation of Korsakoff's psychosis is so distinctive that it probably is recognized as different. From our experience, "wet brain" seems to be used to describe patients who have significant mental impairment and diminished physical capacity due to long-standing alcoholism and who require nursing home care.

Nerve and muscle tissue damage

Nerve tissue other than the brain can also be damaged by chronic alcohol use. The most common disturbance is *alcoholic polyneuropathy* from nutritional deficiencies.

This has a gradual onset and progresses slowly. Recovery is equally slow, taking weeks to months with discontinuation of alcohol, plus appropriate vitamins. Most commonly the distal nerves (those farthest from the body trunk) are affected first. The damage to these nerves seemingly is caused directly by toxic properties of alcohol, as well as by nutritional deficiencies related to chronic alcoholism. Typically, someone with polyneuropathy will have a painful burning of the soles of the feet, yet an absence of normal sensation. Because there is sensory impairment, the individual isn't getting feedback to the brain to tell him how his body is positioned. This loss of position sense may lead to a slapping style of walk because the victim is unsure of where his feet and legs are in relation to the ground.

Muscle damage can go hand in hand with nerve damage. There is often a wasting of muscle tissue in the areas affected by nerve damage because in some fashion muscles are improperly nourished if there is surrounding nerve damage. Other forms of muscle damage and degeneration have been reported even in the absence of neuropathy. The condition is termed *alcoholic myopathy* and involves the proximal muscles (those nearer the body trunk). Another form of muscle damage may result when a person is intoxicated and passes out, lying in the same position for a long time with constant pressure of body weight on the same muscles. Muscle degeneration means certain muscle proteins are released into the bloodstream. If these protein (myoglobin) levels are too high, kidney damage can occur. Potassium is also a product of muscle tissue breakdown. An increase in the level of potassium can disturb mineral balance throughout the body. For reasons that are entirely unclear, alcoholics are known to be very prone to muscle cramps.

Finally, an entity known as *tobacco-alcohol amblyopia* (dimness of vision) is another nervous system disorder. As the name implies, it is associated with chronic, excessive smoking and drinking. It is characterized by slow onset of blurred, dim vision with pain behind the eye. There is difficulty reading, intolerance of bright light, and loss of central color vision. Although eventually blind spots can occur, total blindness is uncommon. The cause is thought to be a vitamin deficiency coupled with the toxic effects of alcohol. Treatment includes B-complex vitamins, plus abstinence, and is usually effective in reversing the eye symptoms, though recovery is typically only partial.

Subdural hematoma

An indirect result of chronic alcoholism is the increased frequency of subdural hematomas. These occur as the result of falling down and striking the head. A blow on the head can cause bleeding of the vessels of the brain lining, the dura. The skull is a rigid box, so any bleeding inside this closed space exerts pressure on the brain. This can be very serious and is often overlooked. Presenting signs and symptoms can vary widely, although fluctuating states of consciousness (i.e., drifting in and out of consciousness) are often associated with this. Treatment involves removal of the blood clot.

■ *Neuropsychological impairment*

Personality change has long been regarded as an aspect of chronic alcohol abuse. Historically this was chalked up to serious underlying psychological problems. Then the emphasis shifted to viewing the "alcoholic personality" as a life-style the alcoholic developed to rationalize his alcohol problems and/or to protect his right to drink. There was little systematic research to explore a physiological basis, if any, and to correlate it to personality changes. This is now changing. Neuropsychological research, using psychometric tests, has uncovered specific impairments associated with alcohol use.

Overall intellectual deterioration is not seen until very late in the course of alcoholism. The IQ of most alcoholics remains relatively intact and normal. Nonetheless, there are other specific deficits, including decreased ability to solve problems, a lessened ability to perform complex psychomotor tasks, and a decreased ability to use abstract concepts. Drinking history is the major factor determining the severity of the impairments. How much alcohol, for how long? These deficits tend to improve with abstinence. The first 2 to 3 weeks bring the most dramatic improvement. After that, improvement is gradual for the next 6 months to a year. It is important to realize that the improvement, while considerable, is not complete.

The areas of the brain that seem to be most affected are the frontal lobes and the right hemisphere. This may help explain the profound personality changes associated with chronic alcohol abuse. In fact, some of the behaviors accompanying alcoholism, such as "inability to abstain" and "loss of control," may partially be a product of organic brain dysfunctions. Most of the impaired functioning being discussed is subtle. It is not readily apparent. In fact, many of the patients in the clinical studies documenting neuropsychological impairment seemed "normal." They often could be described as "young, intelligent, and looking much like any other citizen." That should alert us to the possibility that such alcohol-related brain damage may be more widespread than previously thought.

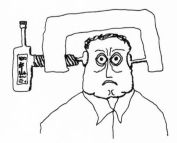

■ *Other miscellaneous effects*

Alcohol is also related to a variety of other signs, symptoms, and conditions that do not fit neatly into a discussion of a particular organ system.

Hodgkin's disease is a form of cancer that, although certainly very serious, is becoming more and more treatable. Many persons with Hodgkin's disease who drink alcohol may experience pain in the regions involved with the disease.

Alcohol abuse is also associated with *Dercum's disease*, which is characterized by symmetrical and painful deposits of fat around the body and limbs.

Alcoholism has for a long time been thought to occur more frequently than would be expected by chance in persons who have manic-depressive illness. Why these are associated is unclear.

An interesting property of alcohol is its ability to relieve tremors in persons with familial tremor. As suggested by the name, this condition runs in families. It may occur in relatively young persons, and the cause is unknown. To account for the heavy drinking not infrequently seen in some patients with this condition, it is hypothesized that such persons might medicate themselves by drinking and thereby invite alcoholism. Fortunately, there are other drugs besides alcohol that are effective with this condition and much safer.

Alcohol abuse is associated with a variety of metabolic disorders:

- Gout, a painful joint swelling caused by increased levels of uric acid due to overproduction by the body or inadequate excretion by the kidneys. In the case of alcohol-induced gout it is the latter factor that is at work. Elevated levels of blood ketones and lactate result from alcohol-induced shifts in liver metabolism and compete with uric acid for the kidney's means of eliminating organic acids. Hence less uric acid is excreted and its levels in blood rise.
- Potassium levels can be diminished because of excess mineral-regulating hormone (aldosterone) associated with cirrhosis and ascites.
- Serum magnesium levels can also go down. This is probably as a direct effect of alcohol on the kidneys' handling of magnesium, as well as decreased oral intake, and increased gastrointestinal loss.
- Lactic acidosis, which results from alterations in the liver's metabolic functioning, may be seen in some alcoholics. This can be a life-threatening situation and requires prompt and vigorous treatment.

In closing, what have been described here are the many

physical and medical complications frequently associated with alcoholism. It is important to realize, however, that health problems can arise from alcohol use, period. One does not have to be an alcoholic first. We predict it will become increasingly popular to discuss alcohol use as a risk factor for the development of a variety of illnesses, rather than to limit the focus to alcoholism and major disease states. The current general notion is that alcohol poses a health hazard "only if you really drink a lot." Evidence indicates this isn't so. A recent study of mortality from all causes over a 10-year period in nondrinkers and persons with varying degrees of alcohol use revealed that persons who used from zero to two drinks per day had the lowest mortality rate of any of the groups. Nondrinkers and persons who used from three to five drinks per day both had a 50% higher mortality rate, whereas those who used six or more drinks per day had a 100% higher rate. Among nondrinkers, the mortality rate from coronary artery disease was significantly higher than in the groups using zero to two drinks per day; moreover, cancer, cirrhosis of the liver, accidents, and a variety of pulmonary conditions were major factors in the increased mortality among heavy drinkers.

*'Tis pity wine should be so deleterious,
For tea and coffee leave us much more serious.*

LORD BYRON

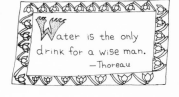

■ *Advice for the moderate drinker*

It probably comes as no great surprise to most people that excessive alcohol use over a long period of time can lead to serious problems. What is unfortunately less well recognized and appreciated is that even in moderate amounts alcohol use can present medical risks.

For some people, in some circumstances, what is usually considered a moderate amount of alcohol is too much. The most striking example is the caution against alcohol use during pregnancy. There are other conditions, many not uncommon, in which even relatively modest alcohol use can have a deleterious effect. Persons at greater risk are those with hypertension; coronary artery disease and/or congestive heart failure; idiopathic epilepsy; particular kinds of hyperlipoproteinemias; diabetes mellitus; gout; osteoporosis; various skin conditions including psoriasis; and gastric and duodenal ulcers. Although none of these conditions may constitute an absolute contraindication, all fall into the category of relative contraindication. A glass of wine with meals once or twice a week may present no problem, but several drinks before dinner, plus wine, or an evening on the town may be ill advised. If you are being treated for any medical condition, you might wish to inquire about the possible temporary modifications of even very moderate drinking behavior. In addition to the possibility of alcohol complicating the medical condition, it is necessary to consider the possibility of any interactions with medications.

■ *Sleep and sleep disturbances in alcoholics*

Many people say they cannot sleep unless they have a drink or two before bedtime, "to relax." On the other hand, alcohol actually interferes with sound sleep. To understand this paradox, we will take a look at how people sleep, how alcohol affects normal sleep, and what can be done for people who cannot sleep after they have stopped drinking.

Scientists have studied sleep by recording brain waves of sleeping subjects on the electroencephalograph (EEG). It is known that everyone sleeps basically in the same way. There are four stages of sleep: stage 1, stage 2, delta, and REM. Each stage has characteristic brain wave patterns. These stages occur in a fairly predictable sequence throughout the night.

Sleep patterns

Before we can fall asleep, we need to relax. This is a fairly individualized affair—one man's relaxant is another man's tension! Some relax best in a dark, quiet bedroom; others need a loudspeaker blasting rock music before they can let go. In either case, as soon as one can become drowsy, the brain will show alpha waves.

Next comes the transition period, a time when one is half asleep and half awake. This is called *stage 1*. One still feels awake, but does not attend to input from the environment. Little dreamlets or pictures may appear in front of the mind's eye. Stage 1 sleep lasts anywhere from 2 to 10 minutes in normal sleepers, but can last all night in some recovering alcoholics.

Finally, there comes the real thing—sleep! The average, nondreaming sleep is called *stage 2*, and we spend about 60 to 80% of our sleep in this stage. Stage 2 is a medium deep and restful sleep, and the first episode of it will last about 20 to 45 minutes.

Gradually, sleep deepens until we are in the soundest sleep of the night: *delta sleep*. The length of time one spends in delta sleep depends on age. This type of sleep lasts only a few minutes for older people, but up to 2 hours for children. Delta sleep is mainly concentrated in the early part of the night; there is rarely any left after about the first 3 hours of sleep.

After delta, we return to stage 2 sleep for awhile. Then, about 60 to 90 minutes after falling asleep, the most exciting sleep begins. This is *rapid eye movement sleep—REM sleep.* The brain waves now resemble a waking pattern. The eyes are moving rapidly under closed eyelids, but the body is completely relaxed and asleep. During REM sleep we dream. The first dream of the night lasts about 5 minutes. Following it, there is a return to stage 2 and then, possibly, some delta sleep again, but it is not quite as deep as the first time. After the few minutes more delta, we return again to stage 2. The second dream of the night occurs about 3 hours after sleep onset and lasts about 10 minutes.

The cycle of alternating nondreaming (stage 2) and dreaming (REM) sleep then continues throughout the night. Dreams occur about every 90 minutes. As the night goes on, nondreaming sleep periods become shorter, and dreaming (REM) sleep periods become longer.

From the above, you can see that you are guaranteed about four dreams in 6 hours of sleep. In fact, you dream for about 20% of an average night. During dreaming, part of the brain is awake, part is not. For example, the long-range memory part of the brain does not function during dreaming. So, in order to remember a dream, you have to wake up from it and think about the dream immediately after you awaken. (Since dreaming is a light state of sleep, one often wakes up from it.) If someone reports he dreams a lot, it means one of two things: either he is not sleeping very well, and therefore wakes up a lot, or he thinks about his dreams a lot just after he does awaken. Someone who says he never dreams is probably a reasonably sound sleeper, with few awakenings. He is probably also one who jumps right out of bed when he wakes up and therefore forgets his dreams. Someone who tells you he is dreaming ''more'' lately has either become more interested in himself and thinks more about his dreams, or he is waking up more because he has developed poorer sleep.

Sleep seems to be good for both body and mind. Stages 2 and delta are thought to be mainly body-recovery sleep. When this sleep functions well, the body feels refreshed on awakening in the morning. Delta sleep appears to be more efficient than stage 2 in refreshing the body. Dreaming sleep, on the other hand, has something to do with our psychological recovery. People do not go crazy if they are deprived of dreams, as was originally believed, but they lose some psychological stability. Someone who is usually very reliable, stable, and punctual may become irresponsible, irritable, and impulsive if deprived of REM sleep. As to the amount of sleep someone needs, the old 7 to 8 hours rule is useless. It depends on the individual. For some of us, 2 or 3 hours are enough; for others, 12 hours are necessary.

Sleep disturbances

Why do we need sleep? Take it away and see what happens! Despite what most of us think, an occasional sleepless night is not all that devastating. Although you might feel awful and irritable, *total loss of sleep for one or two nights has surprisingly little effect on normal performance and functioning.* There are two exceptions: very boring tasks, such as watching radar blips or driving long distances; or very creative tasks, such as writing an essay, are affected by even one night of very little sleep. On the other hand, for most jobs of average interest and difficulty, one can draw upon one's reserves and "rally" to the task even after 2 to 4 totally sleepless nights if one really tries to do so.

There are three brain systems regulating the state of our existence: the awake or arousal system (the reticular activating system), the sleep system, and the REM (dreaming) system. There is a continual struggle among the three, each trying to dominate the other two. The three different systems have different anatomical places in the brain and apparently run on different neurochemicals. If you influence these neurochemicals, then you disturb the balance between the three systems. Alcohol does disturb these neurochemicals.

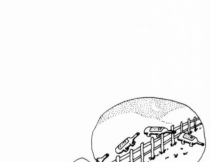

It is not too difficult to disturb the balance between the waking and the sleeping systems for a few days. Stress and stimulants (coffee, Dexedrine) will strengthen the waking system; sleeping pills will help the sleeping system. However, after just a few days or weeks, the brain chemistry compensates for the imbalance, and the chemicals become ineffective. Therefore, after just one month on sleeping pills, an insomniac's sleep will be as poor as ever. There is even some evidence that the continued use of sleeping pills causes poor sleep in itself. Furthermore, when the sleeping pill is withdrawn, sleep will become extremely poor for a few days or weeks because the brain chemical balance is now disturbed in the opposite direction. Many people stay on sleeping pills for decades even though the pills do not really help them because of this "rebound insomnia" when they try to sleep without drugs.

Because one sleeps so poorly for awhile when withdrawing from the chronic use of sleeping pills, caution should be used. Go slow, cutting down the use of sleeping pills in very gradual doses over a period of weeks. Abrupt withdrawal from some sleeping pills can be dangerous and even cause seizures. In addition, practically all sleeping pills, contrary to advertising, suppress dreaming sleep. After stopping the pills, the dreaming sleep increases in proportion to its former suppression. It can then occupy from 40 to 50% of the night. Dreaming sleep, too, takes 10 days or so to get back to normal. During these days there is very little time for deep sleep, as dreaming is taking up most of the night. You feel exhausted in the morning because you had very little time for body recovery. Nevertheless, people who have taken heavy doses of sleeping pills for a long time often sleep better after being withdrawn than they did while taking them. It is all right to take a sleeping pill on *rare* occasions, say before an important interview, or after 3 to 4 nights of very poor sleep. However, it does not make any sense to take sleeping pills regularly for more than a week.

Insomnia

Insomnia can be based on either an overly active waking system or on a weak sleeping system. On rare occasions, this can have an organic or genetic basis. Some people have a defective sleep system from birth. However, most insomnias are based on psychological factors. Any stress, depression, or tension will naturally arouse the waking system. If that is the problem, the cure obviously involves helping the person deal with the psychological stress.

Surprisingly, poor sleep is often little more than a bad habit! Say a person went through a stressful life situation a few years back and, quite naturally, couldn't sleep for a few nights because of it. Being very tired during the day after a few poor nights, he then needed sleep more and more. So the person tried harder and harder to get to sleep, but the harder one tries, the more difficult it is to fall asleep. Soon a vicious cycle develops. Everything surrounding sleep becomes emotionally charged with immense frustration, and the frustration alone keeps you awake.

How do you break this habit? The rules for its treatment are simple, and treatment is effective, provided the individual sticks with it. The first step is for the person to recognize that he or she is misusing the bed by lying in it awake and frustrated! The specific rules for treatment are as follows: (1) Whenever you cannot fall asleep relatively quickly, get up because you are misusing the bed. You can do your "frustrating" somewhere else, but *not* in the bedroom! (2) As soon as you are tired enough and think you might fall asleep quickly, you are to go to bed. If you cannot fall asleep quickly, you are to get up again. This step is to be repeated as often as necessary, until you fall asleep quickly. (3) No matter how little sleep you get on a given night, you have to get up in the morning at the usual time. (4) No daytime naps! If the individual sticks to this regimen for a few weeks, the body again becomes used to falling asleep quickly.

Shortening the time spent in bed is also crucial to many insomniacs. Because they haven't slept during the night, many insomniacs stay in bed for half the morning. They want to catch a few daytime naps, or they feel too tired and sick after not sleeping to get up. Pretty soon they lie in bed routinely for 12, 14, even 20 hours. They sleep their days away, while complaining of insomnia. It is important that one maintain a regular day/night rhythm, with at least 14 to 16 hours out of bed, even if the nights are marred by insomnia.

Alcohol's effects on sleep

What does alcohol do to all this? Many find that a nightcap "fogs up" an overly active waking system. No question, some people can fall asleep faster with a drink. *However, alcohol depresses REM (dreaming) sleep, and it causes more awakenings later at night.* The drinker frequently awakens many times throughout the night, leading to a lack of recovery during sleep. These effects continue in chronic drinkers. In addition, the pressure to dream becomes stronger the longer it is suppressed. The dreaming sleep system will finally demand its due. Thus, after a binge, there is a tremendous recovery need for dreaming. It is thought that part of the DTs and the hallucinations of alcohol withdrawal can be explained by a lack of sleep (many awakenings) and a pressure to dream (lack of REM).

The great fragmentation of sleep and a lack of delta and REM sleep in chronic alcoholics is a serious problem. Even though they think they sleep well, there is little or no recovery value in it. This very poor sleep makes people want to sleep longer in the morning and during the day. This adds to the usual problems of coping.

What happens to sleep when the booze is taken away from a chronic alcoholic? First, there is the rebound of dreaming. Increased dreaming can last up to 10 days before subsiding. Often there are nightmares because dreaming is so intensive. The sleep fragmentation lasts longer. A loss of delta sleep can go on for as long as 2 years after stopping drinking! In sober alcoholics as a group, there are still more sleep disturbances than in nonalcoholics. We don't know why. It could be due to some chronic damage to the nervous system during the binges—as has been produced in alcoholic rats—or it could be that some alcoholics were poor sleepers to start with. In any case, it appears that the longer one can stay on the wagon, the more sleep will improve.

Sweet dreams!

■ *Blackouts*

Having covered a multitude of physical disorders associated with alcohol abuse, it would seem that there is nothing left to go wrong! Yet there remains one more phenomenon associated with alcohol use. It is highly distinctive: the blackout. Contrary to what the name may imply, it does *not* mean passing out or losing consciousness. Nor does it mean psychological blocking out of events, or repression. A blackout is an amnesia-like period that is often associated with heavy drinking. Someone who is or has been drinking may appear to be perfectly normal, and function quite normally with the task at hand. Yet later, the person has no memory of what has transpired. A better term might be *blank-out*. The blank spaces in the memory may be total or partial. A person who has been drinking and who experiences a blank-out will not be able to recall how he got home, how the party ended, how he landed the 747, how he did open-heart surgery, or how the important decisions were made at a business lunch. As you can imagine, this spotty memory can cause severe distress and anxiety, to say nothing of being dangerous in certain circumstances.

What causes blackouts? The mechanisms are not fully understood. Recent research indicates that whereas blackouts may on occasion occur in nonalcoholics who have drunk more heavily than they usually do—that is to the point of intoxication (see below)—they are typically associated with alcoholism that is at a fairly advanced stage. Thus in general the greater the severity of the alcoholism— that is, the heavier the drinking and the greater the number of years over which it has occurred—the more likely the occurrence of blackouts. There is also a positive correlation between the extent and duration of alcohol consumption during any given drinking episode and the occurrence of blackouts. Several other factors correlate with the occurrence of blackouts in alcoholic patients. These include out-of-control drinking, poor diet, ability to consume large quantities of alcohol (i.e., tolerance), a history of a prior head injury, and the tendency to gulp drinks. Up to one third of alcoholics report never having had a blackout at all. Some alcoholics have blackouts frequently, whereas others only have them on occasion.

These findings regarding blackouts differ in some respects from the oft-quoted work of Jellinek done in the 1950s, which suggested that they were an early manifestation in patients who had a high risk of later developing alcoholism. He felt they were of great prognostic significance in predicting eventual alcoholism. Other studies done recently have found that from 30 to 40% of young to middle-aged, light to moderate (social) drinkers have had an alcohol-induced blackout at least once. Typically these occurred on one of the few occasions in their lives when they had been drunk. In fact, among this category of drinkers, blackouts seem to be more frequent among those who generally drank less. From this finding it has been hypothesized that in certain persons the lack of tolerance to the blackout-producing effects of alcohol may be a strong factor in maintaining their moderate use of alcohol. In others (i.e., those who become alcoholic), high tolerance to this effect may prevent its appearance until a relatively late stage of the illness. This interesting, but as yet unproven theory, suggests that though blackouts occurring late in a heavy drinking history are highly associated with alcoholism, those occurring early on in association with a light to moderate drinking history may indicate a relatively low rather than a high likelihood of eventual alcoholism.

What is evident, despite the scanty research, is that for some reason, in some persons, alcohol interferes with the mechanisms of memory. Memory is one of the many functions of the brain. It is a complex process that is in general poorly understood. We can recall and report what happened to us 5 minutes ago. Similarly, many events of yesterday or a week ago can be recalled. In some cases, our memories can extend back many years and even decades. Psychological and neuropsychological research has distinguished between different types of memory. Immediate, short-term or recent, and long-term memory is one way of categorizing the types of memory. Memory of whatever type involves the brain's capacity to handle and store information. According to one popular theory of memory function, the brain has at least two different kinds of "filing systems" for information. Immediate memory is stored for very short periods electrically. Long-term memory involves a biochemical storage system that is relatively stable over long periods. Short-term or recent memory is a way station somewhere between these two and is thought to involve the process of conversion of electrical brain impulses into stable neuronal macromolecules. This is the point at which, it is hypothesized, alcohol exerts its influence. This theory suggests that the presence of alcohol inhibits the brain's ability to move short-term memory into long-term storage, though it does not interfere directly with immediate memory for events occurring during the blackout itself nor for events from before the blackout already stored in long-term memory banks. Thus the superficially normal appearance and function, even with respect to relatively complicated tasks, of the person in a blackout. The amnesia that occurs during a blackout is typically of one of two types. It may be sudden in onset, dense, and permanent—that is without return of memory at any point —or it may lack a definite onset and be something of which the person is unaware until he is reminded of or spontaneously recalls the forgotten event. In the latter instance the recall is usually dim and incomplete, but interestingly may be enhanced by the use of alcohol. This facilitation of recall by alcohol is thought to reflect the phenomenon of state-dependent learning where whatever has been learned is best recalled when the person is in the same state or condition as existed at the time of the original learning.

In conclusion, it might be noted that there has been recent discussion of blackouts being employed as a defense in criminal proceedings. To our knowledge, no such cases have yet been resolved. Although a novel approach, it would appear that there is no support to any contention that a blackout alters judgment or behavior at the time of its occurrence. The only deficiency appears to be in memory of what has occurred. Of course, having no recollection would make it difficult to prepare a case or decide from one's own knowledge whether to plead guilty or innocent.

It is hoped that more can be learned of blackouts in the future. Research is difficult, since it depends almost entirely on self-report. So far, no one has found a way to know that an alcoholic blackout is occurring and to study it with EEGs and other tests at the time it is happening. Other types of brain research may eventually lead to the key to this phenomenon.

▪ *Withdrawal*

Alcohol is an addictive drug. Thus when it is taken in sufficient quantities, the body becomes adapted or accustomed to its presence. Drinking as much as a quart of liquor daily for one week can create a state of physical dependence. After physical dependence is established, if consumption is curtailed, there will be symptoms of withdrawal. These symptoms taken together constitute the so-called abstinence syndrome. One sure way to terminate an abstinence syndrome is to administer more of the addictive drug. Another facet of addiction is that tolerance develops. Over the long haul, increasing amounts of the drug are necessary to achieve the same effects of the drug and to continue to ward off withdrawal. The withdrawal symptoms for any drug are generally the mirror images of the effects induced by the drug itself. Alcohol is a depressant. The alcohol abstinence syndrome has symptoms that are indicative of a stimulated state. A hangover, a kind of miniwithdrawal, testifies to this. Being jumpy, edgy, irritable, hyped-up— these well-known symptoms are the exact opposite of alcohol's depressant qualities.

The basis of withdrawal is related to alcohol's depressant effects on the central nervous system. With regular chronic use of alcohol, the CNS is being chronically depressed. With abstinence, this chronic depressant effect is removed. There is a "rebound" hyperactivity. An area of the CNS particularly affected is the reticular activating system that oversees the general arousal level and CNS activity. The duration of the withdrawal syndrome is determined by the time required for the "rebound" to be played out and a normal baseline level of functioning to be reestablished. Studies of CNS activity with EEGs during heavy drinking, abstinence, and withdrawal support this.

Not everyone physically dependent on alcohol who stops drinking has the same set of symptoms. In part, the severity of the withdrawal state will be a function of how long someone has been drinking and how much. Another big factor is going to be the person's physical health plus his unique physiological characteristics. Therefore, accurately predicting the difficulties of withdrawal is impossible. Despite the phrase abstinence syndrome, withdrawal can occur even while someone continues to drink. The key factor is a *lowering* of the blood alcohol level. *Relative abstinence* is the condition that triggers withdrawal. It is this phenomenon that often prompts the alcoholic's morning drink. He is treating his withdrawal symptoms.

Withdrawal syndromes

Four different major withdrawal syndromes have been described in conjunction with alcohol. Although they can be distinguished for the purposes of discussion, clinically the distinctions are not so neat. In real life, these different syndromes blend together.

The most common syndrome of alcohol withdrawal is *tremulousness*. It is this shakiness that prompts the actively drinking alcoholic to have a morning or midday drink. Recall that increasing amounts of an addictive drug are necessary to ward off withdrawal, and a lowered blood alcohol level (BAL) is sufficient to induce withdrawal. An alcoholic who is used to drinking heavily in the evenings is eventually going to find himself feeling shaky the next morning. A drink will take this discomfort and edge away. With time, further boosts of booze during the course of the day may be necessary to maintain a BAL sufficient to prevent the shakes.

If the physically dependent person abstains completely, there will be a marked increase of tremulousness. The appearance is one of stimulation. The alcoholic startles easily, feels irritable, and in general is "revved up" in a very unpleasant way. There's a fast pulse, increased temperature, and elevated blood pressure, sweating, dilated pupils, and a flushed face. Sleeping will be difficult. Usually these symptoms subside in 2 or 3 days. The shakes will go away, and the vital signs return to normal. However, feeling awful, being irritable, and having difficulty sleeping can persist for 2 to 3 weeks. This syndrome by itself does not require medical treatment. It is important, however, that the person not be alone and that an evaluation be made about the likelihood of DTs. As this acute stage passes, the probability of DTs is greatly lowered. But if the jitteriness does not subside, beware. Be sure the person is evaluated by a physician.

Another syndrome of alcoholic withdrawal is acute and chronic *alcoholic hallucinosis.* This occurs in some 25% of persons withdrawing from alcohol. This syndrome includes true hallucinations, both auditory and visual. It also includes illusions, the misperception or misinterpretation of real environmental stimuli. The individual with hallucinosis is oriented, knows who he is, where he is, and the time. Very bad nightmares often accompany this withdrawal syndrome. It is believed that the nightmares may result from the suppression of dreaming sleep for so long by alcohol. Hence there is a rebound effect. Hallucinosis is not dangerous by itself and does not necessarily require specific medical treatment. This is because in nearly all patients it has cleared by the end of the first week after withdrawal. In a small number of cases, however, a chronic and persistent form of the syndrome may develop and continue for weeks to months.

The chronic form of alcoholic hallucinosis accompanying alcohol withdrawal is often thought of as being a separate syndrome. It is characterized primarily by persistent auditory hallucinations. Usually the hallucinations are of voices familiar to the patient, often of relatives or acquaintances. In the early stages they are threatening, demeaning, or invoke guilt. Since they are true hallucinations, the person thinks they are real and acts as if they were. This can lead to the person doing harm to himself or others. With persistence of the hallucinations over time, they become less frightening and are tolerated with greater equanimity by the patient. Some patients with chronic hallucinosis develop a schizophrenia-like condition and require treatment with antipsychotic medications. In most instances alcoholic hallucinations do not indicate an underlying psychiatric problem. They are simply the central nervous system's reponse to the body's lack of alcohol.

Convulsive seizures, often referred to as "rum fits," also occur in association with acute alcohol withdrawal.

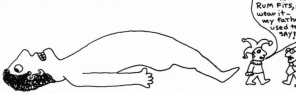

These seizures are major motor seizures; the eyes roll back in the head, the body muscles contract and relax and extend rhythmically and violently, and there is loss of consciousness. After the seizure, which lasts a minute or two, the person may be stuporous and groggy for up to 6 or 8 hours. Although very frightening to watch, seizures in and of themselves are not dangerous. A very uncommon, though serious outcome is the development of *status epilepticus*, in which seizures follow one another with virtually no intervening periods of consciousness. Most typically, only one or two seizures occur with acute alcohol withdrawal. The only long-term treatment of alcohol-withdrawal seizures is abstinence. Anticonvulsants are not routinely prescribed, because further seizures are not expected after withdrawal. It is critical, though, to rule out any other possible source of the seizures and not merely to assume that alcohol withdrawal is responsible. Infections or falls with associated head trauma to which the alcoholic is prone can be causes. Seizures are most likely to occur between 12 and 48 hours after stopping alcohol. But they can occur up to one week after the last drink. Alcohol-withdrawal seizures indicate a moderate to severe withdrawal problem. One third of all persons who have seizures go on to have delirium tremens (DTs), which are serious business.

Withdrawal seizures are thought to be caused by the "rebound" CNS hyperexcitability. Alcohol has an anticonvulsant effect acutely; it raises the seizure threshold. But with abstinence, the seizure threshold is correspondingly lowered. (This has been postulated as the basis for the increased seizures in epileptics who drink, since these seizures tend to occur the morning after, while sobering up.)

Delirium tremens is the most serious form of alcohol withdrawal syndrome. Despite the availability of good medical care, mortality rates of up to 15 to 20% have been reported. As many as one out of every five persons who go into DTs dies. The name indicates the two major components of this withdrawal state. Either of these components can predominate. Delirium refers to hallucinations, confusion, and disorientation. Tremens refers to the heightened autonomic nervous activity, the agitation, fast pulse, elevated blood pressure, and fever. Someone who develops the DTs will have all the symptoms first described with early withdrawal. Instead of clearing by the second or third day, the symptoms continue and get worse. In addition to increased shakiness, profuse sweating, fast pulse, hypertension, and fever, there are mounting periods of confusion and attacks of anxiety. In full-blown DTs there are delusions and hallucinations, generally visual and tactile. The terrifying nature of the hallucinations and delusions is cap-

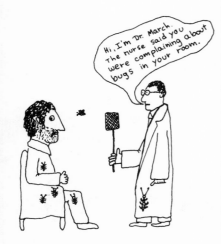

Hi, I'm Dr. March. The nurse said you were complaining about bugs in your room.

tured by the slang phrase for DTs, "the horrors." Seeing bugs on the walls and feeling insects crawling all over the body naturally heighten the anxiety and emotional responses. In this physical and emotional state of heightened agitation, infections, respiratory problems, fluid loss, and physical exhaustion create further difficulties. These complications may substantially hike the mortality rate. The acute phase of DTs can last from one day to a week. In 15% of cases they are over in 24 hours; in 80% within 3 days. The person will then often fall into a profound sleep and, upon awakening, feel better with usually little memory of what has happened.

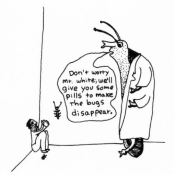

Although predictions cannot be made about who will go into DTs, persons who fit the following description are the most likely candidates. A daily drinker who has consumed over a fifth a day for at least the last week and who has been a heavy drinker for 10 years or more is very susceptible. The occurrence of withdrawal seizures, or the persistence, and worsening with time, rather than improvement of the acute early withdrawal symptoms, should be indicators that the DTs are more likely to occur. If with a prior period of acute abstinence, the person had convulsions, extreme agitation, marked confusion, disorientation, or DTs, they are more likely to occur again. Another ominous sign is recent abuse of other sedatives, especially barbiturates, which also have potentially very serious withdrawal syndromes. Abuse of multiple drugs complicates withdrawal management. If it is anticipated that there is a physical dependence on more than one drug, generally they will not be withdrawn simultaneously, but first one, then the next, and so on.

Some cautions

Not all persons who experience withdrawal symptoms intend to do so by design! Withdrawal occurs by itself whenever a drug is reduced or terminated in physically dependent persons. So circumstances may play their part and catch persons unaware. Addicted persons who enter hospitals for surgery, thereby curtailing their usual consumption, may to their surgeon's (and even their own) amazement develop acute withdrawal symptoms. Another possibility is the family vacation, when the secretly drinking housewife, who has been denying a problem, intends just to sweat it out. She can wind up with more than she bargained for.

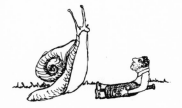

▪ Alcohol-drug interactions

Alcohol is a drug. Thus, not unexpectedly, when it is taken in combination with other medications, there can be undesirable and quite possibly dangerous drug-alcohol interactions. These interactions can vary from individual to individual, but they are largely dependent on the amount and type of alcohol and other medications consumed, as well as the person's drinking history. The nonalcoholic, who has not developed tolerance, will have a very different response than the inveterate drinker. In fact, the consequences may be far more serious.

There are two basic mechanisms that explain virtually all alcohol-drug interactions. One is that the acute presence of alcohol affects the liver's ability to metabolize other drugs. In the nonalcoholic, the MEOS system, which handles a variety of other kinds of drugs (see Chapter 2), may be significantly inhibited by the presence of alcohol. Therefore, drugs ordinarily metabolized by the MEOS system are not being removed as rapidly as usual and are present in higher than expected levels. Obviously this can result in unexpected toxic effects. For those with a long history of heavy drinking, alcohol on board has the opposite effect on the MEOS system. The MEOS action is enhanced or speeded up, through a process known as enzyme induction. Thus drugs are removed (i.e., metabolized) more quickly. The result of this is that the individual will very likely *not* be receiving the intended therapeutic effects of the drug. Because it is being removed more rapidly, its levels in the body will be lower than expected.

The other major source of difficulty results from so-called additive effects. Alcohol is a central nervous system depressant. Other medications may also depress CNS functions. When two depressant drugs are present simultaneously their effects are combined, and are often far greater than would be expected with either alone.

It is also important to be aware that drugs are not metabolized quickly. Recall it takes the body approximately one hour to handle one "drink" (whether the drink is a 12-ounce bottle of beer, or one mixed drink with a shot of 80-proof liquor). Therefore, if someone has had several drinks, an hour or two later alcohol will still be in the system and will still have the potential for significant additive effects with other depressant drugs at that point.

Table 1 outlines many of the potential interactions of alcohol with several commonly prescribed medications. These include both the general types of interactions just described and a variety of other types not specifically discussed. Note, this table is *not* all-inclusive. Because a drug is not listed, do not assume that there is no interaction with alcohol. Anyone who uses alcohol and is taking other medications is well advised to ask his or her physician or pharmacist specifically about possible interactions.

Table 1. The interaction effects of alcohol with other drugs

Type of drug	Generic name	Trade name	Interaction effect with alcohol
Analgesics Nonnarcotic	Salicylates	(products containing aspirin) Bayer Aspirin Bufferin Alka Seltzer	Heavy concurrent use of alcohol with analgesics can increase the potential for gastrointestinal bleeding. Special caution should be exercised by individuals with ulcers. Buffering of salicylates reduces possibility of this interaction.
Narcotic	Codeine Morphine Opium Oxycodone Propoxyphene Pentazocine Meperidine	 Pantopon Paregoric Percodan Darvon Darvon-N Talwin Demerol	The combination of narcotic analgesics and alcohol interact to reduce functioning of the central nervous system (CNS) and can lead to loss of effective breathing function or respiratory arrest: death may result.
Antianginals	Nitroglycerin Isosorbide dinitrate	Nitrostat Isordil Sorbitrate	Alcohol in combination with antianginal drugs will cause the blood pressure to lower— creating a potentially dangerous situation.
Antibiotics Antiinfective agents	Furazolidone Metronidazole Nitrofurantoin	Furoxone Flagyl Cyantin Macrodantin	Certain antibiotics, especially those taken for urinary tract infections, have been known to produce disulfiram-like reactions (nausea, vomiting, headaches, hypotension) when combined with alcohol.
Anticoagulants	Warfarin sodium Acenocoumarol Coumarin derivatives	Coumadin, Panwarfin Sintrom Dicumarol	With chronic alcohol use, the anticoagulant effect of these drugs is inhibited. With acute intoxication the anticoagulant effect is enhanced: hemorrhaging could result.
Anticonvulsants	Phenytoin	Dilantin	Chronic heavy drinking can reduce the effectiveness of anticonvulsant drugs to the extent that seizures previously controlled by these drugs can recur if the dosage is not adjusted appropriately. Enhanced CNS depression may occur with concurrent use of alcohol.
Antidepressants	Nortriptyline Amitriptyline Desipramine Doxepin Imipramine	Aventyl Elavil, Endep Pertofrane Sinequan Tofranil	Enhanced CNS depression may occur with concurrent use of alcohol and antidepressant drugs.
Antidiabetic agents *Hypoglycemics*	Chlorpropamide Acetohexamide Tolbutamide Tolazamide Insulin	Diabinese Dymelor Orinase Tolinase Iletin	The interaction of alcohol and either insulin or oral antidiabetic agents may be severe and unpredictable. The interaction may induce hypoglycemia or hyperglycemia; also disulfiram-like reactions may occur.

References: Lipman, A. G.: "Drug Interactions With Alcohol," *Modern Medicine,* Feb. 15, 1976, pp. 67-69. "Fact Sheet—Drug Interactions with Alcohol," National Clearinghouse for Alcohol Information (Feb. 1976). "It's Dangerous to Mix Alcohol and Drugs," National Clearinghouse for Alcohol Information. *The Whole College Catalog About Drinking,* U.S. Department of Health, Education, and Welfare, NIAAA.
Courtesy of Nebraska Division on Alcoholism, Lincoln, Nebraska.

Continued.

Table 1. The interaction effects of alcohol with other drugs—*continued.*

Type of drug	Generic name	Trade name	Interaction effect with alcohol
Antihistamines	(for example) Chlorpheniramine	(many cold & allergy remedies) Coricidin Allerest	The interaction of alcohol and these drugs enhances CNS depression.
Antihypertensive agents	Rauwolfia preparations Reserpine Guanethidine Hydralazine Pargyline Methyldopa	Rauwiloid Serpasil Ismelin Apresoline Eutonyl Aldomet	Alcohol, in moderate dosage, will increase the blood pressure–lowering effects of these drugs, and can produce postural hypotension. Additionally, an increased CNS-depressant effect may be seen with the rauwolfia alkaloids and methyldopa.
Antimalarials	Quinacrine	Atabrine	A disulfiram-like reaction and severe CNS toxicity will result if antimalarial drugs are combined with alcohol.
CNS depressants Barbiturate hypnotics	Phenobarbital Pentobarbital Secobarbital Butabarbital Amobarbital	Luminal Nembutal Seconal Butisol Amytal	Since alcohol is a depressant, the combination of alcohol and other depressants interact to further reduce CNS functioning. It is extremely dangerous to mix barbiturates with alcohol. What would be a nondangerous dosage of either drug by itself can interact in the body to the point of coma or fatal respiratory arrest.
Nonbarbiturate hypnotics	Methaqualone Glutethimide Bromides Flurazepam Chloral hydrate	Quaalude Doriden Neurosine Dalmane Noctec	Many accidental deaths of this nature have been reported. A similar danger exists in mixing the nonbarbiturate hypnotics with alcohol. Disulfiram-like reactions have been reported with alcohol use in the presence of chloral hydrates.
Tranquilizers (major)	Thioridazine Chlorpromazine Trifluoperazine Haloperidol	Mellaril Thorazine Stelazine Haldol	The major tranquilizers interact with alcohol to enhance CNS depression resulting in impairment of voluntary movement such as walking or hand coordination; larger doses can be fatal.
Tranquilizers (minor)	Diazepam Meprobamate Chlordiazepoxide HCl Oxazepam	Valium Equanil Miltown Librium Serax	The minor tranquilizers depress CNS functioning. Serious interactions can occur when using these drugs and alcohol.
CNS stimulants	Caffeine Amphetamines Dextro-amphetamine Metham-phetamine	(in coffee and cola) Vanquish Benzedrine Dexedrine Desoxyn	The stimulant effect of these drugs can reverse the depressant effect of alcohol on the CNS resulting in a false sense of security. They do not help the intoxicated person gain control over coordination or psychomotor activity.

Table 1. The interaction effects of alcohol with other drugs—*continued.*

Type of drug	Generic name	Trade name	Interaction effect with alcohol
Disulfiram (antialcohol preparation)	Disulfiram	Antabuse	Severe CNS toxicity follows ingestion of even small amounts of alcohol. Effects can include headache, nausea, vomiting, convulsions, rapid fall in blood pressure, unconsciousness, and—with sufficiently high doses—death.
Diuretics (also anti-hypertensive)	Hydro-chlorathiazide Chlorothiazide Furosemide Quinethazone	HydroDIURIL, Esidrix Diuril Lasix Hydromox	Interaction of diuretics and alcohol increases the blood pressure—lowering the effects of the diuretic; and could possibly precipitate postural hypotension.
Monoamine oxidase inhibitors (MAOI)	Pargyline Isocarboxazid Phanelzine Tranylcypromine	Eutonyl Marplan Nardil Parnate	Alcoholic beverages (such as beer and wines) contain tyramine, which will interact with an MAOI to produce a hypertensive, hyper-pyrexic crisis. Common use of alcohol with MAOIs may result in enhanced CNS depression.

▪ *Medications containing alcohol*

Alcohol, in one or another of its many forms, was for centuries virtually *the* pharmacological agent available to physicians. In the twentieth century, alcohol has had rather limited uses. Now, in addition to being used exter-nally as an antiseptic (e.g., to wash the skin before giving an injection or taking a blood sample—except when this is being obtained for a blood alcohol determination), its only other major use is as an "inert" medium or carrier for liquid medications. Alcohol is an almost universal ingredient of cough medicines and liquid cold preparations sold over the counter or by prescription (see Table 2). Furthermore, the percentage of alcohol is often not insignificant. Nyquil, for example, contains 25% alcohol. That's 50 proof! It is also an ingredient in a variety of other kinds of commonly used liquid medications (see Table 3).

Recovering alcoholics in general are well advised to avoid alcohol-containing preparations. For persons taking disulfiram (Antabuse), it is imperative.

There are some preparations containing no alcohol available for coughs and colds. These are listed in Table 4. But some of these contain substances that also have psy-choactive properties. Although using such agents will avoid the danger of disulfiram reactions, the recovering al-

Table 2. Some alcohol-containing preparations for coughs, colds, and congestion

Drug	Manufacturer	Alcohol, %
Actol Expectorant	Beecham Laboratories	12.5
Ambenyl Expectorant	Marion	5.0
Calcidrine Syrup	Abbott	6.0
Chlor-Trimeton Syrup	Schering	7.0
Citra Forte Syrup	Boyle	2.0
Coryban-D Syrup	Pfipharmecs	7.5
Demazin Syrup	Schering	7.5
Dilaudid Cough Syrup	Knoll	5.0
Dimetane Elixir	Robins	3.0
Dimetane Expectorant	Robins	3.5
Dimetane Expectorant-DC	Robins	3.5
Dimetapp Elixir	Robins	2.3
Hycotuss Expectorant and Syrup	Endo	10.0
Lufyllin-GG	Wallace	17.0
Novahistine DH	Dow Pharmaceuticals	5.0
Novahistine DMX	Dow Pharmaceuticals	10.0
Novahistine Elixir	Dow Pharmaceuticals	5.0
Novahistine Expectorant	Dow Pharmaceuticals	7.5
Nyquil Cough Syrup	Vicks	25.0
Ornacol Liquid	Smith Kline & French	8.0
Periactin Syrup	Merck Sharp & Dohme	5.0
Pertussin 8-Hour Syrup	Cheseborough-Ponds	9.5
Phenergan Expectorant, Plain	Wyeth	7.0
Phenergan Expectorant, Codeine	Wyeth	7.0
Phenergan Expectorant, VC, Plain	Wyeth	7.0
Phenergan Expectorant, VC, Codeine	Wyeth	7.0
Phenergan Expectorant, Pediatric	Wyeth	7.0
Phenergan Syrup Fortis (25 mg)	Wyeth	1.5
Polaramine Expectorant	Schering	7.2
Quibron Elixir	Mead Johnson	15.0
Robitussin	Robins	3.5
Robitussin A-C	Robins	3.5
Robitussin-PE and DM	Robins	1.4
Robitussin-CF	Robins	4.75
Rondec-DM	Ross	0.6
Theo-Organidin Elixir	Wallace	15.0
Triaminic Expectorant	Dorsey	5.0
Triaminic Expectorant DH	Dorsey	5.0
Tussar-2 Syrup	Armour	5.0
Tussar SF Syrup	Armour	12.0
Tussi-Organidin	Wallace	15.0
Tuss-Ornade	Smith Kline & French	7.5
Tylenol Elixir	McNeil	7.0
Tylenol Elixir with Codeine	McNeil	7.0
Tylenol Drops	McNeil	7.0
Vicks Formula 44	Vicks	10.0

Modified from Rubinstein, J.: "Beware of These Drugs When You Prescribe for a Recovering Alcoholic." *Resident & Staff Physician,* March 1980, p. 63.

Table 3. Other commonly used drugs containing alcohol

Drug	Manufacturer	Alcohol, %
Alurate Elixir	Roche	20.0
Aromatic Elixir	Circle	22.0
Anaspaz PB Liquid	Ascher	15.0
Asbron Elixir	Dorsey	15.0
Atarax Syrup	Roerig	0.5
Belladonna, Tincture of	Purepac	67.0
Benadryl Elixir	Parke-Davis	14.0
Bentyl-Phenobarbital Syrup	Merrell-National	19.0
Carbrital Elixir	Parke-Davis	18.0
Cas-Evac	Parke-Davis	18.0
Choledyl Elixir	Parke-Davis	20.0
Decadron Elixir	Merck Sharp & Dohme	5.0
Dexedrine Elixir	Smith Kline & French	10.0
Donnagel	Robins	23.0
Donnagel-PG	Robins	3.8
Donnatal Elixir	Robins	5.0
Dramamine Liquid	Searle Labs	5.0
Elixophyllin	Berlex	20.0
Elixophyllin-KI	Berlex	10.0
Feosol Elixir	Smith Kline & French	5.0
Gevrabon	Lederle	18.0
Ipecac Syrup	Lilly	2.0
Isuprel Comp. Elixir	Breon	19.0
Kaon Elixir	Warren-Teed	5.0
Kay Ciel	Berlex	4.0
Kay Ciel Elixir	Berlex	4.0
Kaochlor S-F	Adria	5.0
Marax Syrup	Roerig	5.0
Mellaril Concentrate	Sandoz	3.0
Minocin Syrup	Lederle	5.0
Modane Liquid	Adria	5.0
Nembutal Elixir	Abbott	18.0
Paregoric, Tincture of	(several)	45.0
Parelixir	Rorer	0.69
Parepectolin	Purdue Frederick	18.0
Propadrine Elixir	Merck Sharp & Dohme	16.0
Serpasil Elixir	Ciba	12.0
Tedral Elixir	Parke-Davis	15.0
Temaril Syrup	Smith Kline & French	5.7
Theolixir (Elixir Theophylline)	Ulmer	20.0
Valadol	Squibb	9.0
Vita-Metrazol Elixir	Knoll	15.0

Modified from Rubinstein, J.: "Beware of These Drugs When You Prescribe for a Recovering Alcoholic." *Resident & Staff Physician,* March 1980, p. 64.

Table 4. Some nonalcoholic preparations for coughs, colds, and congestion

Drug	Manufacturer
Actifed-C Expectorant	Burroughs Wellcome
Actifed Syrup	Burroughs Wellcome
Hycodan Syrup	Endo
Hycomine Syrup	Endo
Ipsatol Syrup	Key
Omni-Tuss	Pennwalt
Orthoxicol Syrup	Upjohn
Sudafed Syrup	Burroughs Wellcome
Triaminic Syrup	Dorsey
Triaminicol Syrup	Dorsey
Tussionex Suspension	Pennwalt

Modified from Rubinstein, J.: "Beware of These Drugs When You Prescribe for a Recovering Alcoholic." *Resident & Staff Physician,* March 1980, p. 66.

coholic may wish to carefully monitor exposure to the effects of any such drugs—by carefully measuring the medication, taking it only at specified intervals, or settling for a hot lemonade with honey and figuring that this cold too shall pass.

The medical complications of acute and chronic heavy alcohol use as well as of alcohol withdrawal constitute a broad array of serious and even potentially life-threatening conditions. Moreover, even in relatively moderate amounts, alcohol may have potentially serious effects on a variety of common medical illnesses and conditions, may in specific instances be a significant public health risk factor, and clearly carries a potential risk when used with a wide variety of commonly prescribed medications.

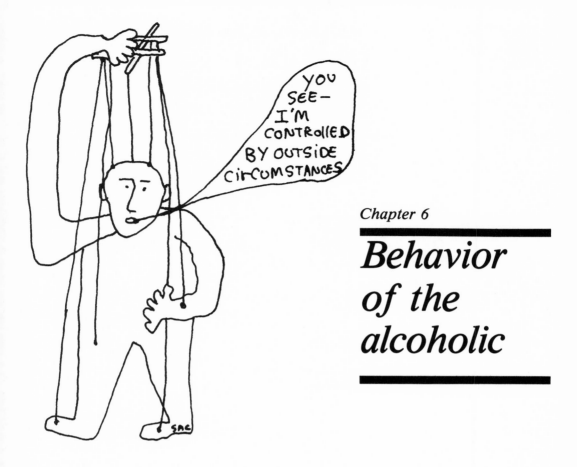

Chapter 6

Behavior of the alcoholic

Leaving aside theories about alcoholic personalities and behavioral or psychological causes, there are some striking similarities in the behavioral "look" of alcoholics. This is true whether the alcoholic is male or female, age seventeen or seventy. From these, a general profile can be drawn. Although *not* applying totally to *all* alcoholics, this profile would cause signal bells to ring when seen by someone familiar with the disease.

▪ *The composite alcoholic*

Our composite alcoholic would be most confusing to be around. The active alcoholic is always sending mixed messages. "Come closer, understand/Don't you *dare* question me!" Jubilant, expansive/secretive, angry, suspicious; laughing/crying. Tense, worried, confused/relaxed, "Everything's fine." Uptight over bills/financially irresponsible (buying expensive toys for the kids, while the rent goes unpaid). Easygoing/fighting like a caged tiger over a "slight." Telling unnecessary lies and having them come to

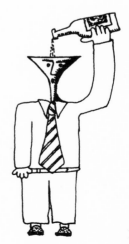

117

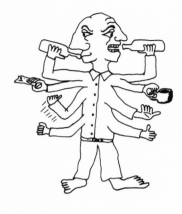

light is not uncommon behavior. She might also spend considerable, if not most, of her time justifying and explaining why she does things. He is hard to keep on the track. He always has a list of complaints about a number of people, places, and things. (If only . . .) She considers herself the victim of fate and of a large number of people who are "out to get" her. He has thousands of reasons why he *really* needs/deserves a drink. She will come in exuberant over a minor success and decline rapidly into an "I'm a failure because of . . ." routine. He's elusive. Almost never where he said he'd be when he said he'd be there, or he's absolutely *rigid* about his schedule, especially his drinking times.

The mood swings are phenomenal! The circular arguments never quite make sense to a sober person, and a lot of hand-throwing-up results. The thought that he might be crazy is not at all unusual from either side because of the terrible communication problems. Perfectionistic at some times and a slob at others. Although occasionally cooperative, he's often a stone wall. Her life is full of broken commitments, promises, and dates that she often doesn't remember making. Most of all, the behavior denotes guilt. The active alcoholic is extremely defensive. This seems to be one of the key behaviors that is picked up early and seen, but not understood, by others. "Wonder why Andy's so touchy? What a short fuse!" Certainly at times a drunken slob is much in evidence, but often the really heavy drinking is secretive and carefully hidden. It would be easier to pin down the alcoholism if the behaviors described only occurred with a drink in hand. This is often not the case. The behaviors are sometimes *more* pronounced when the alcoholic is going through an "on the wagon," or controlled drinking, phase. The confusion, anger, frustration, and depression are omnipresent unless a radical change in attitude toward the drinking takes place.

▪ *How, if not why*

The profile just given is a fair description of alcoholic behavior. This kind of behavior is part of the disease syndrome. Unfortunately, this behavior pattern develops slowly, and the many changes of personality occur gradually, making them less discernable to the alcoholic and the family. So the slow, insidious change of personality is almost immune to recognition as it is happening. Despite the fact that the alcoholic is vulnerable to a host of physical problems, neither current neurological nor physiological data can adequately explain this behavioral phenomenon. Yet, despite the inability to provide a simple answer, *how* the transformation occurs can be described. Vernon Johnson, in *I'll Quit Tomorrow*, has developed a four-step process that neatly sets forth the personality changes that occur in the alcohol-dependent person. His explanations really describe what alcoholism feels like from the inside out. Becoming familiar with these stages will be helpful in dealing with alcoholics and problem drinkers.

Alcohol dependence requires the use of alcohol, an obvious fact. Another obvious fact: for whatever reasons, drinking becomes an important activity in the life of the problem drinker or alcoholic. The alcoholic develops a *relationship* with alcohol. The relationship, with all it implies, is as real and important a bond as with friends, a spouse, or a faithful dog. Accordingly, energy is expended to maintain the relationship. The bond with the bottle may be thought of as an illicit love affair. Long after the thrill, pleasure, and fun are gone, all kinds of mental gymnastics are gone through to act as if it's still great.

The first step Johnson describes is quite simple. The drinker *learns the mood swing.* The learning has a physiological basis. Alcohol is a drug; it has acute effects. It makes us feel good. Someone's mood could be plotted at any time on a graph, on which one end represents pain and the other end euphoria. If someone is feeling "normal" and then has a drink, his mood shifts toward the euphoric end. Then after the effects of the alcohol wear off, he's back where he started.

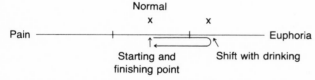

Anyone who drinks learns this pharmacological effect of alcohol and learns that it happens consistently. Alcohol can be depended on.

The second stage in the developmental process is *seeking the mood swing.* This happens *after* someone learns that alcohol can be counted on to enhance or improve mood. Drinking now has this particular purpose. Anyone who drinks occasionally does so to make things better. Whatever the occasion—an especially hard day at work, a family reunion, celebrating a promotion, or recovery from a trying day of hassling kids—the expectation is that alcohol will help. In essence, the person is entering into a contract with alcohol. True to its promise, alcohol keeps its side of the bargain. By altering the dosage, the person can control the mood swing. Still there are no problems.

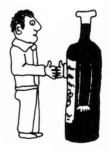

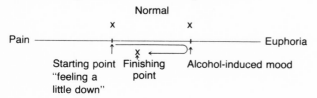

*Wine in excess keeps neither
secrets nor promises.*

CERVANTES, DON QUIXOTE

According to Johnson, only a thin line separates the second and third phases. The third phase is *harmful dependence*, in which, suddenly, alcohol demonstrates a boomerang effect. Alcohol, which previously had only a beneficial, positive effect, now has some negative consequences. These can include such things as a hangover or feelings of embarrassment over last evening's antics. *Emotional costs* are going to be exacted to continue drinking in that fashion. Many people will say: "Forget it, no more nights like last night for me." They really mean it. What's more, there is no problem for them in sticking with that decision. In the future, they are more cautious about drinking. But there are a significant minority of people who react differently. These are the people bound for trouble with alcohol. Unwilling to discontinue their use of alcohol to alter their moods, they are willing to pay the price. In a sense, they remain "loyal" to their relationship with booze. This decision to pay the price isn't a conscious decision, logically thought out. It is based on how the person is feeling. In the pain-euphoria chart, the mood shift initially heads in the right direction, achieves the drinker's purpose, but in swinging back, drops the person off in a less comfortable place than where he began.

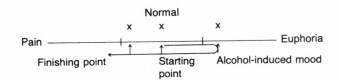

The costs are psychological. The person's drinking behavior and its consequences are inconsistent with his values and self-image. To continue drinking requires revamping the personality. The normal psychological devices will be used to twist reality just enough to explain away the costs. Every person does this every day to some degree. If I'm walking down the street, say hello to a friend and get no response, my feelings are momentarily hurt. Almost automatically, I tell myself, "He must not have seen or heard me." So I shut off the hurt feelings with an explanation that may or may not be true. I pick the "reality" that makes me comfortable. Or another time, if I'm particularly ill-tempered and nasty, acting in a way I don't really like, I become uncomfortable with myself. I could say to myself: "Yep, I sure have been a grouch." More likely it will come out: "I've not been myself. It must be the pressure of work that's gotten to me." In this fashion, each of us attempts to control our discomfort and maintain psychic harmony. This is what the budding problem drinker does to keep harmony in the relationship with alcohol. One way to twist reality to explain away the costs is to suppress emotions. When feeling some negative emotions arising, the alcoholic tries to push this away. "I just won't think about it." So, the fellow who made an ass of himself at last night's party tries to ignore the whole thing. "Heavens, these things happen sometimes. There's no sense in worrying about it." However, pretending your emotions are not there doesn't make them disappear. They simply crop up somewhere else. Since suppression doesn't work totally, other psychological gymnastics are used. Rationalization is a favorite device—coming up with a reason that inevitably stays clear of alcohol itself. "I really got bombed last night because Harry was mixing such stiff ones." Here we see projection at work as well. The reason for getting bombed was that the drinks were *stiff*, and it's *Harry's* fault! No responsibility is laid on the drinker or on alcohol.

Now there might not be any problems if these instances of distortion are only occasional. But they aren't. And what is worse, with continued heavy drinking, the discrepancy between what is expected to happen and what *does* happen gets larger and larger. Proportionately, so does the need for further distortion to explain it. Drinking is supposed to improve the mood, but the budding alcoholic keeps being dropped off further down on the pain side.

A vicious cycle is developing. The mental gymnastics used to minimize the discomfort are also preventing the alcoholic from discovering what is really happening. None of the defenses, even in combination, are completely foolproof. At times, the alcoholic feels real remorse about his behavior. At those times it doesn't matter where the blame lies—on Harry, on oneself, on alcohol—anyway you cut it, the drinker regrets what's happening. So a negative self-image is developing.

For the most part, the drinker truly believes the reality of the projections and rationalizations. Understandably, this begins to screw up relationships with others. There are continual hassles over whose version of reality is accurate. This introduces additional tensions as problems arise with friends, family, co-workers. The alcoholic's self-esteem keeps shrinking. The load of negative feelings expands. Ironically, the alcoholic relies more and more heavily on the old relationship with alcohol. Drinking is deliberately structured into life patterns. Drinking is anticipated. The possibilities of drinking may well determine which invitations are accepted, where business lunches are held, and other life activities. Gradually, *all* of leisure time is set up to include drinking.

The stage is now set for the last developmental phase of the alcoholic personality. The alcoholic now *drinks to feel*

*Boundless intemperance
In nature is a tyranny; it
hath been
Th' untimely emptying of
the happy throne
And fall of many kings.*

SHAKESPEARE, MACBETH

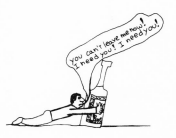

You can't leave me now! I need you! I need you!

normal. By now the alcoholic is in chronic pain, beset by a load of negative feelings, constantly at the negative end of the mood scale. Drinking is now done to enhance the mood, to achieve a *normal* feeling state.

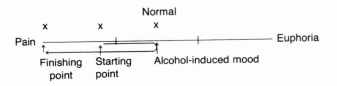

In addition to achieving this normal feeling state, alcohol may assist "normal" functioning in other respects. Psychologists have documented the phenomenon of "state-dependent learning." Things learned in a particular context are most readily recalled under similar circumstances. Thus, things learned when sober are best recalled later when sober. Similarly, learning that occurs while intoxicated will also be more available for recall later when the person is again (or still) intoxicated. Thus, the heavy drinker may have a repertoire of behavior, coping mechanisms, social skills, even information that, if learned during drinking, is less accessible when sober. In fact, drinking may be necessary to tap a reservoir of knowledge. This fact is what sometimes explains the alcoholic's inability to find liquor stashes that were hidden when drunk. Another way in which alcohol may be essential to "normalize" function is to ward off withdrawal symptoms if the drinker has become physically dependent.

Other memory distortions are not uncommon at this point. Blackouts may mean the absence of memory for some events. Repression is a psychological mechanism that also blocks out memory. Further havoc is raised by the alcoholic's "euphoric recall." The alcoholic remembers only good times, and/or the sense of relief he associates with drinking. The problems and difficulties seemingly don't penetrate.

■ *Deteriorating functioning*

Given the transformation of thinking, the distorted view of reality, and the ebbing self-esteem, the alcoholic's functioning deteriorates. Each of us is expected to fulfill various roles in life. For each slot we find ourselves in, there is an accompanying set of expectations about what is appropriate behavior. Some of the typical roles are parent, spouse, worker, citizen, friend. Other roles may be more transient, such as scout leader, committee chairman, patient, or Sunday school teacher. No matter what the role, the alcoholic's performance suffers. There are expectations that others have of someone in a position. The alcoholic does not meet them. Behavior is inconsistent. The active alcoholic cannot be depended upon, sometimes doing what is expected, and doing it beautifully; yet the next time, no show, followed later by the flimsiest excuse. To add insult to injury, he or she gets furious at you for being disappointed, or annoyed, or not understanding. This has a profound impact on the people around the alcoholic. Being filled with the normal insecurities of all humans, those around the alcoholic think it might/must be their fault. Unwittingly others accept the alcoholic's rationalizations and projections. People around the alcoholic are confused. Often they feel left out. They sense and fear the loss of an important relationship, one that has been nourishing to them. In turn, their usual behavior is kinked out of shape. Now, in addition to whatever problems the alcoholic has directly with alcohol, interpersonal relationships are impaired. This adds more tension.

▪ *Family and friends*

Let's focus on the family and friends of the alcoholic for a moment. Applying behavioral learning terms, the alcoholic has those around him or her on a variable-interval reinforcement schedule. There they are, busily trying to accommodate the alcoholic. Everyone feels that somehow if they behave differently, do the "right thing," the alcoholic will respond. One time they're harsh, the next time they try an "understanding" tack. Then another time they might try to ignore the situation. But nothing works. The alcoholic's behavior doesn't respond in any predictable way to their behavior. If he happens to be a "good boy" or she's been a "perfect lady" on occasion, it really has no connection to what the family has, or has not, done. The others, in fact, are accommodating themselves to the alcoholic. Never sure why some times go better, they persist in trying. And trying some more. Meanwhile, the alcoholic remains inconsistent and unpredictable.

Eventually the family as well as close friends give up and try to live around the alcoholic; alternately the drinker is ignored or is driving them crazy. Yet out of love and loyalty, all too long the alcoholic is protected from the consequences of the drinking. In the marital relationship, if one spouse is alcoholic, the other gradually assumes the accustomed functions of the drinking partner. If the wife is alcoholic, the husband may develop contingency plans for supper in case it isn't ready that night. If the father is alcoholic, the wife may be the one who definitely plans to attend Little League games. If the father is up to it, fine; if not, a ready excuse is hauled out. This leads to resentments on both

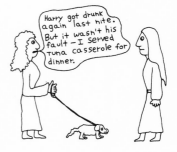

parts. The spouse carrying the load feels burdened; the alcoholic feels deprived and ashamed.

■ *Marital relationships*

In the marital relationship, if one partner is alcoholic, you can count on sexual problems. In American society, concern over sexual performance seems to be the national pastime. Sexual functioning is not merely a physical activity. There are strong psychological components. How someone feels about oneself and one's partner is bound to show up in the bedroom. Any alcohol use can disturb physiological capacity for sex. Shakespeare said it most succinctly: alcohol provokes the desire but takes away the performance. In the male, alcohol interferes with erection, popularly referred to as "brewer's droop." The psychological realm has as strong an impact. Satisfying sexual relationships require a relationship, a bond of love and affection. In the alcoholic marriage, neither partner is able to trust that bond. There are doubts on both sides. Problems result in many ways. A slobbering drunk invites revulsion and rejection. By definition he is an unattractive, inconsiderate lover. Any qualities of love have, for the moment, been washed away by booze. Intercourse can also become a weapon. Wives or husbands can use the old Lysistrata tactic of emotional blackmail: refusing sex unless the partner changes behavior. Or both partners can approach intercourse as the magic panacea. If they can still make love, that can make up for everything else lacking in the relationship. Sexual fears and anxiety, which are rampant in the total population, are compounded in the alcoholic marriage.

■ *At work*

Often, although the alcoholic is deeply mired in the symptoms of deterioration in the social, family, and physical areas of his life, the job may remain intact. The job area seems to be the last part of the alcoholic's life to show the signs of illness. The job is often the status symbol for both the alcoholic and the spouse. He might think or say: "There's nothing wrong with me. I'm still bringing in a good paycheck!" She is likely to make excuses to his boss for him to protect her livelihood. And vice versa.

Much effort is being made to alert employers to the early signs of alcoholism and to acquaint them with the rehabilitation possibilities. The employer is in a unique position to exert some pressure on the alcoholic at a relatively early stage. Recommending that someone go for treatment may well be a precipitating factor in a recovery. The fact that

*Wine makes a man better
pleased with himself;
I do not say that it makes him
more pleasing to others.*

SAMUEL JOHNSON

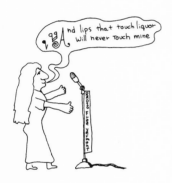

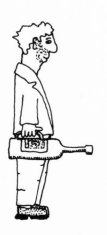

the boss sees the problem and calls a spade a spade can go far in breaking down the denial system. Keeping a job may be important enough to get the alcoholic to begin to see the problem more realistically. Employee Assistance Programs and their impact on earlier intervention and treatment will be discussed at length in a later chapter.

Alcoholics often believe that their cover-up, or diversionary, tactics are successful. Most people are unwilling to confront someone with a drinking problem until it is no longer possible to ignore it. One study found that some person other than a family member had noticed a drinking problem on an average of 7 years prior to an alcoholic's seeking help. Often the alcoholic has no idea how obvious the difficulties are to so many other people. When an alcoholic is finally confronted, it can be a great shock to find out how much of the telltale behavior was in fact observed. The rationalization and denial systems actually convinced the active alcoholic that *no one* on the job or in the community knew about the drinking problem.

All of this disruption causes pain and confusion for alcoholics and those around them, and unfortunately, most of the attempts that all of these people make to alter the situation don't work. With all the best will in the world, alcoholism rarely responds to the more common maneuvers of concerned people. Only special knowledge of the dynamics of the disease, its effects on others, and of the various treatments, can effectively begin to break these destructive patterns.

Who hath woe? who hath sorrow? who hath contentions? who hath babbling? who hath wounds without cause? who hath redness of eyes? They that tarry long at the wine.

PROVERBS 28:31-32

Chapter 7

Effects of alcoholism on the family

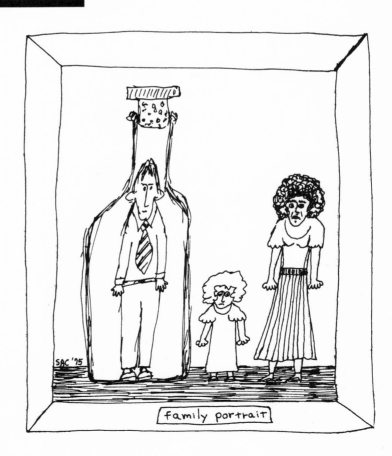

family portrait

127
*Effects of alcoholism
on the family*

Alcoholism is often termed the *family illness*, referring to the tremendous impact an active alcoholic has on those around him. There is no way the family members can escape or ignore the alcoholic. The majority of the alcoholic's impairments are behavioral. So in the day-to-day interactions of family life, the family members are confronted with alcoholic behavior, which initially may appear to have little connection to the drinking. The family is confused, bewildered, angry, and afraid. They act accordingly. Their responses characteristically become as impaired as the alcoholic's.

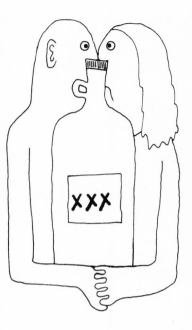

Were we to single out *the* major development in the alcohol field during the last decade, it would be the vastly increased attention to the plight of the alcoholic's family. This is evidenced particularly with involvement of families in alcohol treatment. However, there has been comparatively little formal research on the effects of alcoholism on the family. A recent review of two books purporting to be comprehensive tomes on alcoholism noted the scanty attention paid to the impact of active alcoholism on the family. The reviewer plaintively asked, "Why is so much written about the effects of alcoholism upon a patient's liver enzymes and so little written about the effects of parental alcoholism on the children?" With such questions being raised, combined with increasing attention to family treatment, one may hope that answers will be forthcoming. Maybe in future editions of books like this, the discussion of family issues can be more complete and less speculative.

Certainly no family member ever caused alcoholism. Yet the family may, despite its best intentions, behave in a way that allows the alcoholic to continue drinking. They may protect the alcoholic, make excuses, buy into the alibis, cover up. They might call the employer, pretending the alcoholic has "the flu." Other facilitating behavior can include covering a bad check or retaining a good lawyer to beat a charge of driving while intoxicated. The alcoholic's actions are bound to increase the family's anxiety level. The alcoholic drinks more to relieve his own anxiety, which in turn ups the family's even higher. The higher the anxiety, the more the family members react by anxiously doing *more* of what they were already doing and then the alcoholic drinks more because of the higher anxiety, ad infinitum. The thing can become a spiraling squirrel cage or a collapse. The family is no better able to cope with the alcoholism than is the alcoholic.

▪ Family system

Joan Jackson, in a classic monograph on "Alcoholism and the Family," was the first to describe the stages that occur as a family comes to grips with an alcoholic in its midst. Her stages were initially intended to describe the family in which the husband and father is the alcoholic. With modification, they probably describe any alcoholic family. These stages are sketched out here in order of appearance.

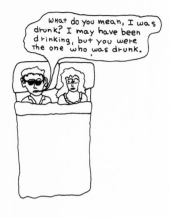

Denial. Early in the development of alcoholism, occasional episodes of excessive drinking are explained away by *both* marriage partners. Drinking because of tiredness, worry, nervousness, or a bad day is not unbelievable. The assumption is that the episode is an isolated instance and therefore no problem. If the couple is part of a group where heavy drinking is acceptable, this provides a handy cover for developing dependency. A "cocktail" before dinner easily becomes two or three, and wine with the meal and brandy afterward don't attract much notice.

Attempts to eliminate the problem. Here the spouse recognizes that the drinking is not normal and tries to pressure the alcoholic to quit, be more careful, or cut down. "If you only pulled yourself together and used a little willpower," or "If you really love me, you won't do this anymore." Simultaneously, the spouse tries to hide the problem from the outside and keep up a good front while continuing to sneak drinks or drinking outside the home. Children in the family may well start having problems in response to the family stress.

Disorganization and chaos. The family equilibrium has now broken down. The spouse can no longer pretend everything is okay and spends most of the time going from crisis to crisis. Financial troubles are common. Under real stress, possibly questioning his or her own sanity, the spouse is likely to seek outside help. Unfortunately, spouses often ask for help from friends who know as little as they of what to do; or they may seek out a member of the clergy who has not had training in dealing with alcoholism. If they do seek trained help at this point or become involved with Al-Anon, the process will take a different course altogether.

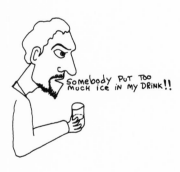

Reorganization in spite of the problem. The spouse's coping abilities have strengthened. He or she gradually assumes the larger share of responsibility for the family unit. This may mean getting a job or taking over the finances. The major focus of energy is no longer directed toward getting the alcoholic partner to shape up. Instead, the spouse takes charge and fosters family life, despite the alcoholism.

Efforts to escape. Separation or divorce may be attempted. If the family unit remains intact, the family continues living around the alcoholic.

Family reorganization. In the case of separation, family

reorganization occurs without the alcoholic member. If the alcoholic achieves sobriety, a reconciliation may take place. *Either* path will require both partners to realign roles and make new adjustments.

As mentioned, Jackson's formulations are focused on the family in which the husband is alcoholic. Families with an alcoholic wife and mother exist, too. An interesting difference is found in marriage outcomes, depending on which partner has the alcohol problem. The female alcoholic is much more likely to be divorced than is the male alcoholic. Several hypotheses are possible to account for the difference. In the past, various authors have speculated that women who marry alcoholics may have unconscious, neurotic needs to be married to weak, inadequate males. The implication is that because they have the need, they'll stay married to the drunk. The more accepted view now is that the difficulties seen in the alcoholic's wife come simply from the stress of living with him. Given the economic realities, it is not unlikely that the nonalcoholic wife stays in her marraige longer than the nonalcoholic husband because she feels the need of the husband's financial support to maintain the family.

On the other side, men in general are less likely to seek outside help for any kind of problem. Therefore, the husband of a female alcoholic may see no option other than divorce to save himself and the children.

The most common approach to the alcoholic family considers the family a system. Central to this view is the belief that changes in any part of the system (any family member), of necessity affect all of the others. The other members, in response, also make changes in an attempt to maintain the family equilibrium. An example might be a circus family specializing in a high-wire balancing act. All six members of the act climb up to the top of the tent. In turn they step out upon the thin wire to begin an intricate set of maneuvers to build a human pyramid high above the audience. Timing and balance are critical. And the interdependence is obvious. Each member is sensitive to even the tiniest movements of the rest in order to keep making the adjustments of balance necessary to maintain the routine. If only one of the six members fails to do what is expected, is not exactly where he is supposed to be, the entire routine fails.

In essence, families with an impaired member do the same thing. The alcoholic's behavior begins to invade the family routine. Everyone else is put off balance. Doing the same things over again doesn't work, so each member scrambles around to find some place, or role, that will restore the equilibrium. In fact, most families do achieve a precarious, though unhealthy, new balance based on the

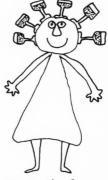

Portrait of a woman who can't understand why her husbands were all alcoholics.

drinking behavior. If the alcoholic starts to get well and returns to more normal behavior, or leaves the family system, the balance is again thrown off. Either way, outside help is strongly recommended to short-circuit the probability of continuing an unhealthy balance in the family. Because each family member has come to relate to the others on the basis of the inappropriate roles, it is virtually impossible to make corrections from inside the system. To return to the circus family, were one member to leave, those remaining would have to regroup as a new act. Conversely, having adjusted over a period of time to altered performance by an impaired member, should that person return in an unimpaired role again, yet another adjustment would be necessary. They would in either case for the moment stop performing, and call another aerialist to help them develop and supervise their practice of new routines. The old relationships, timing, and patterns would be set aside, as they learned to work in new ways.

In terms of the kinds of accommodations that alcoholic families make, there can be a range of responses; there is no single "routine." At one extreme the drinking alcoholic is almost like a "boarder" in the family's household. The family isolates and walls off the alcoholic, expects little, gives little. In this way the nonalcoholic family members maintain some stability and continuity. At the other extreme the entire family life is alcohol centered, responding to the crises of the moment. And families can vacillate between patterns of accommodating to the alcoholic, depending on whether the alcoholic is drinking or on the wagon.

■ *Children of alcoholics*

The children in an alcoholic family deserve some special attention. In an atmosphere of conflict, tension, and uncertainty, their needs for warmth, security, and even physical care may be inadequately met. In a family where adult roles are inconsistently and inadequately filled, children lack good models to form their own identities. It is likely that such children will have a hard time as they enter into relationships outside the home, at school, or with playmates. A troubled child may be the signal of an alcohol problem in a family. Although alcoholics comprise only 2% of the American population, their children account for approximately 20% of all referrals to child guidance clinics. In fact, put the book down for a moment. Take five minutes to imagine what life is like for a child with an alcoholic parent.

As a preschooler. What's it like to lie in bed listening to your parents fight? Or having Daddy disappear for periods unexpec-

131
*Effects of alcoholism
on the family*

tedly? Or being spanked *really* hard, and sent away from dinner, because your milk spilled? Or having a succession of sitters because mommy works two jobs? Or get lots of attention sometimes and be in the way the next moment?

As an elementary school child. What's it like when your mom forgets to pack a lunch? Or you wait and wait, after scout meeting for a ride, long after the other kids have been picked up? Or your Dad cancels out on the cub scout hike, 'cause he's sick? Or you're not allowed to bring friends home to play? Or your friends' moms wouldn't let them ride in your car? Or you're scared to tell your mom you need a white shirt to be a pilgrim in the class Thanksgiving play?

Or as an adolescent. What's it like if you can't participate in school functions because you must get home to care for your younger brothers and sisters? Or, the money you make mowing lawns is missing from your room? Or, your dad's name is regularly featured in the court column of the newspaper? Or your mother asks you to call her boss, because she has a black eye, from falling down. Or there's no one from your family to come to the athletic awards banquet. . . . or . . .

The family environment is not the only potential trouble spot for the child of an alcoholic. As discussed in Chapter 5, maternal alcohol use can influence fetal development. So the risk to a child can extend to earliest childhood, even before birth. In addition to the direct impact of the drug, behaviors associated with alcoholism may have direct effects on fetal development. Physical trauma, falls, malnutrition, or abnormalities of glucose metabolism are not uncommon in alcoholics. Any of these could have an impact on the developing baby.

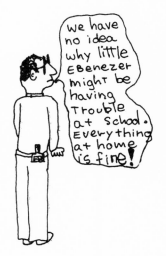

The emotional state of the expectant mother probably influences fetal development. It certainly has an influence on the course of labor and delivery. The emotional state of the alcoholic expectant mother might differ dramatically from that of a normal, healthy, nonalcoholic expectant mother and be a source of problems. An alcoholic expectant father may exert some indirect prenatal influences. If he is abusive or provides little emotional and financial support, this could cause anxiety in the mother. Lack of support and consequent anxiety during pregnancy is associated with more difficult deliveries. In a similar vein, stress at certain times during pregnancy increases fetal activity. This, in turn, is linked to colicky babies. There are no specific data available on labor and delivery for either female alcoholics or wives of male alcoholics. It is known that increased maternal anxiety may precipitate problems of labor and delivery. Furthermore, it is known that these difficulties are related to developmental disorders in the children. One particular difficulty that children of alcoholics have more frequently than children of nonalcoholics is hyperactivity.

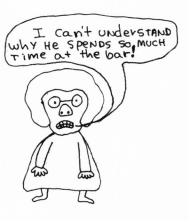

Another crucial time in any infant's life comes shortly after delivery. The very early interactions between mother and infant are important influences in the mother-child relationship. Medications that may be required for a difficult delivery may make the "bonding" more difficult. Both mother and infant, under the effects of the drug, are less able to respond to each other. A new mother needs emotional and physical support to help her deal with the presence of the baby in her life. At a minimum, the baby requires food, warmth, physical comfort, and consistency of response from the mother. In the case of a family with an active alcoholic, one can't automatically assume everything is going smoothly.

Some children of alcoholics may be having quite apparent and obvious problems. Yet, given the environment of the alcoholic family, what is sometimes more striking is how well the children do cope with alcoholism. Drawing upon a family systems approach to the alcoholic family, family counselors have identified several distinctive coping styles children adopt.

One of these is to be *the responsible one.* This role usually falls to the oldest or to an only child. The child may assume considerable responsibility for himself or herself, but also younger brothers and sisters—taking over chores, keeping track of what needs to be done. In general this child compensates as much as possible for the instability and inconsistency introduced by the parental alcoholism.

Another role is that of *the adjuster.* This child doesn't take on the responsibilities of managing; instead the child follows directions and easily accommodates to whatever comes along. This child is remarkable for how much is taken in stride.

The other possible role is to be *the placater.* This role involves managing not the physical affairs, as the responsible one does, but the emotional affairs. This child is ever attuned to being concerned, and sensitive to others. It may include being sympathetic to the alcoholic, and alternately the nonalcoholic parent, always trying to soothe ruffled feathers.

What these roles have in common is that each in its own way is a model for survival, a coping strategy. These roles can also provide the child with support, and approval from persons outside the home. The "responsible one," for example, probably is a good student, Mommy's little helper, and gets praise for both. The danger to the child is that he becomes frozen in these roles, that the roles become the lifetime pattern. What is helpful in childhood can become a deficiency as an adult. The "responsible one" can become an adult, who always needs to be on top of things, in control, destined to the stress of attempting to be a lifetime

133
*Effects of alcoholism
on the family*

superachiever. "The flexible one" may be so tentative, so unable to trust as to be unable to make the long-term commitments that are required to succeed in a career or intimate adult personal relationships as a spouse or parent. Likely as not, the "adjuster" adults are so attuned to accommodating to others that they allow themselves to be manipulated. An ever-present option for the adult "adjuster" is to marry someone with a problem, such as an alcoholic, which allows the continuation of the adjuster role. The adult "placaters" are continually caring for others, often at the price of being unaware of their own needs, or being unable to meet them. This can lead to large measures of guilt and anger, neither of which a placater can easily handle.

A different but similar typology set forth of the roles that children adopt in response to parental alcoholism includes "the Family Hero," "the Lost Child," "the Family Mascot," and "the Scapegoat." The first three have much in common with "the responsible one," "the adapter," and "the sensitive one." The specific labels are less important than the fact that children do develop coping styles in response to the family stress of alcoholism, and for the majority of children the coping may not elicit external attention and invite intervention. The exception is the "Scapegoat," who is likely to be acting out—be in trouble in school, or trouble with the authorities—who, usually acting angry and defiant, may be the only one clearly seen as having a problem. If the child is a teenager, the trouble may take the form of drug or alcohol abuse. (This is discussed in the section on adolescents in Chapter 10.) Frequently through the attention focused on this child by outsiders or the family, the family alcohol problem may first surface. Of course, the family will initially see the child as the central problem. The myth the family may have established for itself is that the drinking is the parent's coping response to the child's behavior. The child may be held responsible for aggravating the parent's drinking.

Further insight into the effects on children of parental alcoholism is becoming available from the very recent emergence of self-help groups for adult children of alcoholics. Presumably because attention and help for the alcoholic is such a recent phenomenon, they as children received no help in confronting these issues, no matter what the fate of the alcoholic parent. Whether the alcoholic parent died from the disease, left the home, or recovered, the grown children are experiencing difficulties that developed from the experiences in the alcoholic family.

There are several common themes, or "holes" worth commenting on. An extreme fear of abandonment is one. Because the alcoholic parent may have been so often absent, late picking them up, or indeed "left them" through death, divorce, or true abandonment, no amount of assurance from other loved ones is ever enough to dispel this anxiety. "I know you *say* you love me, but someday you'll leave me too," is the underlying motive for a lot of clutching, dependent behavior that often does push people away, fulfilling the terrible prophecy. The fear may even be so great that they remain unable to form any deep attachment, "knowing" it will only cause them pain.

Some may have spent a lot of time trying by various behaviors to control or change the drinking pattern of their parent and, inevitably failing, often come to feel as though they are "failures" ahead of time. Life seems overwhelming, especially because the behaviors developed in an attempt to cope with the alcoholic aren't usually effective elsewhere. They feel caught in a "no win" situation and very often choose to live out their lives considerably below the level of their abilities and talents. An easy job, in an easy place, with superficial relationships is another way to avoid pain.

Others may receive so little approval at home that they work intensively for outside approval. They may become obsessive overachievers, courting success at any cost to relationships of any kind. They may become "workaholics," competitive and defensive. Unfortunately, this choice often achieves high rewards and regard in this work ethic-oriented society, and no one attends to the personal destruction around them. Their expectations of themselves, and consequently of others, often destroy their relationships with those around them much as alcoholism does.

One deeply buried and usually unacknowledged theme is intense guilt feelings. A young child suffering from neglect or outright abuse from an alcoholic parent feels anger and hatred in response to such treatment. A perfectly natural momentary "I wish she were dead!" can become a habitual thought—and added to it, the horror of thinking such a thing. The cruelty of other children who know about the "drunk" at home may have left deep scars and the inevitable feeling that if only the parent had not been around, life would have been better. No matter *what* the outcome of the problem, such feelings were and are felt to be abnormal, "sinful," not allowed, and therefore never discussed. Couple with this the guilt at having failed to change the situation by being a "better" or "different" child! The anger at the parent can spill over throughout life, even long after the parent is dead, creating even more buried guilt. These are only examples of some of the far-reaching effects that can be encountered by adults of any age who lived with an active alcoholic when growing up.

135
*Effects of alcoholism
on the family*

Another way in which the child of an alcoholic is vulnerable is in terms of genetic endowment. The issue of the causes of alcoholism is far from settled; yet a genetic component is suspected, and children of alcoholics are considered people at risk for development of the disease in an approximate 4/1 ratio to those without a biological alcoholic parent.

The effects of alcoholism are not limited to the alcoholic. This only scratches the surface of possible complications in the nuclear family. All the people directly involved with an alcoholic need information and help to combat these effects.

Chapter 8

Treatment

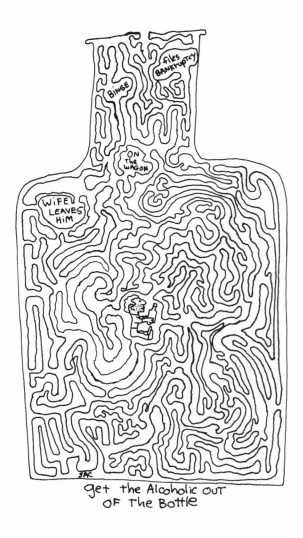

get the Alcoholic out
of The Bottle

When one is acutely aware of alcohol problems and alcoholism, the question arises: "How do you treat them?" Or perhaps your question is more personal: "How can I help?" The first step is to consider how people get better and what treatment or intervention is about. An understanding of what happens in treatment is important to anyone who cares about an alcoholic and wants to be supportive.

It is important to keep in mind that alcoholism is a chronic illness. From the perspective of medicine, the key to successful management of any chronic disease is to intervene as early as possible in order to arrest the disease and reduce the associated disabilities. This is the approach whether the disease is hypertension, diabetes, or arthritis. Consider the example of high blood pressure (hypertension). A patient who comes into the physician's office has a family history of hypertension. The patient is 40 pounds overweight, consumes considerable "junk food," a diet just loaded with cholesterol and salt, is a heavy smoker, and exercises little. This patient is such an obvious candidate for developing hypertension that the physician will undoubtedly initiate some preventive measures. Even though the patient's present blood pressure may be normal, the physician will educate the patient about hypertension, pointing out the benefits of changing diet and improving health habits, versus the risks of taking no action. The physician certainly will not sit back and wait for an elevation of blood pressure, much less wait for the patient to suffer a stroke before assuming that it is the responsibility of a medical professional to do something! How does this apply to alcoholism? As a chronic disease, alcoholism develops slowly and has well-demonstrated warning signs. As a chronic illness it would probably be impossible ever to pinpoint an exact time at which a nonalcoholic "turns" alcoholic. Even to think in such terms makes little sense and is unproductive. The proper frame of reference is to consider whether someone is "developing alcoholism." If a possibility exists, preventive measures should be instituted with as much concern as in the case just described.

To be quite candid, in practice this approach to alcoholism has not yet become the norm. All too often, in the presence of a possible alcohol problem, usually behavior consists of a lot of hand-wringing and waiting. The family, physician, everyone too often waits until the "possible problem" has progressed to the point where it is unequivocably and unquestionably the "real thing," alcoholism.

Consequently, most of the alcohol-treatment resources are now directed toward treating alcoholism. Treatment of persons with early alcohol problems is more an ideal than a reality. However, we are confident that the situation is changing. Compared to a generation ago, the professional training of physicians, clergy, nurses, social workers, and teachers has vastly changed with regard to alcohol, alcohol problems, and alcoholism. Also, prevention of disease and maintenance of health are getting more attention than ever before. The impact of diet, health habits, and life-style are more commonly concerns of the physician. The changes that have occurred over the last 20 years in attitudes toward smoking have been nothing short of dramatic. Questions about smoking are now a standard part of any medical history. Probably exceedingly few smokers are unaware that smoking may cause or aggravate medical problems. When seeing a physician a smoker expects to be asked questions about smoking and awaits the associated comments that smoking is ill-advised. Along with this, the attitudes of the general public have changed. On one hand there is a vocal antismoking lobby composed of people who do not wish to put up with secondhand smoke. There are also the concerned family members and friends of smokers, who more often are expressing their concerns directly to the smoker. Although the smoker may well continue to puff away it isn't without the nagging awareness that there are definite health risks. It is our prediction that within 20 years we will see a similar stance toward alcohol use. Though we do not expect to see the routine cautioning of total abstinence for all drinkers, we do expect to see, in medical situations, an alcohol-use history alongside a smoking history. We do expect that physicians will routinely be discussing the contraindications to moderate alcohol use when the individual's medical picture warrants it. We do expect that the general public will be more aware that alcohol is a drug and therefore potentially problematic. We do expect that drunkenness will become less socially acceptable. All of this, in turn, we believe, will lead to both earlier identification of alcohol problems and earlier treatment. We expect that future alcohol treatment will not be so exclusively directed toward treatment of alcoholism. Nonetheless, we are not there yet. So the majority of this chapter is directed toward a description of alcoholism treatment.

Treatment is nothing more (or less) than the interventions designed to short-circuit the alcoholic process and introduce the alcoholic to a sober, drug-free existence. Alcoholism is the third leading cause of death in the United States. It shouldn't be. In comparison with other chronic disease, it is significantly more treatable. Virtually *any* alcoholic who seeks assistance and is willing to participate actively in rehabilitation efforts can realistically expect to lead a happy, productive life. Sadly, the same is not true for a victim of cancer, heart disease, or emphysema. The realization that alcoholism is treatable is becoming more widespread. Both professional treatment programs and AA are discovering that the alcoholic today is often younger and in the early or middle stages of alcoholism when seeking help. It is imperative to keep firmly in mind the hopefulness that surrounds treatment.

Just as people initially become involved with alcohol for a variety of reasons, there is similar variety in what prompts treatment. For every person who wanders into alcoholism, there is also an exit route. This exit is most easily found with professional help. Typically the professional is an alcohol counselor or therapist who serves as a guide, to share knowledge of the terrain, to be a support as alcoholics regain their footing, and to provide encouragement. The counselor cannot make the trip *for* the alcoholic but can only point the way. The counselor's goal for treatment, the destination of the journey, is to assist the alcoholic in becoming comfortable and at ease in the world, able to handle his life situation. This will require the alcoholic to stop drinking. In our experience, a drinking alcoholic *cannot* be happy, at peace with himself, healthy, or alive in any way that makes sense, not to us, but to him. The question for all others—counselor, friends, and associates of the alcoholic is never "How can I make him stop?" The only productive focus will be "How can I create an atmosphere in which he is better able to choose sobriety for himself?"

▪ Obstacles to recognition and treatment

If alcoholism is so highly treatable, what has been going wrong? Why aren't more people receiving help? The obstacles do need to be looked at. One big handicap remains society's attitude toward alcohol and its use. Despite all the public education and information, there still lurks the notion that talking about someone's drinking is in bad taste. It seems too private, somehow, none of anyone's business. Most of us have a good feel for the taboo topics—sexual behavior, people's way of handling their children. The way someone drinks is a large taboo. This is to be expected. An alcoholic has a stake in keeping *his* drinking and its associated problems off limits. Should the drinking behavior be discussed, the alcoholic's rationalization combined with the tendency to "psychologize," analyze, and get to the why would spring another trap. The notion that someone drinks alcoholically *because* he is an alcoholic sounds circular and simpleminded. Thus everyone scurries around to find the "real" cause. Alcoholism as a phenomenon, a fact of life, gets pushed aside and forgotten in the uproar.

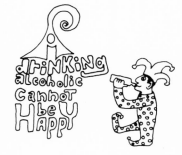

Another obstacle is the confusion introduced for the alcoholic and his family by the behavioral symptoms of alcoholism. If there is one hallmark characteristic of alcoholic behavior, it is the extreme variation, the lack of consistency,

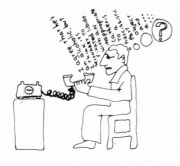

sometimes good mood, sometimes foul mood, sometimes sloshed, sometimes sober. This inconsistency invites a host of explanations. This very inconsistency is what allows the alcoholic, his family, and friends to hope things will get better on their own. It permits them to delay seeking assistance. It almost seems to be human nature to want, and wait, for things to get better on their own. Consider for a moment the simple toothache. If the toothache comes and goes, you probably will delay a trip to the dentist. After all, maybe it was something hot you ate—or maybe it was caused by something cold—or maybe, or maybe . . . ? On the other hand, if the pain is constant, if it doesn't go away, if it is clearly getting worse, if you can remember wicked toothaches in the past, you'll probably call immediately for an emergency appointment with your dentist. The total time you are actually in pain in the latter case may be much less that what you would have put up with in the former example, but you are spurred into action because it doesn't look like it will improve by itself.

Unfortunately, even when alcoholism treatment is instituted, it can be seriously unbalanced, zeroing in on only a part of the symptomatology. When this happens, the alcoholism treatment can end up looking a lot like treatment for depression, or cirrhosis, or just a "rest cure." These one-sided approaches are major sources of recidivism and failure, and not infrequently give the impression that alcoholism treatment doesn't work.

Factors in successful treatment

Having alluded to failure and some sense of what to avoid—on to success. Likelihood of success is greatly enhanced if treatment is tailored to the characteristics of the disease being treated. Awareness of the following factors, always present in the alcoholic, should guide the treatment planning and treatment process.

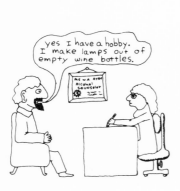

Alcohol-centered life. The alcoholic's life has become centered on alcohol. If this is not immediately evident, it is because the particular alcoholic has done a better-than-average job of disguising the fact. Thus one cannot expect a large repertoire of healthy behaviors that come automatically. Treatment should help build these, as well as dust off and rediscover behaviors from the past to replace the warped "alcoholic" responses. This fact is what may make residential treatment desirable. Besides cutting down the number of easy drinking opportunities, it provides some room to make a new, fresh beginning.

Few experiences of handling stress without alcohol. Alcohol has been the alcoholic's constant companion. It is used to anticipate, get through, and then get over stressful

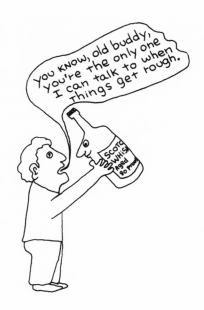

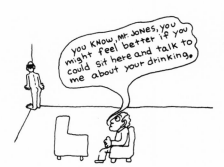

times. The alcoholic, to his knowledge, is without any effective tools for handling problems. Effective treatment programs will be alert to what may be stressful for a particular client, and provide supports.

Psychological wounds. Alcohol is the alcoholic's best friend and worst enemy. The prospect of a life without alcohol seems either impossible, or so unattractive as to be unworthwhile. The alcoholic feels lost, fragile, vulnerable, fearful. No matter how well put together the person can appear, or how much strength or potential others can see, the alcoholic, by and large, is unable to get beyond feelings of impotence, nakedness, nothingness. Others need to have a gentle awareness of this.

Physical dysfunctions. Chronic alcohol use takes its toll on the body. Even if spared the more obvious physical illnesses, there will be other subtle disturbances of physical functioning with which the alcoholic must contend. Sleep disturbance can last up to 2 years. Similarly, a thought impairment would not be unusual on cessation of drinking. The alcoholic in the initial stage of recovery will have trouble maintaining his attention. There will be diminution of adaptive abilities. During treatment, education about alcohol and its effects can help allay fears.

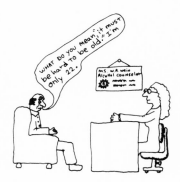

Chronic nature of alcoholism. A chronic disease requires continuing treatment and vigilance about the conditions that can prompt a relapse. This continued self-monitoring is essential to success in treatment.

Deterioration in family function. As described in Chapter 7, the family is in as great a need of help as is the alcoholic. Better outcomes result when they have a treatment program of their own in conjunction with the alcoholic's.

■ *Recovery as a process*

Recall how the progression of alcoholism can be sketched out. Similarly, recovery is a process that doesn't happen all at once. Gradually, in steps, the alcoholic becomes better able to manage his life. Recovery is a process that takes time. Alcohol treatment should be designed to facilitate the process. For the purpose of this discussion we have distinguished three stages of treatment: evaluation and assessment, the intensive initial treatment phase, and follow-up care. There is no clear-cut beginning or end point to each. But each of these has its observable hallmarks.

■ *Preludes to treatment*

Every alcoholic has some moments when the problems of drinking come to the foreground. This is happening when the alcoholic lets those nagging suspicions rise up that there is something wrong with his drinking, and he is unhappy and worried. On his own initiative he may make some initial inquiries. These may be directed to friends and associates.

You know, Jim was really mad at me for getting a bit tipsy when we went out last Friday night. You were there. I don't see anything wrong with letting go after a long hard week, do you? He's always on my back about something these days.

Often others may not recognize these queries as a disguised, or tentative "cry for help."

What can friends, co-workers, or colleagues do if they are the recipients of these initial queries? First, listen. Listen carefully, especially to find out the basis for the concern. Second, don't offer false reassurance. Don't unwittingly reinforce denial with an "Oh, you're just imagining it," or "It's probably nothing, just the holidays," or "If I had your problems, I'd probably drink a bit more, too!" Share the information that people can get into trouble with alcohol, that alcohol use can be a significant health problem. Recommend and strongly support seeking a professional opinion. Do what you can to see the person gets there. Unless you are in the habit of removing your friend's appendix or treating diabetes or otherwise providing medical advice, you will try to see that they seek advice from a professional. Rarely do people *not* having problems with alcohol worry about their drinking. Consider it as serious as the comment by a woman who thinks she *may have* a small lump in her breast.

Since there are growing numbers of recovering alcoholics successfully sober in AA, it is likely you have a friend or acquaintance in AA. It is possible also to suggest that your troubled friend speak with the AA person. Mention of AA might alarm the drinking alcoholic; simply describing the AA person as "someone who's been in a similar situation," and therefore more knowledgeable than you, may be the better tactic. The important point is never to minimize the concern, and always to try to get the person to see someone else. Don't let it drop. Later, find out if they've done anything. You may feel that you are being pushy, but likely as not the potential alcoholic on his own is immobilized and confused, and therefore needs the "pressure" to act. If you really care, take the time to get the name of an alcohol-treatment program to which you can refer the person if necessary.

The first overture may instead be made to the alcoholic by a member of the clergy, family member, friend, or perceptive physician—someone who is sufficiently concerned to speak up and take the risk of being accused of meddling. Suspecting an alcohol problem, any one of them might request that the alcoholic seek an alcohol expert to explore the possibility. In other situations, a court may "sentence" an individual convicted of driving while intoxicated to alcohol treatment.

It is increasingly common for a spouse of the alcoholic to seek counseling, as a result of the chaos of living with an alcoholic; or, the employer may notice developing problems and attempt to intervene.

Though anyone may attempt to persuade a person to check out his drinking with a professional, the dynamics of denial present in the disease itself often doom these individual efforts to failure. A method of confronting alcoholics early in their disease and increasing the chances of success has been developed by the staff of the Johnson Institute in Minneapolis and is now being taught all over the country.

Briefly, intervention, as it is called, requires the cooperation of a number of people close to an alcoholic person. With the aid of a trained counselor, employers, family, and/or friends come together to share evidence of the alcoholic's deteriorating function that is tied directly to drinking. Working with them, the counselor helps them to assess their evidence and prepare for a meeting with the alcoholic. Preparation also includes sorting out feelings so the participants can present their concerns concretely and objectively. The goal is to supply information, not make accusations. Because one of the important features of the disease is the inability of the alcoholic to see the connection between alcohol and life problems, it is up to those concerned to present the facts in a way that the alcoholic can accept. If a group of people who obviously care deeply present to the alcoholic the reality of the drinking behavior as each one has experienced it, the mounting evidence often breaks through the denial system. It is vitally necessary for those who intervene to agree on the need for and importance of what they propose to do. They also must agree totally on what options they plan to present to the drinker. An alcoholic is usually well able to immobilize an individual who attempts to "interfere" with the drinking, but a group of people is quite another matter.

A word of caution is necessary here. Intervention is a tricky business and should *not* be attempted without a professional helper specifically trained in intervention techniques. The process is described in much more detail in Vernon Johnson's *I'll Quit Tomorrow* and depicted in the film of the same name.

▪ *Evaluating the problem*

Suppose an alcoholic has entered the door of an alcohol-treatment program, or a counselor's office; then what happens? Before treatment for any medical condition can be initiated, several important preliminary steps must be taken. First, there must be a careful evaluation of the problem, to assess its nature and severity. Following that, a tentative treatment plan will be devised, possibly using outside expert opinions. These treatment recommendations will then be discussed with the patient. This discussion will explain the recommendations, including any possible risks of treatment versus the dangers of not initiating treatment.

The assessment process for an alcohol problem or alcoholism, just like any other evaluation process, is intended initially to collect data. The counselor in a very general way will be endeavoring simply to get a clear picture of what is going on in the client's life. The questions the counselor will typically ask in an initial interview are as follows:

1. What brings the person in now?
2. What is going on in his life—in terms of family, job, marriage?
3. What problems does the individual see?
4. Alcohol use—What, where, when, how much, and what does it do for you?

Counselors do their work by observing, by listening, and by asking questions to gain a picture of the situation. The image of a picture being sketched and painted is quite apt to capture the idea of the counseling process. The space below is the canvas. The total area includes everything that is going on in the client's life.

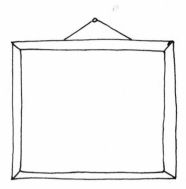

In the course of their meeting, this space gets filled in. Now the counselor is getting a picture of the situation. Not only does he or she have the "facts" as the client sees them, he or she can see the client, his mood and feelings, and also get a sense of what the world and picture *feels* like. As this happens, the empty space gets filled in and begins to look like this:

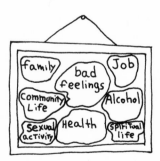

The counselor has a notion of the various areas that make up the person's life: family, physical health, work, economic situation, community life, how the person feels about himself, and so on. He or she will also be aware of how alcohol may affect these areas. As necessary, the counselor will guide the conversation to ensure a total picture of what is happening. The counselor is also aware that if someone is experiencing difficulty, having a problem, it means the pieces are not fitting together in a way that feels comfortable. Maybe some parts have very rough edges. Maybe one part is exerting undue influence on the others. So the counselor attempts to see the relationship and interaction between the parts.

The counselor in an initial interview will also be assessing whether there is an emergency—medical or psychiatric—requiring that the person receive immediate attention from a doctor or psychiatrist. Some examples of this would be a person who hasn't been feeling well and reports bleeding; the individual who has stopped drinking the day before and is shaky, perspiring, and apparently undergoing withdrawal; or someone who is very despondent and contemplating suicide.

The assessment process may take one interview or it may take four or more. It may be completed in half an hour or it may occur over the span of a week or two. Commonly the counselor will seek permission from the client to speak with family members, or contact the client's physician, or others who may have important information that will be useful in understanding the picture.

During this evaluation phase, the counselor will not only gather information, but will also try to develop a therapeutic relationship with the client, knowing that despite the title "Alcohol Counselor," the alcoholic did not come in to have the counselor do the "treatment routine." What the alcoholic desperately wants is a clean bill of health. The hope is to figure out why drinking isn't working anymore.

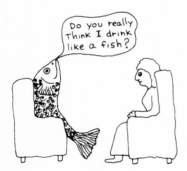

You will recall that the alcoholic's perception of the world is inaccurate. Also, he is beset by fears and anxieties. In his initial contacts with the counselor he is a fish nibbling at the bait. He moves close and backs off. He wants to know, but doesn't want to (is scared to) stop. What he really wants to learn is how to drink well. He wants to drink without the accompanying problems. The chances are pretty good he wants the counselor to teach him how. This represents an impossible request, and the counselor knows that. Hopefully, others concerned for the alcoholic's well-being also know this and refuse to buy into "cutting down" as the way to go.

At this point the counselor will move gingerly, neither holding out any false hopes nor sternly lecturing the alcoholic about how obviously stupid he is. That would be guaranteed to drive the alcoholic away. There is, however, a mutual goal "to have things be okay." The counselor can buy into this without accepting the client's means of achieving it. The counselor realizes that the only thing that may be clear to the alcoholic is the presence of drinking. The alcoholic is often unaware of the relationship of his drinking to the problems in his life. As the client paints a picture of what's going on in his life space, the counselor will certainly see things the client is missing or ignoring.

Client's view of his world

Counselor's view of client's world

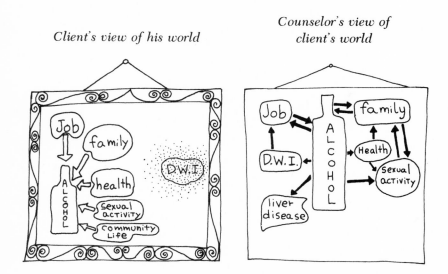

Often the counselor can see that the client is alcoholic, and may be of the opinion that the person needs a rehabilitation facility. However, at the moment, the alcoholic is unable to *use* the treatment. First it is necessary for him to make some connections—that is, get his arrows pointed in the right direction. As this occurs, the alcoholic begins to see the impossible nature of his hope for "good drinking" again.

▪ *Confrontation*

The counselor endeavors to help the client make the essential connections. Confrontation is one technique. Confrontation does *not* equal attack. According to *Webster's*, to confront means "to cause to meet: bring face to face." Several examples of what the counselor may do to bring the client face to face with the consequences of his behavior are through a family meeting, so that the family's concerns can be presented; or clarifying others' views, or reminding the alcoholic of the physician's findings.

In assisting the alcoholic to "see" what is going on, the counselor's observation skills pay off. The alcoholic has a notoriously warped perception of reality. The ability of the counselor "merely" to provide accurate feedback to the client, giving specific descriptions of behavior, of what the client is doing, is very valuable. The alcoholic has lost the knack of self-assessment. It is quite likely that the feedback from family members has also been warped and laced with threats, so that it is useless to the alcoholic. In the counseling situation, it may go like this: "Well, you say things are going fine. Yet, as I look at you, I see you fidgeting in your chair, your voice is quavering, and your eyes are cast down toward the floor. For me, that doesn't go along with someone who's feeling fine." *Period.* The counselor simply reports his or her observations. There isn't any deep interpretation. There's no attempt to ferret out hidden unconscious dynamics. The client isn't labeled a liar. The willingness and ability simply to describe what is seen is the therapeutic tool. The alcoholic can begin to learn how he does come across, how others see him. Thus the counselor's observations serve to educate the client about himself.

The goal of all this is certainly not for the alcoholic to gain total insight. It is intended to help make the one critical connection—that alcohol is a major difficulty and to go it alone is a certain, possibly literal, dead end.

Alcoholism is a disease that requires the sufferer to make a self-diagnosis for successful treatment. Treatment, full steam ahead, cannot begin until the alcoholic, inside himself, attaches that label to cover all that is going on with him. A head, or intellectual, understanding doesn't suffice. It must come from the heart. In fact, the whole thing can be confusing. He certainly doesn't have to be happy. He simply needs to know it's true. Then without hope of his own, he borrows others' belief that things can change.

At this point of acknowledgment, seeing alcohol as the culprit, and with a desire to change, the alcoholic by himself is lost. If he knew what to do, he'd have done it. Thus he, in essence, needs to turn the steering of his life over to someone else.

The assessment period is a time when the evidence gathering can begin to cement the diagnosis. This assessment period may be very disconcerting for families. The family —very worried, concerned, frustrated—wants something to happen, *now*. The family—relieved because the alcoholic is finally seeing someone—wants definitive action. How long they have waited to have someone else shape him or her up! If that doesn't appear to be happening, the family may feel panic. It is not uncommon for the family to wonder about the counselor's competence. They'll question their own judgment. Should they have urged seeing a psychiatrist instead, and so on. The family may fear the counselor will fall for the alcoholic's warped view of the world, and be conned.

A family meeting is becoming a routine part of any assessment process. At this time, the counselor will be seeking the family's view of what is happening. When this meeting is held will be determined by the alcoholic's status, the severity of the alcohol problem, what is going on with the family, the receptivity and/or resistance to treatment. Say alcoholism is clearly evident; at such a stage, it is diagnosable even by the parking lot attendant. In this situation, the family may be the only reliable source of even the most basic information, such as how much alcohol is being consumed, past medical history, prior alcohol treatment. Or the alcoholic's judgment may be so severely impaired that realistically others will have to make the decision about admission for treatment. The postponement of formal family involvement is most likely when the alcoholism is in the early stages, and the alcoholic's life still has some semblance of order. In such circumstances the counselor may want to explore with the alcoholic his view of the world and develop a working relationship, before introducing possibly opposing views.

Of course, a family member can always offer to go with the alcoholic initially and see the counselor as a family or couple. If the family is not approached by the counselor, they must make the first overture. They should be wary if the alcoholic reports that the counselor doesn't want to see them. That is almost always untrue. Counselors want to see families at some point in the process. But it isn't productive to become involved in an argument with the alcoholic about what the counselor supposedly does or doesn't want. By making an offer to contact the counselor themselves to make arrangements, the family can successfully skirt the argument.

Based on the information that has surfaced during the evaluation, the counselor will be ready to move ahead quickly with recommendations for treatment. The major considerations for making this determination will be the alcoholic's physical state and the extent of alcohol-induced impairment. To put that more simply, the basic issue is "How extensive is alcohol's interference in the person's life?"

Indications for inpatient or residential treatment are few family or social supports; a long history of an alcohol-centered life-style; the serious disruption of family, job, and social spheres; and strong ambivalence about need for treatment.

Outpatient care may be possible if the individual has strong family support, has less social, family, or occupational dysfunction, or if this is a first alcohol-treatment effort.

In almost every area of the country, there are certain to be several facilities that provide the necessary treatment. The family and alcoholic may well be given several choices.

▪ *Intensive initial treatment*

Treatment could be defined as all the interventions intended to short-circuit the alcoholism process and to introduce the alcoholic to effective sobriety. This could be put in equation form as follows: Treatment = individual counseling + client education + family therapy + family education + group therapy + medical care + AA + Alanon + Antabuse + vocational counseling + activities therapy + spiritual counseling + ...

Meanwhile, the first and immediate concern will be to return the alcoholic safely to a drug-free state. This detoxification process is a medical matter and ought to be accomplished under medical supervision. If there is significant physical dependence (see Chapter 5), the alcoholic may be admitted to a hospital or possibly a special detoxification unit of an alcohol-treatment center. In this setting, the alcoholic can be closely monitored and be given the appropriate medications to ease withdrawal. These medications replace the alcohol and then are gradually tapered off over a period of several days. Detoxification can be accomplished on an outpatient basis, depending on the drinking history and the availability of support, and if the alcoholic has no major medical problems or prior history of difficulties with withdrawal.

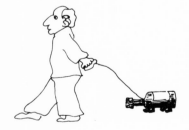

This detoxification period is the part of alcoholism treatment that most resembles what we usually consider to be "treatment" of illness. There are physicians in white coats, temperature and blood pressure checks, pills, and so on. If the alcoholic has been feeling ill physically, there will be a dramatic improvement within a week. He will look and feel better. It may be quite tempting for the alcoholic at this point to say "Gee, you've really helped me to see exactly what I have to do. I'll _____, _____, _____, and _____, and everything will be just fine. Thanks so much. You've made my life for me," and leave. It is important not to equate detoxification with treatment of alcoholism and buy into what the alcoholic is saying. All detoxification does is to prepare or enable the alcoholic to start the rehabilitation process that is the essence of alcoholism treatment.

As the alcoholic begins treatment, he badly needs to have a rehabilitative regimen set forth for him. He needs his environment simplified. The number of decisions he is confronted with must be pared down. He is able to deal with little more than "How am I going to get through this day (or hour) without a drink?" Effort needs to be centered on doing whatever is necessary to buy sober time. To quote the old maxim: "Nothing succeeds like success." A day sober turns on the light a little. It has become something that is possible. For the alcoholic, this is an achievement. It doesn't guarantee continued sobriety, but it demonstrates the possibility. In the sober time, the alcoholic is gaining skills. He is discovering behavior that can be of assistance in handling those events that previously would have prompted drinking.

Although we are not attempting to discuss specific techniques of treatment here, a mention of AA is nonetheless in order. Anyone in the alcoholism-treatment field will acknowledge that clients who take up AA have a much better chance of recovery. This is not accidental. AA has combined the key ingredients essential for recovery. It provides support, it embodies hopes. It provides concrete suggestions without cajoling. Its slogans are the simple guideposts needed to reorder a life. And its purpose is never lost.

The necessity for a direct and uncluttered approach to the alcoholic cannot be overstressed. He isn't capable of handling anything else. This is one of several reasons for the belief that alcoholism has to be the priority item on any treatment agenda. The only exceptions are life-threatening or serious medical problems. For the alcoholic to work actively and successfully on a list of difficulties is overwhelming. Interestingly enough, when alcoholism treatment is undertaken, the other problems often fade. Furthermore, waiting to treat the alcoholism until some other matter is settled invites the alcoholic's ambivalence to surface. This waiting feeds the part of him that says, "Well, maybe it isn't so bad after all," or "I'll wait and see how it goes." Generally the matters are unsolvable because an active drinking alcoholic has no inner resources to tackle anything. He's drugged.

▪ Common themes during recovery

Early in the recovery process, many alcoholics have a tendency to become quite upset over very small matters. They look well, feel well, and sound well. But they really aren't quite there yet. This can be very trying for the alcoholic and his family. Remembering and reminding them of how sick they have recently been makes this less threatening. The steps after any major illness seem slow and tedious. There are occasional setbacks. Yet, eventually, all is well. It works that way with alcoholism, too. It is simply harder to accept, since there are no bandages to remove, no scars to point to, no clear signs of healing to check on. It cannot be emphasized enough that it *takes time.*

One point often overlooked is the alcoholic's plain in-

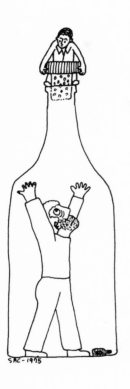

ability to function on a simple daily basis. It is almost inconceivable to anyone else that a person who seems reasonably intelligent, looks fairly healthy after detoxification, and is over 21 can have problems with when to get up in the morning or what to do when he *is* up! Along with family, work, and social deterioration caused by the alcoholic lifestyle, the simple things have gotten messed up too. Alcoholics may have gargled, brushed their teeth, and chewed mints continually while drinking in an effort to cover up. They may, on the other hand, have skipped most mealtimes and eaten only sporadically with no eye to their nutritional needs. They may have thrown up with some regularity. But as we have seen in Chapter 5, their sleep is not likely to be normal. Getting dressed without trying to choke down some booze to quell the shakes may be a novel experience. It may have been years since the person has performed the standard daily tasks in a totally drug-free state.

Alcoholics are rather like Rip Van Winkles during the early weeks of their recovery. Everything they do is likely to feel strange. The face looking back at them from the mirror may even seem like a stranger's. They became used to the blurred perceptions they had experienced while drinking. It is terribly disconcerting to find virtually every task one faces a whole new thing. Whereas it used to take 2 very careful days to prepare Thanksgiving dinner, it now requires only a few hours. The accompanying wine for the cook, trips back to the store for forgotten items (and by the way, a little more booze), the self-pity over *having* to do it, the naps necessary to combat the fatigue of the ordeal, the incredible energy devoted to control the drinking enough to get everything done . . . all these steps are eliminated.

The newly sober alcoholic is continually being faced with the novelty of time. It's either time left over, or the experience of not enough time, or near panic over "what to do next." Many will need help in setting up schedules. After years of getting by on the bottle, they have to regain a sense of the "real" time it takes to accomplish some tasks. He may plan to paint the entire house in 2 days or, conversely, decide that he can't possibly fit a dentist appointment, a luncheon engagement, and a sales call into one. She may believe that it's all she can manage to make the beds, do the dishes, and dust today. Tomorrow she intends to make new living room drapes in time for that evening's dinner party! The perception of time is as distorted as other areas of perception. Reassurance that this is a common state of affairs, along with assistance in setting realistic daily goals, is greatly needed. This is one reason newcomers to AA find the slogans "Keep it simple" and "First things first" so helpful.

The alcoholic may not mention the dilemmas over time and schedules. There may be a sense of shame over such helplessness in the face of simple things. But a gentle question from a counselor or an AA sponsor may open the floodgates. He can offer the alcoholic some much-needed guidance in remastering the details of daily living. All too often the wail is heard, "I don't know! The house was a mess . . . I was a mess . . . I just couldn't handle it, so I drank!"

Another area in which the counselor has to reorient the alcoholic who needs reorientation to reality involves the misperception of events. The faulty memories caused by the drugged state will have to be reexamined. One cannot always wait for some sudden insight to clear things up. For example, the difficulties he has had with his wife. He remembers her as a nagging bitch on his back about a "few little drinks." He might be reminded that on the occasion in question, he was picked up for driving while intoxicated with a blood alcohol content of 0.20—clearly not a few. It can be pointed out that because he has misperceived the amount he was drinking to such an extent, he may have misperceived his wife's behavior. The opportunity is there, if indicated, to educate the alcoholic briefly on the distortions produced by the drug, alcohol, and to suggest that sober observations of his wife's behavior are more valid.

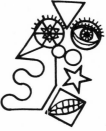

Portrait of a man who has had 4 drinks and thinks someone has insulted him

At a point, after about 3 months, when the sober alcoholic reaches some level of comfort with his new state, the focus can shift. Earlier the attention was virtually at the level of the "mechanics" of daily living. With that out of the way, or reasonably under control, the focus can move on to sorting out the alcoholic's stance in the world, feelings, and relationships.

Though 3 months is a somewhat arbitrary designation, it is not wholly so. Recall the subacute withdrawal syndrome (Chapter 5). The alcoholic may have passed the acute withdrawal period in 5 days, but a longer period is required to regain the ability to concentrate, for example. So there is a physical basis for what the alcoholic can focus on productively. This doesn't mean all the problems previously discussed are totally overcome or that work is not proceeding along some of the above paths. It simply means that other problems may now be surfacing. Some are fairly common. Most of these basically require finding a balance point between two extremes of behavior that are equally dangerous. John Wallace, a psychologist who has had considerable experience working with alcoholics in a major New York City treatment program, has neatly described his observations. He compares these extremes to rocks and whirlpools that must be avoided in the recovery "voyage."

One of the first difficulties is the *denial problem*. The

tendency for others, when faced with the alcoholic's massive rejection of reality, is to want to force him to face all the facts *right now*. The trouble with this approach is that self-knowledge is often bought at the price of anxiety, and anxiety is a drinking trigger. What to do? First, provide support to counteract the initial anxiety caused by the acceptance of the reality of the drinking itself. Don't underestimate how painful it is for the alcoholic to look at the drinking behavior and its consequences. Then, gradually, keep supporting the small increments in awareness that occur in the sober experience. It is difficult, but necessary, to remember that the denial of some particular issue is serving a useful purpose at the time, keeping overwhelming anxiety at bay until more strength is available. Continued involvement with a counselor can be of immense value when these problems begin to crop up. The counselor can be central to deciding how much anxiety the alcoholic can tolerate. The question facing the counselor is whether the denial is still necessary to ward off anxiety or whether it has become counterproductive, blocking further progress.

Other problems occur over the issue of *guilt* and its fraternal twin, *self-blame*. It is clearly desirable to mitigate the degree of both. It is also necessary to avoid the pitfalls of their opposites, rejection of social values and blaming others. Although excessive guilt leads to the guilt/drinking spiral, some degree of conscience and sense of responsibility are necessary to function in society. The objective, therapeutic role permits a counselor to point out unnecessary burdensome guilt on the one hand and yet allow honest guilt to be expressed. Dealing with both kinds, appropriately, is essential. On the blame issue the alcoholic needs help in accepting personal responsibility where necessary. However, it can be helpful to point out that the disease itself, rather than self/others, may be the true cause of some of the difficulties.

Another unhealthy extreme is often seen, particularly early in treatment: *compliance or rebellion*. The compliant alcoholic becomes a "model" of grateful acceptance of his recovery program; the rebellious one says: "Aha! I was right. You *are* against me," and drinks. Moderation is again the key. The aim is to help him to acknowledge the alcoholism and truly accept the facts of his situation.

Feelings, and what to do with them, provide another dual obstacle to be faced. The dry alcoholic is likely to repress feelings entirely. He does this to counteract their all too uncontrolled expression during the drinking experiences. Respect for this need to repress the emotions should prevail in the initial stages of recovery. But the eventual goal of the helper is to teach the alcoholic to recognize emotions and deal with them appropriately. Alcoholics need to learn, or relearn, that feelings need not be repressed altogether or, conversely, wildly acted out. Instead, a recognition and acceptance of them can lead to better solutions.

Another key concern is *dependency issues.* Many articles, and indeed whole books, have been written about dependency and alcoholism. Sometimes the alcoholic is depicted as a particularly dependent type who has resolved his conflict inappropriately by the use of alcohol. Whether this helps promote or "cause" alcoholism isn't the point. It must be noted that many alcoholics do tend toward stubborn independence versus indiscriminate dependence in their relationships. They seem to have an evil genius for attracting the very people they don't need—ones who, in fact, are harmful to them. The need for loving relationships, the development of unsatisfactory ones, and the consequent pain and misery are responsible in an unusually large number of instances for relapses. The alcoholic needs, maybe more than most, to realize that people are all interdependent to some degree. The trick is to recognize the dependent need and ask, as Wallace so aptly states: "1. Upon *whom* should I be dependent? 2. For *what*? 3. At what *cost* to me?" These questions should be asked in regard to all the relationships, not simply the primary love one. It may well turn out that dependency is being channeled into one relationship instead of spread out more effectively. Once these questions are squarely faced, selectivity and judgment stand a better chance; the extremes, with their threat to sobriety, can be more successfully avoided.

There is another issue that may well be encountered by single alcoholics, or those caught in unhappy marriages. It is not uncommon for them to find themselves "suddenly" involved in an affair or an extramarital relationship. With a little bit of sobriety, they are very ripe to fall in love. This may have several roots. They may be questioning their sexuality, and the attentions of another may well provide some affirmation of attractiveness. Also possible is that with sobriety comes a sense of being alive again. There's the reawakening of a host of feelings that have long been dormant, including sexual feelings. In this sense, it may be like the bloom and intensity of adolescence. A romantic involvement may follow very naturally. Unfortunately, it can lead to disaster, if followed with abandon. Knowledge of this potential trouble spot, while helpful in some cases, is not always enough to ward off trouble. The help of people who have successfully dealt with such issues can be of vital importance in handling these feelings in a positive, healthy manner. Participation in groups of other recovering alcoholics is one option to keep feelings in perspective.

But if the "love bug" bites particularly hard in the early days of recovery (up through the first year or so), professional help is certainly recommended to deal with this issue.

The alcoholic's counselor is going to be a very central person in the alcoholic's life. It is important for family and friends to recognize this and not feel personally rejected during this phase. Whereas individual counseling is only one component of alcohol treatment, it is the time, space, and place in which the rest of treatment is organized and planned. Counseling sessions are where the counselor and alcoholic will be working on many of the issues just described—defining problems, exploring solutions, identifying resources. The counselor provides objective support, encouragement, and feedback to the alcoholic.

It should be made explicit that material shared by either the alcoholic or family with a counselor is considered confidential information. A counselor is always ethically bound and in some cases legally bound not to discuss a client's case with any party outside the immediate staff of a particular treatment program, without the client's express permission. (Treatment team members working together with an alcoholic have to share relevant information. Confidentiality then applies equally to the team.) This ethical standard is common to all helping professions.

Practically, what does this mean for the alcoholic or family in treatment? They can be assured that what is discussed in the professional setting is not something that becomes the basis for idle chatter or gossip. It also means that if an alcohol counselor wishes to receive information from the alcoholic's doctor, or some outside agency, the alcoholic will have to sign a permission form allowing others to provide the information. By the same token, if anyone ever requests information from the counselor—be it an insurance company, a physician, or a friend—the same procedure will be necessary.

Often what the alcoholic or family members are most concerned about is that what each one may say will get back to the other. There, too, confidentiality prevails; the counselor will not be divulging information to those not present without permission from those who are. At times this can be a stress and a relief. The spouse wants to know what the alcoholic said and vice versa. Though the counselor will never provide verbatim accounts, this does not mean there will not be a sharing of the general situation.

Sometimes individuals are reluctant to share information unless they can get the counselor to promise explicitly that "so-and-so" will not be told. For the alcoholic, this often centers around some drinking behavior that may be especially embarrassing or shameful—possibly an affair or a legal problem. For the family it is more likely to be a secret, behind-the-alcoholic's-back reporting: most commonly, "I'm sure he's drinking, but don't tell him I told you." Probably in both instances the counselor is going to help the individual to share the information and to deal with it openly.

It must be noted that confidentiality is *not* absolute. Situations, admittedly not common, *do* occur in which it is the counselor's responsibility to share information. Such situations involve a serious likelihood of there being physical harm to self or others. An example of this is a client who comes in very despondent, with a well-thought-out plan for suicide. In another case, a client may call up from a tavern drunk, raving about his wife—a client who has a history when intoxicated of physical assault against his family. In these instances the counselor's obligation is to intervene.

Though the counselor may be a larger-than-life figure for the recovering alcoholic and family members, it is worth commenting on what in fact are the essential "tricks of the counselor's trade." Counselors aren't magical, they have no special powers to divine the darkest, deepest recesses of clients' minds. Despite suspicions to the contrary, there is no T-shirt with a big letter "S" underneath the button-down oxford-cloth collar. The counselor's skills may seem unspectacular, but they are what is desperately needed.

The counselor is objective, that alone distinguishes him or her from everyone else in the alcoholic's world. In addition, although the counselor cares, it isn't the same kind of deep emotional investment that friends and family have. If there is one quality that characterizes the counselor, it is curiosity. This is not to be confused with the voyeurism associated with enjoying hearing about what the alcoholic did while drinking—that is, listening to true confessions. Drinking alcoholics, though very unique to themselves and families, are for the counselor monotonously similar. No, the curiosity lies in awaiting the emergence of the "real" person during recovery, as the alcohol-induced personality is shrugged off.

These factors, combined with the counselor's knowledge of alcoholism and clinical experience with treatment, enable a straightforward, honest telling-it-like-it-is approach. The counselor can challenge, confront, give feedback in a way the recovering alcoholic experiences as supportive, even when it is painful.

Finally, the counselor is very clear on an issue that is likely to trip up the family: responsibility. The counselor is not apt to get caught up either in protecting the alcoholic or in trying to manipulate him. The counselor expects the alcoholic to assume responsibility for his actions. He or she does not buy into the alcoholic's view of himself as either a pawn of fate or a helpless victim. An ironic twist is present. The counselor makes it clear that the alcoholic is an adult who is accountable for his choices. Simultaneously, the counselor is aware that an alcoholic, when he consumes alcohol, is abdicating control of his life to a drug. By definition an alcoholic cannot be responsible for what transpires after even one or two drinks. Therefore, being responsible ultimately means that the attempt to manage alcohol must be abandoned. Here hard facts about the drug alcohol, and the disease alcoholism, are important. A large chunk of the alcoholic's work will be to examine the facts of his own life in light of this information. People's ability to alibi, to rationalize, and otherwise to explain away the obvious varies. But the counselor consistently holds up the mirror of reality, playing back to the alcoholic his drinking history.

Likewise it is the alcoholic's responsibility to learn to deal with the illness. No one else can do it for him. The counselor—in subtle and at times not so subtle ways—supplies this essential message.

As the recovering alcoholic comes to grips with sobriety, so too he simultaneously begins to assume the primary responsibility for managing his life. As this occurs, there is a corresponding shift in the relationship with the counselor. They collaborate in a different way. The counselor will be alert to potential problematic situations, but the alcoholic increasingly takes responsibility for identifying the potential rough spots and selecting ways to deal with them. Rather than being a guide, the counselor becomes a resource, someone to check things out with. At this point, the alcoholic's follow-up treatment has begun.

■ *Follow-up care*

For a period of time the recovering alcoholic may well stay in regular contact with the counselor even when things seem to be well under control, as do other chronically ill persons. It is not uncommon for treatment programs to continue contact for a 2-year period. Appointments may be scheduled at 3-month intervals, with the option of the individual's making other contacts if this seems indicated. It is the responsibility of the individual to self-monitor and reach out for reinforcements as required.

"Why do I drink?" or "Why does he drink?" are the recurrent themes of alcoholics and their family members at the outset of treatment. To focus on that question then, when it seems most pressing, is usually of little value. It looks to the past and to causes "out there." The more important question for either the alcoholic or family facing the nitty-gritty of the present is, "What can be done, now?" However, if there is a productive time to deal with the "whys," it comes well after sobriety has been established, often in the context of the follow-up treatment. Don't misunderstand. Long hours spent on what went wrong, way back are never helpful. Rather, the why can be discerned from the present, daily life events, on the occasion when taking a drink would be most tempting. Dealing with such instances provides insight and a wealth of practical information for immediate use.

The recovering alcoholic needs to be aware of particular situations and personal responses to them that may signal trouble. In any chronic illness there are ups and downs, rough spots, and smooth sailing. Adjustments must be made to accommodate these variations. Some stressful periods, such as holidays, may be predictable. Others may take the recovering alcoholic by surprise. When rough spots arise, the recovering alcoholic should have a variety of options available. We do not wish to imply that forever and ever the recovering alcoholic is connected to the counselor by an umbilicus. Far from it; other options are attending AA more frequently, or clearing one's schedule for a day or two, using the supports available through family. However, the recovering alcoholic needs to maintain some awareness of his alcoholic status, and the elements essential to recovery, if sobriety is to continue.

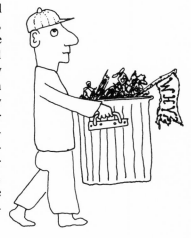

■ *Getting stuck*

It is not uncommon to hear the following comments in reference to recovering alcoholics: "Reformed drunks are as bad as ex-smokers." "Sending someone to AA just creates another dependency." "It seems the treatment is as bad as the disease." In many instances, such comments represent nothing more than mere ignorance. Of course, in affiliating with AA the newly sober person shifts his dependency from alcohol to AA, and at that point that's a plus. The newly recovering alcoholic may also be seeing a counselor, attending an alcohol-treatment group, be very involved in AA, and be pleased that the family is attending Al-Anon and Al-Ateen. Great.

It is true, however, that some people do become stuck in the recovery process. By this we mean in a life just as alcohol-centered as before. The only difference is that the center is "not drinking" instead of "how to keep drinking." Granted, physical health is less threatened, traumatic events less frequent, and maybe even job and family stability have been established. Nonetheless, it is a recovery rut, maybe even a trench!

There are probably many factors that account for the "stuckness." One might be an "I never had it so good, so I won't rock the boat" feeling—a real fear of letting go of the life preserver even when safely ashore.

Another factor is that some recovering alcoholics—particularly those who began drinking as teenagers—have spent the bulk of their adult lives as active alcoholics. Therefore, they have no baseline of adult healthy behaviors to which they can return. They are confronted with gaining sobriety, growing up, and functioning as adults simultaneously. Such a tall order can be an overwhelming prospect. To make it more manageable, it may well be tempting for these recovering alcoholics to keep their world narrowed down to alcoholism recovery. The only thing they now feel really competent to do, the only area where they have had support and a positive sense of self, is in getting sober. Giving up the status of "newcomer" to be replaced by "sober, responsible adult" may be scary, so a relapse or drinking episode may ensue. They then can justify and ensure that they can keep doing the only thing they feel they do well: being a patient, an AA newcomer, a recovering alcoholic.

Another factor could be that some counselors and some AA members—as well as some family members—are better equipped to deal with the crisis period of getting sober than with the later issues of growth and true freedom. They may simply be unable to guide the alcoholic onward to the next phase of recovery. If this is the source of "stuckness," other types of therapy or groups that promote personal exploration and growth may be indicated. This is a delicate situation; the adjunctive treatments are not to be seen as substituting for whatever has worked so far. Rather, they are an addition to it, whether it is AA, individual counseling, or some other form of assistance.

People in the alcoholic's life should beware of getting stuck in back-patting behavior. The phrase, "Well, I didn't do much today, but at least I stayed sober" is OK once in a while. When it becomes a recovered alcoholic's standard refrain, over a long period of time, it should be questioned and certainly not encouraged. Those who work around treatment facilities are all too aware of groups of alcoholics who hang around endlessly, drinking coffee, talking to other alcoholics exclusively, and clearly going nowhere, year after year. For some, who for instance may have suffered brain damage or some other disability, this may be the best that can be hoped for. However, we suspect that others are there simply because they are not being helped and prodded to proceed any further.

■ *Relapses*

Any individual with a chronic disease is subject to relapses. For the alcoholic, relapse means the resumption of drinking. Why? The reasons are numerous. For the relatively newly sober person it probably boils down to a gross underestimation of the seriousness and severity of the disease. Thus the alcoholic fails really to come to grips with his or her own impotence to deal with it single-handedly. Hence, while going through the motions of treatment, one may harbor the lingering notion that though other alcoholics may need to do this or that, somehow it's not applicable to him or her. This may show up in very simple ways, such as the failure to change the little things that are likely to make drinking easier than not drinking. "Hell, I've always ridden home in the bar car, after 20 years that's where my friends are," "What would people say if _____," "There's a lot going on in my life, getting to the couples group simply isn't possible on a regular basis." If families and close friends are not well informed about alcoholism treatment, and willing to make adjustments too, they can unwittingly support and even invite this dangerous behavior.

This type of thinking is common for persons with diabetes or heart disease as well. Diet is one important part of their treatment, but the temptations of "just a little potato, or cholesterol-laden goodie, etc." proves too much to resist. And those of us who are families and friends have a difficult time keeping temptations at a minimum for anyone. We provide salted and oiled snacks, and cheeses, red meat, and egg dishes (to be avoided by heart disease patients), starches, sumptuous breads, rich desserts, sugar galore (problem foods for diabetics); and we press alcohol on all comers (especially a problem to the alcoholic, but probably contraindicated in generous amounts for the other two categories as well). We need to be aware that our hospitable instincts can really be harmful to others. Comparing this to our own efforts to diet or exercise or stop smoking may help us to be more compassionately aware of our neighbor's problems.

For the recovering alcoholic with more substantial sobriety, relapse is commonly tied to two things. One is that relapse may be triggered by the recovery rut, already described. On the other hand, if things have been going really well, with the recovering alcoholic's life proceeding quite swimmingly, there is the trap of thinking the alcoholism is a closed chapter.

As an aside, probably as a response to this danger, one sometimes hears alcohol counselors, AA members, or those well acquainted with alcoholism stating a preference for the phrase recover*ing* alcoholic, rather than recover*ed*. It serves as a reminder that one is not cured of alcoholism. From a medical standpoint, this is in fact seemingly accurate. The evidence does point to biological-biochemical changes that occur during the course of heavy drinking.

Even with long-term abstinence, in this respect there is no return to the "normal" or prealcoholic state. The body's biological memory of alcoholism remains intact, even if the recovered alcoholic has "forgotten."

A drinking episode need not be the end of the world, but it should not be taken lightly. Whether it's one drink, or an evening of drinking, or a weekend or a month, the alcoholic needs to be immediately reinvolved with a treatment center, a counselor, or—if active or previously active in AA—an AA member, or do several of these things. The important thing is not to sit back and do nothing. It is critical that a drinking cycle not be allowed to develop. Active intervention is needed to prevent this. If the alcoholic is still involved in treatment at the time of relapse, it is a clear signal that more needs to be done. If the alcoholic is currently trying to become sober, on an outpatient basis, while continuing to hold down a job and handle all the usual obligations, the drinking episode clearly shows that the approach is not working. A residential inpatient experience, which allows and indeed forces the alcoholic to put full attention to alcoholism treatment, may well be what is needed.

The alcoholic may have "played" at treatment, seen someone a few times, and decided things were under control. Fully resolved not to drink again, counseling was terminated. Since willpower and determination even with a dash of counseling didn't accomplish what the alcoholic had intended, the answer is a commitment by the alcoholic to engage in more substantive treatment.

Seasoned alcohol counselors often say that the most dangerous thing for a recovered alcoholic is "a successful drunk." By this they refer to the recovering alcoholic who has a drink, doesn't mention it to anyone, and suffers no apparent ill effects. It wasn't such a big deal. A couple of evenings later, it isn't a big deal, either. And so forth. Almost inevitably, if this continues the alcoholic is drinking regularly, drinking more, and on the threshold of being reunited with all the problems and consequences of active alcoholism. The danger, of course, is that as the drinking continues, the less able the alcoholic is either to recognize the need for help or to reach out for it. The alcoholic who had a difficult withdrawal in the past may also be terrified of the prospect of stopping again.

For the recovering alcoholic who has possibly attained substantial sobriety, reentry into treatment after relapse may be especially difficult. There is embarrassment, remorse, guilt, a sense of letting others down, and so on. Recognition that alcoholism is a chronic disease, that it can involve relapses, may ease this. Following a relapse it is necessary to look closely at what led up to it, what facilitated its occurrence. Dealing with a relapse openly is important also because the alcoholic can gain some valuable information about what is critical to maintaining his or her own sobriety.

How should others respond? This is potentially a very ticklish situation for the family on a number of counts. If prior to treatment an alcoholic has made repeated unsuccessful attempts on his own to stop drinking, the family may be fearful and waiting for drinking to begin again. Everyone in the home is being hypervigilant. They may even act like virtual police officers: looking for bottles, double-checking on the alcoholic—everything but having a breathalyzer at the front door. After all, their trust level has been pushed to the limit and then some! At the other end of the spectrum, the family may think everything is fine. Optimism reigns. The possibility of a relapse to them is infinitesimal. A healthier attitude lies somewhere in the middle. If the possibility of a relapse is a family's preoccupation, this must be dealt with. Family or couples group sessions are a good place to deal with this problem. On the other hand, a return to drinking can occur. If there is real reason to suspect drinking, this must be confronted. If the family members and the recovering alcoholic are engaged in treatment, the suspicions can be dealt with there. Ideally the alcoholic volunteers the information to the spouse. Of course, real life isn't always ideal. It is often up to the family to make a move. For the moment, and we emphasize *the moment*, the family too may be thrown back into functioning just as it did during the old days of active drinking. The old emotions of hurt, anger, self-righteous indignation, to hell with it all, may spring up as strongly as before. This is true even if—or especially if—the family scene has vastly changed and improved. All of that progress suddenly evaporates. There also may well be the old embarrassment, guilt, and wish to pretend it isn't so. If the family is unable because of the alcoholic's behavior or their own emotional overload to deal with the situation directly with the alcoholic, the family needs to make contact with professional help.

Maintaining sobriety

The reason for the emphasis on lots of treatment over a fairly long period throughout this treatment section is simple. The people most successful in treating alcoholism are those who recognize that anywhere from 18 to 36 months are necessary for the alcoholic to be well launched in a healthy life-style. It might be said that recovery requires an alcoholic to become "weller than well." To maintain sobriety and avoid developing alternate harmful dependencies, the alcoholic must learn a range of healthy alternative

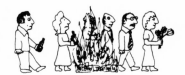

behaviors to deal with tensions arising from living problems. Nonaddicted members of society may quite safely alleviate such tensions with a drink or two. Because living, problems, and tensions go hand in hand, the alcoholic may well need to grow to a higher level of health than might be necessary for the general population.

■ *Alcoholism-treatment techniques*

The relationship with a counselor can be a central part of any recovering alcoholic's treatment. Individual sessions will likely be a combination of the typical regularly scheduled 50-minute counseling hour (initially scheduled several times a week), peppered with less-structured contacts, telephone calls, a brief chat over a cup of coffee. Exactly how these are organized will depend on whether the setting is an in- or outpatient one.

Alcoholism treatment ideally involves multiple modalities. The most common will be described in this section. Again, how these are organized within a particular alcoholic's treatment program will depend on the type of setting, as well as the needs of that particular alcoholic. The alcoholic who enters a residential rehabilitation program will undoubtedly be exposed to a wide array. The analogy may not seem very apt, but one could compare the experience to summer camp. (Be assured very few alcoholics mistake their inpatient stay for a summer camping experience!) However, time is structured, and there are multiple activities—some of which may be particularly helpful, others merely interesting. Some of the "merely interesting" at some future point may in retrospect be seen as the most valuable. The intention is to provide the alcoholic with the tools and information needed to readjust and recenter his life comfortably without alcohol.

■ *Group work*

One of the tools is group work. Group therapy has become an increasingly popular form of treatment for a range of problems, including alcohol abuse. Of course, with AA dating back to 1935, alcoholics have been working toward recovery in groups for over 40 years. This was long before group therapy became popular or alcohol treatment was even known. Why the popularity of group-treatment methods? The first response often is, "It's cheaper," or "It's more efficient; more people can be seen." These statements may be true, but a more fundamental reason exists. Group therapy works. It works very well with alcoholics. Some of the reasons for this can be found in the characteristics of alcoholism, in addition to normal human nature.

For better or worse, people find themselves part of a group. And whatever being a human being means, it does involve other people. We think in terms of our family, our neighborhood, our school, our club, our town, our church. On the job, at home, on the playground, wherever, it is in group experiences that we feel left out or, conversely, find a sense of belonging. Through our contacts with others, we feel OK or not OK. As we interact, we find ourselves sharing our successes or hiding our supposed failures. It is through groups we get strokes on the head or a kick in the pants. There's no avoiding the reality that other people play a big part in our lives. Just as politicians take opinion polls to see how they're doing with the populace, so do each of us run our own surveys. The kinds of questions we ask ourselves about our relationships are "Do I belong?" "Do I matter to others?" "Can I trust them?" "Am I liked?" "Do I like them?" To be at ease and comfortable in the world, the answers have to come up more ayes than nays. The practicing alcoholic doesn't fare so well when taking this poll. For the myriad reasons discussed before, relationships with other people are poor. Isolated and isolating, rejecting and rejected, helpless and refusing aid: With such a warped view of the world, alcoholics are oblivious to the fact that it's been the drinking causing the trouble. When one is wed to the bottle, other bonds cannot be formed. Attempts to make it in the world sober will require reestablishing real human contacts. Thus groups, the setting in which life must be lived, become an ideal setting for treatment.

Group as therapy

Being a part of a group can do some powerful therapeutic things. The active alcoholic is afraid of people "out there." The phrase "tiger land" has been used by alcoholics to describe the world. That's a fairly telling phrase! Through group treatment, the alcoholic will ideally *reexperience* the world differently. The whole thing need not be a jungle—other people can be a source of safety and strength. Another big bonus from a group experience is derived from alcoholics' opportunities to become *reacquainted* with themselves. A group provides a chance to learn who they are, their capabilities, their impact on and importance to others. Interacting honestly and openly provides opportunity to adjust and correct the mental pictures of themselves. They get feedback. Group treatment of persons in a similar situation reduces the sense of *isolation*. Alcoholics tend to view themselves *very* negatively and have an overwhelming sense of shame for their behavior. Coming together with others proves one is not uniquely awful. Yet mere confession is not therapeutic. Something else must happen for healing to occur. Just as absolution occurs in

the context of a church, in a group that functions thera-
peutically, the members act as priests to one another.
Members hear one another's confession and say, in essence, "You are forgiven, go and sin no more." (A short
lesson in linguistics: "sin" is derived from the Greek word
meaning "to miss the target." It's what the person standing by the target called back to the archer, so the archer
could readjust his aim. It doesn't imply evil, or bad, as is
so often assumed.) That is to say, group members can see
one another apart from the alcoholic behavior. They can
also often see a potential that is unknown to the individual.
This is readily verified in our own lives. Solutions to other
people's problems are *so* obvious, but not so solutions to
our own. Members of the group can see that people need
not be destined to continue their old behaviors. Old "sins"
need not be repeated. Thus they *instill hope* in one another. Interestingly enough, one often finds that people are
more gentle with others than with themselves. In this regard, the group experience has a neat boomerang effect. In
the process of being kind and understanding of others, the
members are in turn forced to accord themselves similar
treatment.

What has been discussed is the potential benefit that can
be gleaned from a group exposure. How this group experience takes place can vary widely. Group therapy comes in
many styles and can occur in many contexts. Being a resident in a halfway house puts the alcoholic in a group, just
as the person who participates in outpatient group therapy.
Group therapy means the use of any group experience to
promote change in the members. Under the direction of a
skilled leader, the power of the group processes is harnessed
for therapeutic purposes.

Group work with alcoholics

In group work with alcoholics, there are many possible
emphases. Experience shows that *not* all can be met simultaneously. Therefore, different types of groups may be
available, with members participating in several, rather
than lumping everything into one group and accomplishing
nothing.

Some of the more common groups are educational, self-
awareness, problem-solving, and activity.

Educational groups attempt to impart factual information about alcohol, its effects, and alcoholism. There is a
complex relationship between knowledge, feelings, and behavior. Correct facts and information do not stop alcoholic drinking. But they can be important in breaking down
denial, which protects the alcoholic drinking. Information
provides an invaluable framework for understanding what
has happened and what treatment is about. In an educa-

tional group alcoholics acquire some cognitive tools to participate more successfully in their own treatment. Educational groups may be organized around a lecture, film, or presentation by a specialist in the alcohol field, followed by a group discussion. Topics such as a description of AA and how it works, alcohol's effects on the body, and the recovery process may be included.

Self-awareness and support groups are intended to assist the members to grapple honestly with the role of alcohol in their lives. The group function is to support sobriety, to identify the characteristic ways in which people sabotage themselves. In these groups, the emphasis is on the here and now. The participants are expected to deal with feelings as well as facts. The goal is not intellectual understanding of why things have, or are, occurring. Rather, the hope is to have members discover how they feel and learn how feelings are translated into behavior. They then *choose* how they would prefer to behave, and try it on for size.

A *problem-solving* group is directed at tackling specific problem or stress areas in the group members' lives. Either discussion, role play, or a combination may be used. For example, how to say no to an offer to have a beer or how to handle an upcoming job interview could be appropriate themes. The goal is to develop an awareness of potential stress situations, to identify the old response pattern and how it created problems, and then to try new behaviors. These sessions thus provide practice for more effective coping behaviors.

Activity groups are least likely to resemble the stereotype of group therapy. In these groups an activity or project is undertaken, such as a ward or patient government meeting or a planning session for a picnic. The emphasis is on more than the apparent task. The task is also a sample of real life; thus it provides a practice arena for the group to identify areas of strength and weakness in interpersonal relationships. Here, too, is a safe place to practice new behaviors.

Group functions

No matter what the kind of group, a number of functions will need to be performed. For any group to work effectively, there are some essential tasks, regardless of the goal. Initially the leader may need to be primarily responsible for filling these roles.

- Initiating—suggesting ideas for the group to consider, getting the ball rolling
- Elaborating or clarifying—clearing up confusions, giving examples, expanding on other person's contribution
- Summarizing—pulling together loose ends, restating ideas

- Facilitating—encouraging others' participation by asking questions, showing interest
- Expressing group feelings—recognizing moods and relationships within the group
- Giving feedback—sharing and responding to what is happening
- Seeking feedback—asking for others' responses to what is happening

As time goes on the leader teaches the group members to share the responsibility for these functions.

Different types of group therapy can be useful at different times during recovery. During the course of an inpatient stay, alcoholics might well attend an educational group, an AA Training Group, a problem-solving group, and a self-awareness group. In addition, they could attend outside AA meetings. In this example, they would be participating in five different types of groups. On discharge from the residence, they might return for weekly group sessions as part of follow-up, and with their spouses might join a couples group. None of these group experiences would be intended to substitute for AA. The most effective treatment plans will prescribe AA *plus* alcohol-related group therapy. They are no more mutually exclusive than is AA or group therapy, along with medical treatment of cirrhosis.

Groups as a fad

Group experiences have become something of a fad. There is a bandwagon phenomenon. Marathon, encounter, TA, gestalt, sensitivity, EST, what have you are seemingly offered everywhere: school, church, job, women's clubs. The emphasis placed on groups here does not imply the alcoholic should ride the group-therapy circuit! On the contrary, alcoholics seeking *alcohol* treatment in a group *not* restricted to alcoholics are likely to waste their own and other peoples' time. As was stated earlier, until an alcoholic has taken some step to combat the alcohol problem, there is little likelihood of working on other problems successfully. Inevitably, an alcoholic will raise havoc in a mixed group. The prediction we would make is that the alcoholic will have others running in circles figuring out the whys, get gobs of sympathy, and remain unchanged. Eventually the other group members will wear out, end up treating the alcoholic just as the family does, and experience all the same frustrations as the family. But in a group with other alcoholics and a leader used to the dynamics of alcoholism, it's a different story. The opportunity to maintain the charade is diminished to virtually zero because everyone knows the game thoroughly. The agenda, in this latter instance, is clearly how to break out of the game.

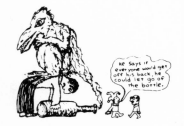

He says if everyone would get off his back, he could let go of the bottle.

A word of caution to family members is in order. Say you are concerned about a possible alcohol problem, but do not believe you can confront it directly. It might seem reasonable to try to get the alcoholic into some group, under the supposition that it is the next best thing to alcohol treatment, or in the hope that someone else will pick up on the alcohol problem and do something. This tactic has multiple flaws. First, there is no such thing as "the next best thing" for alcoholism treatment. To make the point clearly, is gallbladder surgery the next best treatment for a hernia!? Second, it is highly unlikely the group or leader will spot what is going on. Then you are stuck with a situation that is even further complicated. You are still unhappy and concerned. Yet, the alcoholic has gone along with your suggestion. It's a perfect setup. The dialogue would sound something like this:

"Aren't you ever satisfied?"

"You must not have done much with that group, you're still drinking."

"The group didn't see anything wrong with me, you are the only one," and so on, and so on.

▪ *Family treatment*

Members of an alcoholic's family need treatment as much as the alcoholic. Often they will come to this conclusion themselves and seek help. They deserve as much compassion, aid, and assistance as the drinker. However, their energy should be directed toward *their* problems, *not* the alcoholic's. What do they need? Education about alcoholism the disease will be one thing. Another is some aid in sorting out their behavior to see how it fits into, or even perpetuates, the drinking problem. Most importantly, family members require support to live their own lives *despite the alcoholic*. Paradoxically, by doing this, they enhance the actual chances of short-circuiting alcoholism.

Al-Anon may be their first attempt (see p. 174). Both individual counseling and group work can be useful. Family therapy is another possibility. Here the family is seen as a total group and counseled as a unit. The basic notions behind this approach are that the family behaves as a unit, has characteristic ways of interacting (see Chapter 7). No matter how sick it looks, these interactions and behaviors are the family's attempt to minimize pain and disruption. The family is trying to maintain a balance. When one person is identified as "sick" or "the one with a problem," other family members may allow the illness to continue. Working with the family as a group allows a therapist to see the family together. Ineffective behaviors can be identified as they occur, and support provided for desired change. Family therapy is a special skill similar to, yet different from, group work, and qualified family therapists should be sought by those wishing to pursue this approach.

Once the alcoholic does seek help, it is equally important for the family to be helped as well. Unfortunately, what is more probable in treatment centers designed primarily for the alcoholic person, is that the family will be called in to give background information and then ignored. Attention will be paid again only if problems arise and counselor or treatment staff feel the spouse or family isn't being supportive or sympathetic. The staff may not be trained to deal with the problems the spouse or family has had or is having. The alcoholic's entering treatment, especially residential treatment, may itself impose immediate problems. The spouse may be concerned about more unpaid bills, fears of yet more broken promises, and so on. When there are immediate concerns, long-range benefits may offer little consolation. Counseling for the family may help them weather the immediate storm and look forward to the future with hope. Many treatment programs now run separate groups for family members in conjunction with the alcoholic's treatment program. For example, a residential treatment program may sponsor family weekends. The family comes Friday evening, is housed on the premises, and remains through Sunday. The program includes educational sessions, family counseling, and groups. The purpose is to provide information on alcoholism and education about the disease, and also to help the family critically examine the effects of the alcoholism on their lives. There is growing recognition of the families' difficulties and their need for help and support in the recovery process. With a program devoted to the alcoholic *and* the family, the entire family again can become supportive of each other and the prospect of recovery for all will be greatly enhanced.

A major objective of the family counselor in family-counseling sessions or family meetings is going to be to assist the family in regaining a healthy balance. Doing that requires a recognition of the family's "unhealthy" style of functioning. The family counselor is probably the first objective person the family has encountered whose job it is to assist the entire family. The counselor is not on a particular person's side. Nor is the counselor going to serve as a referee. If an argument erupts, the counselor will not focus on the content and who's "right" or "wrong." The counselor's concern will be with the interactions, what is going on in the interaction, what is going on that interferes with members seeing one another's point of view.

In family sessions, the family will be provided with some basic tools that they will need if they are to deal with one another and their family problems more effectively.

They will be taught to *check things out.* People tend to guess at other peoples' meanings and motivations. They then respond as though the guesses were accurate. This causes all kinds of confusion and misunderstandings and can lead to mutual recriminations. The counselor will try to put a stop to these mind-reading games, and point out what is going on.

The family will be helped to see when they are "scape-goating." A common human tendency is to lay it all on George. This is true whatever the problem is. The alcoholic family tends to blame the drinker for all the family's troubles, thereby neatly avoiding any responsibility for their own actions. The opposite is equally true: the drinker lays it all on others.

Any good therapy stresses *acceptance of each person's right to his own feelings.* One reason for this is that good feelings get blocked by unexpressed bad feelings. The focus has been on the problems for so long that they have lost sight of the good points. However, negative feelings—be they fears or specific memories of hurts—may have to be expressed so the positive side can emerge.

Avoidance transactions should be pointed out. This includes such things as digressing to Christmas 3 years ago in the midst of a heated discussion of Daddy's drinking. In a similar vein, the family may need the objective, impartial outsider to "speak the unspeakable" to bring out into the open the obvious but unmentioned facts.

While these unhelpful patterns are becoming clearer to the family, they can be *guided into more effective problem-solving techniques as alternatives.* As these alternatives are practiced and used in the therapy, the family can then begin to use them on their own.

After a time of success, when things seem to be going better, there may be some resistance to continuing therapy. The family fears a setback and wants to stop while they're ahead. It is to everyone's advantage to continue beyond this point and try for a more thorough and therefore more lasting balance in spite of the temporary fears.

Pregnancy in the alcoholic family

You may recall some of the particular family problems that relate to pregnancy and the presence of young children in the family. A few specific words should be said about these potential problematic areas. Pregnancy is not a cure for alcoholism in either partner. A couple in which one or both partners is actively drinking would be well advised to make provision for the prevention of pregnancy until the drinking is well controlled. It is important to remember that birth control methods that are adequate for an ordinary

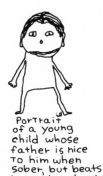

PorTrait of a young child whose father is nice To him when sober, but beats him when drunk.

couple may not be adequate when alcoholism is present. Methods that require planning or delay of gratification are likely to fail. Rhythm, foam, diaphragms, or prophylactics are not wise choices if one partner is actively drinking. A woman who is actively drinking is not advised to use the pill. So the alternatives are few: the pill or IUD for the partner of an active male alcoholic, an IUD for the sexually active female alcoholic. In the event of an unwanted pregnancy, the possibilities of placement or therapeutic abortion should be considered. If the woman is alcoholic, a therapeutic abortion certainly should be considered. At the moment, no amniotic fluid assay test exists that can establish the presence of fetal alcohol syndrome, but the possibility is there when the mother is actively drinking.

Should pregnancy occur and a decision be made to have the baby, intensive intervention should be sought out by those concerned. If the expectant mother is the alcoholic, every effort should be made to get her to stop drinking. Regular prenatal care is also important. Counseling and support of both parents if alcohol is present are essential to handle the stresses that accompany any pregnancy. If the prospective father is the alcoholic, it is important for the mother to have additional supports.

Children in the alcoholic family

A few words are in order on behalf of older children in an alcoholic family. In many cases, children's problems are related to stress in the parents. Children may easily become weapons in parental battles. With alcoholism, children may think their behavior is the cause of the drinking. A child needs to be told that this is *not* the case. In instances where physical or severe emotional abuse has occurred, child welfare authorities must be notified by everyone with this knowledge. (Some states have laws that call for prosecution of any person who fails to report such abuse, and these laws *are* being enforced.) Additional parenting persons may be brought into the picture: grandparents, aunts and uncles, good friends. Going to a nursery school or day-care center may help the child from a chaotic home.

What cannot be emphasized too strongly is that children not be "forgotten" or left out of treatment. Sometimes parents consider a child too young to understand, or feel the children need to be "protected." What this can easily lead to is the child's feeling even more isolated, vulnerable, and frightened. Children in family sessions tend to define an appropriate level of participation for themselves. Sometimes the presence of children is problematic for adults not because they will not understand, but because of their uncanny ability to see things exactly as they are—for exam-

ple, without self-consciousness saying what the rest are only hinting at, or by asking the most provocative questions.
Along the same line, while a parent is actively drinking,
those around the child should allow the child's concerns
and questions to be expressed. Children may not need all
the details, but pretense by adults that everything is okay is
destructive. Many child welfare agencies or mental health
centers conduct groups for children around issues of concern to children, such as a death in the family, divorce, or
alcoholism. Usually, these groups are set up for children of
roughly the same age, and run for a set period, such as 6
weeks. The goal is to provide basic information, support,
and the chance to express feelings the child is uncomfortable with or can't bring up at home. The subliminal message of such groups is, your parents' problems are not your
fault, and talking about it is okay.

Occasionally there may be a child who seems to "be doing well." In fact, the child may reject efforts by others to
be involved in alcohol discussions or treatment efforts. If
the alcoholic parent is actively drinking the resistance on
the child's part may be part of the child's way of coping.
Seeing someone may be perceived by the child as taking
sides or forcing the child to look at things he's trying to
pretend are not there. Resistance to joining in family treatment may also surface when the alcoholic has become
sober, for many of the same reasons. How this should be
handled is best determined by the professionals involved.
Listening to the child's objections will probably provide
clues to the child's concerns. But what is important is not
to let a child's assertion that "everything is fine" pass
without some question.

Recovery and the family

It might be expected, if one considers the family as a
unit, that there are stages or patterns of a family's recovery
from alcoholism. This has not yet been adequately studied.
No one has developed a "valley chart" that plots family
disintegration and recovery. Counselors who have had
considerable involvement with families of recovering alcoholics have noticed and are now beginning to discuss some
common themes of the family's recovery.

One observation suggests that the family unit may experience growth pains that parallel those facing the alcoholic.
It has long been a part of the folk wisdom that the alcoholic's psychological and emotional growth ceases when the
heavy drinking begins. So when sobriety comes, the alcoholic is going to have to face some growing-up issues that
the drinking prevented him from attending to. In the family system, what may be the equivalent of this Rip Van
Winkle experience? Consider an example of a family in

which the father is an alcoholic, whose heavy drinking occurred during his children's adolescence, and who begins recovery just as the children are entering adulthood. If he was basically "out of it" during their teenage years, they grew up as best they could, without very much fathering from him. When he "comes to," they are no longer children but adults. In effect, he was deprived of an important chunk of family life. There may be regrets. There may be unrealistic expectations on the father's part about his present relationship with his children. There may be inappropriate attempts by him to "make it up," regain the missing part. Depending on the situation, he may need help to grieve. On the other hand, it may be necessary to help him recognize that his expectations are not in keeping with his children's adult status. Ideally he may be able to find other outlets to experience a parenting role or reestablish and enjoy appropriate contacts with his children.

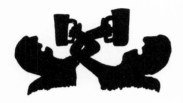

Divorced or separated alcoholics

Issues of family relationships are not important just for the alcoholic whose family is intact. For the alcoholic who is divorced and/or estranged from the family, one task during the early, active treatment phase will be to make it without family supports. Other family members may well have come to the conclusion long ago that cutting off contacts with the alcoholic was necessary for their welfare. Even if contacted when the alcoholic enters treatment, they may refuse to have anything to do with him or his treatment. However, with many months or years of sobriety, the issue of broken family ties may emerge. The recovered alcoholic may desire a restoration of family contacts and have the emotional and personal stability to attempt it, be it with parents, siblings, or the alcoholic's own children.

If the alcoholic is successful, it will still involve stress; very likely many old wounds will be opened on both sides. Professional help may again be needed to guide the family and the alcoholic through the process of reaffiliation. If the attempt is unsuccessful, a counselor could provide support and help the person find a new adjustment in the face of his unfulfilled hopes. As family treatment becomes an integral part of treatment for alcoholism, the hope is that fewer families will experience a total disruption of communications in the face of alcoholism. A more widespread knowledge of the symptoms of alcoholism may hopefully facilitate reconciliation of previously estranged families.

Al-Anon

Long before alcoholism was widely accepted as a disease —much less one that also affected family members—wives of the early members of AA recognized disturbances in their own behavior. They also encountered problems living with their alcoholics whether sober or still drinking. A structured program based on self-knowledge, reparation of wrongs, and growth in a supportive group helped the alcoholic to recover from his disorder—so why not a similar program for spouses and other family members?

Al-Anon was formed and soon became a thriving program in its own right. The founders were quick to recognize that patterns of scapegoating the alcoholic and trying to manipulate the drinking were nonproductive. Instead, they based their program on the premise that the only person you can change or control is yourself. Family members in Al-Anon are encouraged to find an acceptable life-style for themselves *regardless* of the actions of the alcoholic.

Using the Twelve Steps of AA (described in detail on pp. 178–180) as a starting point, the program also incorporated the AA slogans and meeting formats. The major difference lies in Al-Anon members' powerlessness over others' alcohol use rather than powerlessness over their own personal alcohol use. Effort is directed at gaining an understanding of their own inappropriate responses and substituting behavior that will lead them to health. They are *not* encouraged to dodge responsibility for themselves by continuing to focus on the alcoholic as "the problem." Instead they can see, by shared example, the effectiveness of changing themselves, of "detaching with love" from the drinker. Although no promises are made that this will have an impact on a still-drinking alcoholic, there are many examples of just such an outcome. At the very least, when family members stop behaviors that tend to perpetuate the alcoholic drinking, not only will their lives be better, odds are increased for a breakthrough in the alcoholic's denial system.

Through education about the disease and its impact on families, the shared experiences of many who have lived with the shame and grief caused by alcoholism and the stigma attached, and a program for personal change and growth, many people have found support and hope.

Al-Ateen

Al-Ateen is an outgrowth of Al-Anon set up for teenagers with an alcoholic parent. Their problems are different from those of the spouse of the alcoholic and they need a group to deal specifically with these. Under the sponsorship of an adult Al-Anon or AA member, they are taught to deal with their problems in much the same manner as the other programs.

Even though currently more information about alcoholism is widely available, alcoholics and their families still feel a sense of stigma. Most of them feel completely alone.

It's such a hush-hush issue that anyone experiencing it thinks they are unique in their suffering. The statistics mean little if your friends and neighbors never mention it and seem "normal" to you. It is very painful to have a problem you fear even to voice because of the shame of being "different." One of the greatest benefits of both Al-Anon and Al-Ateen is the lessening of this shame and isolation. Hard as it may be to attend the first meeting, once there, people find many others who share their problems and pain. This alone can begin a healing process.

Although Al-Anon can be a tremendous assistance to the family, we should point out what Al-Anon is *not* designed to do. Frequently confusion is introduced because all family-treatment efforts may be erroneously referred to as "Al-Anon." Al-Anon is a self-help group. It is not a professional program whose members are trained family therapists, any more than AA members are professional counselors. Therefore, an Al-Anon member would not be the person to turn to to lead an intervention, or to provide family-counseling sessions for individual families. Al-Anon participation can nicely complement other family-treatment efforts, however.

■ *Alcoholics Anonymous*

Volumes have been written about the phenomenon of AA. It has been investigated, explained, and defended by laypeople, newspaper and magazine writers, book authors, psychologists, psychiatrists, doctors, sociologists, anthropologists, and clergy. Each has brought a set of underlying assumptions and a particular vocabulary and professional or lay framework to the task. The variety of material on the subject reminds one of trying to force mercury into a certain-sized, perfectly round ball.

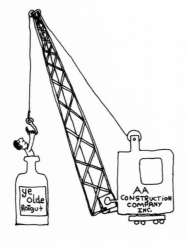

In this brief discussion, we certainly have a few underlying assumptions. One is that "experience is the best teacher." This book will be relatively unhelpful compared to either attending AA meetings over a period of time, or watching and talking with people in the process of recovery actively using the program of AA. AA is more than willing to have interested people attend open meetings. Another assumption is that AA works for a wide variety of people caught up in the disease and for this reason deserves attention. AA has been described as "the single most effective treatment for alcoholism." Certainly AA is the treatment resource most widely available. Virtually every community has several meetings including daytime and evening meetings, up to 7 days a week. There are no dues or fees, so cost is not a barrier to participation.

AA had its beginnings in 1935 in Akron, Ohio, with the meeting of two alcoholics. One, Bill W., had had a spiritual experience that had been the major precipitating event in beginning his abstinence. On a trip to Akron after about a year of sobriety, he was overtaken by a strong desire to drink. He hit upon the idea of seeking out another suffering alcoholic as an alternative. He made contact with some people who led him to Dr. Bob, and the whole thing began with their first meeting. The fascinating story of this history is told in *A. A. Comes of Age.* The idea of alcoholics helping each other spread slowly in geometric fashion until 1939. At that point, a group of about 100 sober members realized they had something to offer the thus-far "hopeless alcoholics." They wrote and published the book *Alcoholics Anonymous,* generally known as the Big Book. It was based on a retrospective view of what they had done that had kept them sober. The past tense is used almost entirely in the Big Book. It was compiled by a group of people who, over time, working together, had found something that worked. Their task was to present this in a useful framework to others who might try it for themselves. This story is also covered in *A. A. Comes of Age.* In 1941, AA became widely known after the publication of an article in a national magazine. The geometric growth rapidly advanced; 1981 figures estimate an active membership of a million alcoholics attempting to loosen their grip on the bottle.

I drink when I have occasion, and sometimes when I have no occasion.
—Cervantes

Goals

AA stresses abstinence and contends that nothing can really happen for a drinker until "the cork is in the bottle." Many other helping professionals tend to agree. A drugged person—and an alcoholic *is* drugged—simply cannot comprehend, or use successfully, many other forms of treatment. First the drug has to go.

The goals of each individual within AA vary widely; simple abstinence to a whole new way of life are the ends of the continuum. Individuals' personal goals may also change over time. That any one organization can accommodate such diversity is in itself something of a miracle.

In AA, the words "sober" and "dry" denote quite different states. A "dry" person is simply not drinking at the moment. "Sobriety" means a more basic, all-pervasive change in the person. Sobriety does not come as quickly as dryness and requires a desire for, and work toward, a contented, productive life without reliance on mood-altering drugs. The Twelve Steps provide a framework for achieving this latter state.

The Twelve Steps

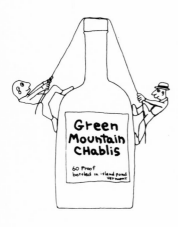

The Twelve Steps function as the therapeutic framework of AA. They were not devised by a group of social scientists, or derived from a theoretical view of alcoholism. The Twelve Steps of AA grew out of the practical experience of the earliest members, based on what they had *done* to gain sobriety. And they do represent a doing. AA is not a passive process.

The initial undrugged view of the devastation can, and often does, drive the dry alcoholic back to the bottle. But the Twelve Steps of AA offer the possibility of another solution: hope for a road out of the maze.

Step 1, "We admitted we were powerless over alcohol—that our lives had become unmanageable," acknowledges the true culprit, alcohol, and the scope of the problem, the whole life. Step 2, "Came to believe that a Power greater than ourselves could restore us to sanity," recognizes the craziness of the drinking behavior, and allows for the gradual reliance on some agent outside (God, the AA group, the therapist, or a combination) to aid an about-face. Step 3, "Made a decision to turn our will and our lives over to the care of God as we understood Him," enables the alcoholic to let go of the precious life preserver, the bottle, and accept an outside influence to provide direction. It has now become clear that as a life preserver, the bottle was a dud, but free floating can't go on forever either. The search outside the self for direction has now begun.

Step 4, "Made a searching and fearless moral inventory of ourselves," allows a close look at the basic errors of thinking and acting that were part of the drinking debacle. It also gives space for the positive attributes that can be enhanced in the sober state. An inventory is, after all, a balance sheet. Number 5, "Admitted to God, to ourselves, and to another human being the exact nature of our wrongs," provides a method of cleaning the slate, admitting just how awful it all was, and getting the guilt-provoking behavior out in the open instead of destructively "bottled up."

Steps 6 and 7, "Were entirely ready to have God remove all these defects of character," and "Humbly asked Him to remove our shortcomings," continue the mopping-up process. Step 6 makes the alcoholic aware of the tendency to cling to old behaviors, even unhealthy ones. Step 7 takes care of the fear of repeated errors, again instilling hope that personality change is possible. (Remember, at this stage in the process, the alcoholic is likely to be very short on self-esteem.)

Steps 8 and 9 are a clear guide to sorting out actual injury done to others and deciding how best to deal with such situations. Step 8 is "Made a list of all persons we had harmed and became willing to make amends to them all." Step 9 is "Made direct amends to such people wherever possible, except when to do so would injure them or others." They serve other purposes, too. First they get the alcoholic out of his bag of blaming others for life's difficulties. They also provide a mechanism for dealing with presently strained relationships and for alleviating some of the overwhelming guilt the now-sober alcoholic feels.

Steps 10 to 12 are considered the continuing maintenance steps. Step 10, "Continued to take personal inventory and when we were wrong promptly admitted it," ensures that the alcoholic need not slip back from his hard-won gains. Diligence in focusing on his own behavior and not excusing it keeps the record straight. Step 11, "Sought through prayer and meditation to improve our conscious contact with God as we understood Him, praying only for knowledge of His will for us and the power to carry that out," fosters continued spiritual development. Finally, Step 12, "Having had a spiritual awakening as a result of these steps, we tried to carry this message to alcoholics and to practice these principles in all our affairs," points the way to sharing the process with others. This is one of the vital keys Bill W. discovered to maintain sobriety. It also implies that a continued practice of the new principles is vital to the sober life.

A word can be said here about "Two Steppers." This phrase is used to describe a few individuals in AA who come in, admit they are alcoholics, dry out, and set out to rescue other alcoholics. However, it is often said in AA that "you can't give what you don't have." This refers to a quality of sobriety that comes after some long and serious effort applying the entire Twelve Steps. It is interesting to note that "carrying the message" isn't mentioned until Step 12.

No AA member serious about the program and sober for some time would ever imply that the Steps are a one-shot deal. They are an ongoing process that evolves over time (a great deal of it) into ever-widening applications. When approached with serious intent, the Steps enable a great change in the individual. That they are effective is testified to not only by great numbers of recovering alcoholics, but also by their adoption as a basis for such organizations as Overeaters' Anonymous, Gamblers' Anonymous, and Emotions Anonymous. These other organizations simply substitute their own addiction for the word alcohol in Step 1.

A therapist/counselor/friend should be alert to the balance required in this process. The newly dry alcoholic who wants to tackle all Twelve Steps the first week should be counseled "Easy does it." The longer dry member hopelessly anguished by Step 4, for instance, could be advised that perfection is not the goal and a stab at it the first time through is quite sufficient. The agnostic having difficulty with "the God bit" can be told about using the group or anything else he chooses for the time being. After all, the spiritual awakening doesn't turn up until Step 12 either.

Organization

AA has very little structure as an organization. It describes itself as a Fellowship, and functions around the Twelve Steps and Twelve Traditions. The Traditions cover the organization as a whole, setting forth the purpose of the fellowship—to carry its message to the still-suffering alcoholic—and defining principles of conduct: For example, AA does not affiliate with other groups, nor lend its name; it should not be organized and should remain forever nonprofessional. Individual groups are autonomous and they politely refuse outside contributions. Thus all care has been taken not to obscure or lose sight of the organization's purpose. The individual groups function in accord with these principles; their focus is on sobriety, anonymity, and individual application of "The Program," which includes meetings, attempting to work the Twelve Steps, and service to other alcoholics.

Before discussing the meetings, a special word about anonymity.

AA's Tradition 12 reads, "Anonymity is the spiritual foundation of all our traditions ever reminding us to place principles above personalities." This concept evolved out of the growth pains of the organization. Early members admit candidly that fear of exposure of their problem was their *original* motivation for remaining anonymous; the need "to hide from public distrust and contempt." The practice of anonymity that was introduced out of that fear began to provide evidence of its value on a totally different level.

This evolutionary process tends to occur for most individual members of AA. At first, the promise of anonymity is viewed as a safeguard against exposure. The stigma attached to alcoholism has not yet disappeared. Added to this are the alcoholic's own guilt, sense of failure, and low self-esteem. It is vital to maintain this concept to encourage fearful newcomers to try out the program while assuring them of complete confidentiality. As they progress, in sobriety, fear gives way to the deeper understanding revealed in the practice. To be simply Joe or Mary, one alcoholic among many has therapeutic value.

In practice, anonymity takes the form of first names only during the meetings, not identifying oneself through the media as a member of AA, and being careful not to reveal anyone else's attendance at meetings. Some meetings end with the reminder that "Whom you see here and what is said here, stays here."

It is important to the ability of AA to continue its healing mission to suffering alcoholics, that this principle of anonymity be respected.

In terms of AA organization, there are different kinds of meetings. There are open meetings (open to any spouses, interested parties, etc.) and closed meetings (only professed alcoholics attend the latter). Both types divide into speaker or discussion meetings. The former format has one to three speakers who tell what it was like drinking (for the purpose of allowing newcomers to identify), what happened to change this, and what the sober life is now like. A discussion meeting is usually smaller. The leader may or may not tell his or her story briefly as above, or "qualify" in AA jargon. The focus of the meeting is a discussion of a particular Step, topic, or problem with alcohol, with the leader taking the role of facilitator.

Attendance at meetings is not all there is to AA. An analogy to medical care may help. The AA meeting might be like a patient's visit to a doctor's office. The office visit doesn't constitute the whole of therapy. It's a good start; but how closely the patient follows the physician's advice and recommendations and acts on what is prescribed make the difference. Sitting in the doctor's office doesn't do it. So too with AA. The person who is seriously trying to use AA as a means of achieving sobriety will be doing a lot more than attending meetings. Persons successful in AA will spend time talking to and being with other more experienced members. Part of this time will be spent getting practical tips on how to maintain sobriety. Time and effort go into learning and substituting other behaviors for the all-pervasive drinking behavior. AA contacts will also be a valuable resource for relaxation. It is a place a newly recovering alcoholic will feel accepted. It is also a space in which the drinking possibilities are greatly minimized. A new member of AA may spend a couple of hours a day phoning, having coffee with, or in the company of, other AA members. Although it is strongly recommended that new members seek sponsors, they will be in touch with a larger circle of people. Frequent contact with AA members is encouraged, not only to pass on useful information. Another key reason is to make it easier for the new members to reach out at times of stress, when picking up a drink would be so easy and instinctively natural. The new member's contacting a fellow AA member when a crunch time comes makes the difference in many cases between recovery and relapse.

Slowly the new member's life is being restructured

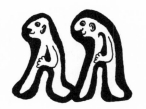

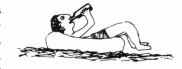

around *not* drinking, and usually the slogans are the basis for this: "One day at a time," "easy does it," "keep it simple," "live and let live," "let go and let God," etc. Although they sound trite and somewhat corny, remember the description of the confused, guilt-ridden, anxious product of alcoholism. Anyone in such a condition can greatly benefit from a simple, organized, easily understood schedule of priorities. A kind of behavior modification is taking place in order that a growth process may begin. Some new members feel so overwhelmed by the idea of a day without a drink that their sponsor and/or others will help them literally plan every step of the first few weeks. They keep in almost hourly touch with older members. Phone calls at any hour of the day or night are encouraged as a way to relieve anxiety.

Resistance

Some alcoholics and their families may be quite resistant to AA. In working with a counselor they may agree to anything, as long as it isn't AA. This resistance probably has a number of sources. It may be based on very erroneous information and myths about AA. Quite likely it's embarrassment, plain and simple. The alcoholic may have been notorious at office parties, or been a regular in the newspaper court column for drinking and driving offenses, or almost single-handedly been keeping the neighborhood general store solvent with beer purchases; but heaven forbid being seen entering a building where an AA meeting is held! Also going to an AA meeting represents, if not a public admission, at least a private one, that alcohol is a problem. Seeing a physician or a counselor, or even going for alcohol treatment, may allow the alcoholic multiple interpretations, at least for a while. Going to AA is clear-cut and in that respect a big step.

Sometimes alcoholics will have had some limited prior exposure to AA, which they use as the basis of their objections. Commonly this is coupled with the similarly "negative" experiences of their best drinking buddies, who also agree that AA doesn't work. Usually these alcoholics say they tried it once, but it wasn't for them, and they didn't like it. Any examination of what was going on in their lives generally reveals at best a very half-hearted "try." The liking or not liking isn't an issue. Usually, we care little if people "like" any other prescribed treatments as long as the treatment produces positive results. No one "likes" braces or casts on broken limbs or hospital stays for any reason, but they are accepted as necessary to produce a desired result.

The alcoholic may find some professionals who will support these resistances. This is unfortunate and we suspect it is because these professionals are not in touch with what the disease is really like. The literal hell that is the life of the active alcoholic is forgotten. That is who AA is for; the primary purpose of AA is to help people escape their hell. Overlooking or underrating that, some professionals may act as if AA were supposed to do other things—for example, be a growth group or handle marital problems—and downgrade it when it fails to provide these. One gets the sense that AA isn't considered to be "real" treatment. Finally, professionals sometimes have mistakenly gotten the impression that AA, as an organization, holds AA and other therapies to be incompatible. This is not the case. Nothing in the AA program supports this idea. Any individual who believes this needs to check the facts.

View of recovery

One thing assumed in AA is that recovery is a serious, lifelong venture. Safety does not exist, and some kind of long-term support is necessary. This seems to be the case, and a lot of experience supports the assumption. Alcoholics, like all of us, have selective memories and are inclined, after varying periods of dryness, to remember only the relief of drinking and not the consequent problems. Some kind of reminder of reality seems to be necessary. Any alcoholic of long-term sobriety will be able to tell about the sudden desire to drink popping up out of nowhere. Those who don't succumb are largely grateful to some aspect of their AA life as the key to their returning stability. No one knows exactly why these moments occur, but one thing is certain: they are personally frightening and upsetting. They can reduce the reasonably well-adjusted recovering alcoholic to a state very like his first panic-ridden dryness. The feelings could be compared to the feelings after a particularly vivid nightmare. Whatever the reason for the phenomenon, these unexpected urges to drink do spring up. This is one reason continued participation in AA is suggested. Another is the emphasis (somewhat underplayed from time to time) on a continued growth in sobriety. Certainly, groups will rally round newcomers with a beginner's focus and help them learn the basics. But in discussion meetings with a group of veterans, the focus will be on personal growth within the context of the Twelve Steps. AA may advertise itself as a "simple program for complicated people," but an understanding of it is far from a simple matter. It involves people, and people are multifaceted. Its simplicity is deceptive and on the order of "Love thy neighbor as thyself." Simple, and yet the working out of it could easily take a lifetime.

In closing, we again strongly urge you to attend AA meetings and speak at some length with veteran members if

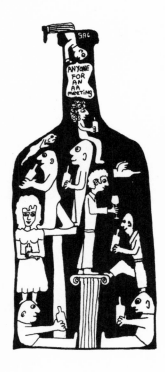

you care about an alcoholic. So much has been written about AA, and in some respects it's so understandable an approach, that people assume they know what it's about without firsthand knowledge.

A few words about suggesting AA to an alcoholic friend or family member. Simply telling someone to go probably won't work in most cases. AA is a self-help group. What AA can do and offer is by far best explained and demonstrated by its members. People can assist by making arrangements for the alcoholic to speak to a member of AA or can arrange for the person to be taken to a meeting. One can always contact AA directly. AA is as close as your telephone. Look under Alcoholics Anonymous in the white pages. Even the most rural areas often have an answering service. Ask to speak with a member of AA, and someone will be in contact with you, and can arrange to take you to a meeting.

▪ *Spiritual counseling*

There is increasing effort to educate and inform clergy about alcohol abuse and alcoholism. This section on spiritual counseling is not about this educational outreach to clergy. Instead, we wish to discuss the contribution that clergy members, priests, or rabbis may make to the recovery process in their pastoral roles. Alcoholics may have a need for pastoring, "shepherding," or spiritual counseling as do other members of the population. In fact, their needs in this area may be especially acute. Attention to these needs may play a critical part in the recovery process.

It is not easy to discuss spiritual matters. Medical, social work, psychology, or rehabilitation textbooks do not include chapters on spiritual issues as they affect prospective clients or patients. The split between spirituality and the "rest of life" has been total. In our society, that means for many it has become an either/or choice. Because defining crisply what we mean by spiritual issues is not easy, let us begin by stating what it is not. By spiritual we do not mean the organized religions and churches. Religions can be thought of as organized groups and institutions that have arisen to meet spiritual needs. But the spiritual concern is more basic than religion. In our view, the fact that civilizations have developed religions throughout history is evidence of a spiritual side to human beings. There are also experiences, difficult to describe, that hint at another dimension different from but as real as our physical nature. They might be called "intimations of immortality" and occur among sufficient numbers of people to give more evidence for the spiritual nature of humankind.

In a variety of ways we can see an awakened interest in

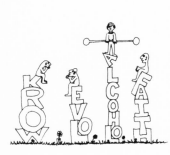

spiritual concerns in contemporary America. This is especially true among younger persons. Whether it is transcendental meditation, Zen Buddhism, Indian gurus, Jesus "freaks," the "Moonies," mysticism, the Moral Majority, or the more traditional Judeo-Christian Western religions, people are flocking in. They are attempting to follow these teachings and precepts, with the hope that they will fill a void in their lives. It is being recognized that "making it," in terms of status, education, career, or material wealth, can still leave someone feeling that something is missing. This "something" is thought by many to be of a spiritual nature. This missing piece has even been described as a "God-shaped hole."

Alcoholism as spiritual search

How does this fit in with alcohol and alcoholism? First, it is worth reflecting on the fact that the very word most commonly used for alcohol is "spirits." This is surely no accident. Further, look how alcohol is used. It is often used in the hope it will provide that missing something or at least turn off the gnawing ache. From bottled spirits, a drinker may seek a solution to life's problems, a release from pain, an escape from circumstances. For awhile it may do the job. But eventually it fails. To use spiritual language, you can even think of alcoholism as a pilgrimage that dead ends. Alcohol is a false god. To use the words of the New Testament, it is not "living water."

If this is the case, and alcohol use has been in part prompted by spiritual thirst, the thirst remains when the alcoholic sobers up. Part of the recovery process must be aimed at quenching the thirst. AA has recognized this fact. It speaks of alcoholism as a threefold disease, with physical, mental, and spiritual components. Part of the AA program is intended to help members by focusing on their spiritual needs. It is also worth noting that AA makes a clear distinction between spiritual growth and religion.

Clergy assistance

How can the clergy possibly be of assistance? Ideally, the clergy are people within society who are the "experts" on spiritual matters. (Notice we say *ideally*.) In real life, clergy are human beings, too. The realities of religious institutions may have forced some to be fund raisers, social directors, community consciences, almost everything but spiritual mentors. But there are those out there who are, and maybe many more who long to act as spiritual counselors and advisors.

One of the ways the clergy may be of potential assistance is to help the alcoholic deal with "sin" and feelings of guilt, worthlessness, and hopelessness. Many alcoholics, along with the public at large, are walking around as adults with virtually the same notions of God they had as a 5-year-old. He has a white beard, sits on a throne on a cloud, checks up on everything you do, and is out to get you if you aren't "good." This is certainly a caricature but also probably very close to the way most people really feel if they think about it. The alcoholic getting sober feels remorseful, guilt-ridden, worthless, endowed with a host of negative qualities, and devoid of good. In his mind, he certainly does not fit the picture of someone God would like to befriend or hang around with. On the contrary, he probably feels that if God isn't punishing him, He ought to be! So the alcoholic may need some real assistance in updating his concept of God. There's a good chance some of his ideas will have to be revised. There's the idea he has that the church, and therefore (to him) God, is only for the "good" people. A glance at the New Testament and Christian traditions doesn't support this view, even if some parishes or congregations act that way. Jesus of Nazareth didn't exactly travel with the smart social set. He was found in the company of fishermen, prostitutes, lepers, and tax collectors! Whether a new perspective on God or a Higher Power leads to reinvolvement with a church, assists in affiliation with AA, or helps lessen the burden of guilt doesn't matter. Whichever it does, it is potentially a key factor in recovery.

Again to use spiritual language, recovery from alcoholism involves a "conversion experience." The meaning of conversion is very simple: "to turn around" or "to transform." Contrasting the sober life to the alcoholic's drinking days certainly testifies to such a transformation. A conversion experience doesn't necessarily imply blinding lights, visions, or a dramatic turning point, although it might. If it does involve a startling experience of some nature, the sober alcoholic will need some substantial aid in dealing with or understanding this experience.

It is interesting to note that an eminent psychiatrist recognized this spiritual dimension of alcoholism and recovery over 50 years ago, in the days when alcoholism was considered hopeless by the medical profession. The physician was Carl Jung. Roland H., who had been through the then standard treatment route for alcoholism, sought out Jung in 1931. He saw Jung as the court of last resort, admired him greatly, and remained in therapy with him for about a year. Shortly after terminating therapy, Roland lapsed back into drinking. Because of this unfortunate development, he returned to Jung. On his return, Jung told Roland his condition was hopeless as far as psychiatry and medicine of that day were concerned. Very desperate and grabbing at straws, Roland asked if there was any hope at all. Jung replied that there might be, provided Roland could have a spiritual or religious experience—a genuine conversion experience. Although comparatively rare, this had been known to lead to recovery for alcoholics. So Jung advised Roland to place himself in a religious atmosphere and hope (pray) for the best. The "best" in fact occurred. The details of the story can be found in an exchange of letters between Bill W. and Jung, published in the AA magazine, *The Grapevine.*

In recounting this story many years later, Jung observed that unrecognized spiritual needs can lead people into great difficulty and distress. Either "real religious insight or the protective wall of human community is essential to protect man from this." In talking specifically of Roland H., Jung wrote: "His craving for alcohol was the equivalent on a low level, of the spiritual thirst of our being for wholeness, expressed in medieval language; the union with God."

You would be hard pressed to find a drinker who would equate his use of alcohol with a search for God! Heaven only knows they are too sophisticated, too contemporary, too scientific for that. Yet an objective examination of their use of alcohol may reveal otherwise. Alcohol is viewed as a magical potion, with the drinker expecting it to do the miraculous.

If convinced that there is a spiritual dimension that may be touched by both alcoholism and recovery, what do you do?

Some residential programs include a member of the clergy as a resource person. He or she may simply be available to counsel with clients, or may take part in the formal program, for example, by providing a lecture in the educational series. If there is no chaplain available, an alcohol counselor may be able to suggest someone. Many communities have at least one member of the clergy who has stumbled into the alcohol field—and we do mean stumbled. It wasn't a deliberate, intellectual decision. It may have occurred through a troubled parishioner who got well; or one whom the clergyman couldn't tolerate watching drink himself to death any longer and so blundered his way through an intervention; or he has gotten involved with alcoholics and finds more and more showing up on his doorstep for help. This is the one you want. If you cannot find him, find one you are comfortable talking with about spiritual or religious issues. That means one with whom you don't feel silly or awkward and, equally important, who doesn't squirm in his seat either at talk of spiritual issues. (Mention of God and religion can get people, including some clergy, as uncomfortable as talk of drinking can!)

For whom may spiritual counseling be useful? First off, if you have any inclinations in that direction, do it. A chat

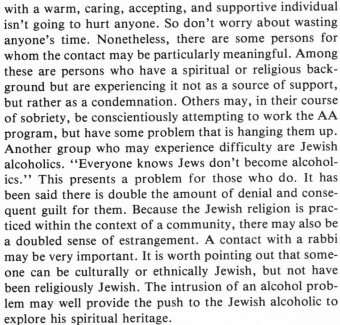

with a warm, caring, accepting, and supportive individual isn't going to hurt anyone. So don't worry about wasting anyone's time. Nonetheless, there are some persons for whom the contact may be particularly meaningful. Among these are persons who have a spiritual or religious background but are experiencing it not as a source of support, but rather as a condemnation. Others may, in their course of sobriety, be conscientiously attempting to work the AA program, but have some problem that is hanging them up. Another group who may experience difficulty are Jewish alcoholics. "Everyone knows Jews don't become alcoholics." This presents a problem for those who do. It has been said there is double the amount of denial and consequent guilt for them. Because the Jewish religion is practiced within the context of a community, there may also be a doubled sense of estrangement. A contact with a rabbi may be very important. It is worth pointing out that someone can be culturally or ethnically Jewish, but not have been religiously Jewish. The intrusion of an alcohol problem may well provide the push to the Jewish alcoholic to explore his spiritual heritage.

Whether or not we are personally convinced of the need for spiritual exploration, we do need an awareness of the possibility of this dimension's importance to those seeking support for their recovery from alcoholism.

■ *Behavioral approaches*

Temperate temperance is best. Intemperate temperance injures the cause of temperance.

MARK TWAIN

The terms *behavioral therapy* and *behavior modification* have been bandied about by many folks, some of whom are poorly informed about them. Here we would like to give you a brief rundown of the pertinent factors, also pointing out some of the things that have muddied the waters.

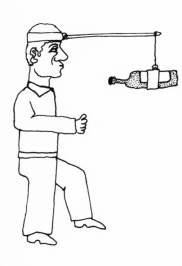

Obviously, any therapy has as its goal the modification of behavior. However, behavioral therapy is the clinical application of the principles psychologists have discovered about how people learn. The basic idea is that if a behavior can be learned, it can also be changed. This can be done in several ways. To put it very simply, one way is to introduce new and competing behavior in place of the old or unwanted behavior. By using the principles by which people learn, the new behavior is reinforced (the person experiences positive results), and the old behavior is in effect "squeezed out." Another technique is negative reinforcement (punishment) of the unwanted behavior; therefore it becomes less frequent. Recall the discussion of Johnson's model for the development of drinking behavior in Chapter 6. That explanation was based on learning principles. People *learn* what alcohol can do; alcohol can be counted on in anyone's early drinking career to have dependable consequences. Therefore, drinking is reinforced and drinking behavior continues.

Behavioral therapy is a field of psychology that has been developing rapidly over the past 20 years. In the course of this development, several techniques have been devised that have been used in the treatment of alcoholism.

Historically, one of the first behavioral methods to be used in alcohol treatment was *aversion therapy.* In this case, a form of punishment was used to modify behavior. The behavior was drinking and the goal was abstinence. Electric shock and chemicals were the things primarily used. The alcoholic would be given something to drink and as he swallowed the alcohol, the shock would be applied. Or a drug similar to disulfiram would induce sickness. The procedure was repeated periodically until it was felt that the drinking was so thoroughly associated with unpleasantness in the subject's mind that he would be unlikely to continue drinking alcohol. Although short-term success was assured, the results over the long haul have been questioned. Aversion therapy of this form is now used very rarely.

As the field became more sophisticated, it became clear that an effective behavioral treatment program cannot be based on a single behavioral technique. One cannot expect all patients to be successfully treated by the routine application of the same procedure. Just as not all patients are given the same kind and dose of a medication, neither can they be given the same behavioral treatment; a careful individual assessment is required for both. Thus efforts were made to devise total alcohol-treatment programs based on a variety of behavioral techniques. However, this approach also was rather short-lived. To succeed it required a very careful behavioral assessment to ascertain all the relevant behaviors related to drinking and their reinforcements; and then the development of a complicated, comprehensive individualized behavioral program to interrupt old patterns and introduce and mold new behaviors. Although theoretically possible, this requires multiple specially trained personnel. The expense is considerable, and the results achieved no better than those with more eclectic programs.

What has become far more commonplace now is the use of behavioral methods to treat particular aspects of an alcohol problem. These will be described next.

A recovering alcoholic is likely to face a multitude of problems. One of these is a high level of anxiety. It can be of a temporary nature, the intitial discomfort with his nondrinking life, or more chronic if he is the "nervous" type. Whether temporary or chronic, it is a darned uncomfortable state, and the alcoholic has a *very* low tolerance for it. Many alcoholics have used alcohol for the temporary and quick relief of anxiety. What is now remembered (and longed for!) is the almost instant relief of a large swig of booze. When alcohol or drugs are no longer an option, the alcoholic has quite a problem: how to deal with anxiety. Many simply "sweat it out"; some relapse over it. There are some positive things that can be done to alleviate their anxiety, or anyone's, for that matter. One is *relaxation therapy.* It is based on the fact that if the body and breathing are relaxed, it is impossible to *feel* anxious. The mind rejects the paradox of a relaxed body and a "tense" mind. Working with this fact, some techniques evolved to counter anxiety with relaxation. Generally, the therapist vocally guides a person through a progressive tensing and relaxing of the various body parts. The relaxing can start with the toes and work up, or with the scalp and work down. The process involves first tensing the muscles, then relaxing them at the direction of the therapist. These directions are generally given in a modulated, soft voice. When the client is quite relaxed, a soothing picture is suggested for him to hold in his mind. The client is then given a tape of the process to take home, with instructions on its use, as an aid in learning the relaxation. With practice, the relaxed state is achieved more easily and quickly. In some cases, he may finally learn to relax totally with just the thought of the "picture." Once thoroughly learned, the relaxation response can be substituted for anxiety at will. The response can then be used by the recovering alcoholic to deal with those situations in which taking a drink might be almost second nature.

Another behavioral approach to deal with anxiety is *systematic desensitization.* It builds on the relaxation response. It is a technique that has been found quite useful in treating people with phobias. This is an appropriate approach for recovering alcoholics who may feel panic at the mere thought of a particular situation. We mean real panic, so that even the idea gets them so uptight that the temptation to drink may be overwhelming.

In this process, with the aid of a therapist the recovering alcoholic in his imagination approaches the situation that leads to anxiety. As the anxiety builds up, he is directed to use relaxation techniques he has been taught. Gradually, going step by step, he uses the relaxation to turn off the anxiety, and eventually the situation itself becomes much less anxiety provoking. In alcohol treatment, this approach has been used for persons whose drinking has been partially prompted by stressful, anxiety-producing situations. Given another option, they are better equipped to avoid drinking when such situations arise.

Assertiveness training, another technique that has evolved from behavioral methods, is also sometimes used in alcoholism treatment. One of the more common applications is to help recovering alcoholics learn how to say no comfortably to a drink in social situations, or say no to other things that might threaten sobriety.

Record keeping is another tool borrowed from behavioral psychology that is used in alcoholism treatment. Not uncommonly, recovering alcoholics may report finding themselves with some regularity "suddenly" in the midst of some kind of troubling situation (e.g., an argument with a spouse) with no idea what led up to it. There may be periods of inexplicable despondency. Often there is a pattern, but what the key elements are may not be apparent. Record keeping, a personal log or diary of one's daily routine, sometimes is used to help identify the precursors that lead up to difficult moments. Recovery requires all kinds of readjustments to routines. By keeping a daily log, over time, one may have a far better sense of which areas need attention.

∎ *Meditation*

Meditation is frequently suggested as an aid in achieving and maintaining sobriety. Any number of approaches are available to those wishing to try it, and many treatment centers include an introduction to one or more. Although meditation has different goals, depending on the type practiced, the process of reaching a meditative state is somewhat similar to relaxation. A fairly relaxed state is necessary before meditation can begin. Some schools of meditation use techniques quite similar to relaxation methods as a lead-in to the meditation period. In yoga, there are physical exercises coupled with mental suggestions as a precursor. Studies have shown that altered physiological states accompany meditation or deep relaxation. Altered breathing patterns and different brain wave patterns are examples. These changes are independent of the type of meditation practiced. The real physical response in part accounts for the feelings of well-being after meditation periods. Those who practice meditation find it, on the whole, a rewarding experience. Many also find in the experience some form of inspiration or spiritual help.

A word of caution: Alcoholics tend to go overboard. Meditation should never be a substitute for their other prescribed treatment. Also, there are extremists in every area of life, and meditation is no exception to exploitation. Meditation is only helpful if it alleviates the alcoholic's anxiety and allows him to continue learning how to function better *in* the world, not out of it.

What is meditation?

Perhaps a meditation is a daydream, a daydream of the soul as the beloved and God, the lover, their meeting in the tryst of prayer, their yearning for one another after parting; a daydream of their being united again.

Or perhaps a meditation is the becoming aware of the human soul of its loneliness and the anticipation of its being united with the One who transcends the All and is able to come past one's own defenses.

Or perhaps, again, it is a standing back with the whole of the cosmos before one's mind's eye as one's heart is being filled with the sheer joy of seeing the balance of the All and one's own self as part of it.

Or perhaps a searching into one's own motives, values, and wishes, with the light of the Torah against the background of the past.

Or perhaps . . .*

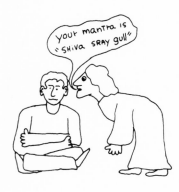

■ *Disulfiram (Antabuse)*

In the late 1940s, by a series of accidents, a group of Danish scientists discovered that a drug they were testing for other purposes, disulfiram, led to a marked reaction when alcohol was ingested by a person exposed to it. Disulfiram chemically alters the metabolism of alcohol by blocking out an enzyme necessary for the breakdown of acetaldehyde, an intermediate product of alcohol metabolism. Acetaldehyde is normally present in the body in small amounts, in somewhat larger ones when alcohol is ingested, and in toxic amounts when alcohol is taken into the body after disulfiram medication.

This adverse physical reaction is characterized by throbbing in the head and neck, flushing, breathing difficulty, nausea, vomiting, sweating, tachycardia (rapid heartbeat), weakness, and vertigo. The intensity of the reaction can vary from person to person and varies with the amount of disulfiram present and the amount of alcohol taken in. Disulfiram is excreted slowly from the body, so the possibility of a reaction is present for 4 to 5 days after the last dose and in some cases longer. Because of this reaction, Antabuse, the trade name for disulfiram, has been widely used in the treatment of alcoholism.

Prescription, administration, and use

Over the years since disulfiram's discovery, trial and error and research have led to some suggestions for its prescription, administration, and use in alcohol treatment. Disulfiram is not a *cure* for alcoholism. At best, it can only postpone the drink for the alcoholic. If the recovering alcoholic chooses to use disulfiram as an adjunct to AA, psy-

*From Siegel, R., Strassfeld, M., and Strassfeld, S. *The Jewish Catalogue.* Philadelphia, The Jewish Publication Society of America.

chotherapy, group therapy, it can be most useful in helping *not* to take an impulsive drink. Because it stays in the system for such a long time, whatever caused the impulsive desire for a drink can be looked at. It possibly could be worked through during the 5-day grace period to forestall the need for the drink entirely.

The alcoholic who wishes to use disulfiram should first be thoroughly examined by a physician to determine physical status. Some conditions contraindicate disulfiram usage. In some cases physicians consider the risks of a disulfiram reaction not as dire as continued drinking certainly would be.

The person taking disulfiram needs to be thoroughly informed of the dangers of a possible reaction. A variety of substances (such as cough syrup, wine sauces, paint fumes, etc.) that contain some alcohol can cause a reaction. A listing of such substances is included in Chapter 5. The person should carry a card or wear a med-alert disk stating he is taking disulfiram. Some medications given to accident victims or in emergency situations could cause a disulfiram reaction compounding whatever else is wrong. There is no way to be able to tell if an unconscious person has been taking disulfiram without such a warning.

There have been several approaches to the administration of disulfiram. Some persons believe it is preferable, at least for a while, to have the disulfiram administered to the alcoholic. For instance, the person may stop by an outpatient clinic to receive the medication, or the employee's health clinic might dispense it. Preferably the spouse should *not* be the one expected to do this. The thinking behind this approach is that it further removes from the alcoholic the decision of ''to or not to,'' also it ensures that the individual will maintain regular contact with outside persons. This may be an issue especially for those persons whose alcoholism led to a rather isolated existence.

Disulfiram seems to free the alcoholic's mind from the constant battle against the bottle. When someone decides to take the pill on a given day, he has made one choice that will postpone that drink for at least 4 or 5 days. If the pill is taken daily, that fourth or fifth day is always well out ahead. The recovering alcoholic can then begin to acquire or relearn behaviors other than drinking behaviors, and the habits of sobriety can take hold. Disulfiram has been described as a crutch (which is not really out of place when one's legs are impaired!). Instead, one might think of it as a way of buying sober time until the alcoholic's ''legs'' are steadier and other healthy supports are found. The supports may be available already, but the alcoholic has to be able to use them successfully. Until then, these supports would fit him no better than a basketball player's crutch would fit a 10-year-old boy!

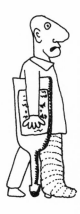

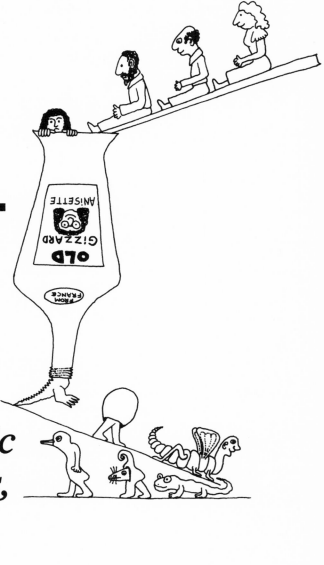

Chapter 9

A dash of bitters: suicide, psychiatric illness, psychotropic medications, polydrug abuse

194

Alcohol problems, alcoholism, and indeed alcohol use can be complicated by other issues. Important among these are suicide, polydrug use with possible multiple addiction, and psychiatric illness. For this reason we wish briefly to discuss each of these in turn. Although these potentially "complicating features" are not routinely present, nonetheless if they are, attention must be paid. In such cases one can little afford the luxury of focusing only on the alcohol issues. To be oblivious to the connection between alcohol use and suicide can invite disaster. Similarly, poly-drug use can cause serious consequences, especially as the numbers of persons using/abusing multiple substances seems to be growing.

The issue of psychiatric illness and alcohol use in various forms is a bit more complicated. Alcoholics and their families may well come into contact with the mental health system. If so, an understanding of psychiatric terminology can be useful. In such encounters, the concern will be two-fold: (1) Not to diagnose alcoholism mistakenly as some other problem; and (2) equally important, not to miss the presence of a possible concurrent psychiatric illness. Alcoholics in approximately the same proportion as the non-alcoholic population do have psychiatric illnesses. To fail to identify and treat these conditions adequately may also doom the alcohol treatment.

An additional concern for alcoholics centers on the use of psychotropic medications, commonly used in treating certain psychiatric disorders. Here, too, there are two sides to the issue. The active alcoholic may welcome any chemical relief, and use psychotropic medications in a way that can lead to problems. The recovering alcoholic, on the other hand, may be so leary of any medication that he may refuse to use any, including those that are very much needed and would probably not lead to difficulties. Thus some familiarity with the types of psychotropic medications and their appropriate use is important. They are not alike, in terms of either their actions or their potential for abuse. Any recovering alcoholic probably needs to develop some sophistication with regard to psychotropic medications. Although these preparations may have been developed to treat specific psychiatric disorders, their use has become quite widespread and they may be prescribed for nonpsychiatric conditions.

■ *Suicide*

Alcohol use and suicide go together. Recall from Chapter 1 that in 65% of all suicide attempts the individual had been drinking, and that 40% of all successful suicides are alcohol-related. The suicide rate for alcoholics is 55 times that of the general population. Because of this, it is important to consider why alcohol use and suicide go hand in hand. The relationship is relevant not only for the alcoholic, but anyone who uses alcohol.

Types of suicide: succeeders, attempters, and threateners

For practical purposes, there are several different groups to be considered when examining suicide. *First* are the *suc-*

ceeders, those who succeed *and intended to.* Classically, these are lonely white men over 50 years of age or lonely teenagers. They use violent means such as a gun or hanging, and their methods are calculated and secretive. *Second* are those who succeed but *did not* intend to. These are the *attempters.* Classically they are white women, ages 20 to 40, often with interpersonal conflicts, whose "method" is pills, and whose action is an impulsive response. Attempters die by mistake or miscalculation. For example, they lose track of dosage, or something goes wrong with their plans for rescue. The attempter's intent is not so much to die, as to elicit response from the environment. Emergency room psychology, which often dismisses this patient with a firm kick in the pants, is inappropriate. Someone who is trying to gain attention by attempting suicide is in reality quite sick and deserves care. *Third* are the *threateners,* who use suicide as a lethal weapon: "If you leave me, I'll kill myself." They are often involved in a pathological relationship. These people usually do not follow through, but are frightened and guilt-ridden and also are in need of professional help.

Statistics and high-risk factors

The real statistic to keep in mind is that suicide is the second leading recorded cause of death in people under 18 or over 65. Sixty percent give some prior indication of their intent, thereby making it preventable. Typical indications might be "I have a friend . . .," "What would you think if . . .," stockpiling drugs, or giving away possessions. Take note of new behaviors as cues. People doing things they have never done before may often indicate they have suddenly decided to commit suicide and are now at peace. Examples might be *suddenly* playing cards, dancing, or taking out the garbage when they have never made a practice of this before.

Certain high-risk factors should be identified if present: recent loss of a "loved" person; single, widowed, and/or childless people; people living in urban areas; being unemployed, nonreligious, or "oppressed." High-risk emotional factors include anger plus hopelessness, broken or pathological family/friend communications, and marital isolation. Verbal high-risk cues take the form of both direct statements: "I'm going to kill myself," or indirect indications: "I won't be around to give you any more trouble." People entering and *leaving* a depression are especially vulnerable, as are those with chronic illnesses like arthritis, high blood pressure, ulcers, and malignancies.

Over 50% of all suicides are alcohol-related. Several reasons explain this correlation. First, the chemical nature of alcohol tends to release certain brain areas from control. The guarding mechanisms are let down. Hidden thoughts and impulses are released. (You may have witnessed incidents such as the intoxicated guy calling the boss an S.O.B.) Second, because of the chemical action of alcohol, a state is created wherein the integrative capacity of the brain is diminished. It is a condition in which aspects of memory and concentration are lost. Third, when alcohol is used as a medicine, it is unfortunately a good one to produce an initial mood of relaxation and pseudostability. In this state, people may think things are just the way they should be. They feel cool, calm, and collected. Suicide at this point may seem relevant and a good idea: "I'll just jump. It's the rational solution." More alcohol acts as a true depressant with obvious potential consequences. Finally, alcohol may also bring out psychological weakness. It may place people on the edge of reality, tip the scales, lead to loose associations, bring out psychosis, loosen normal fears, produce voices saying: "The thing to do is rid the world of you," or "The world is better off without you." In all these cases, alcohol acts as a catalyst, both physically and psychologically.

The most fertile ground for suicide is in cases of clinical depression. Most people who have the "blues" are not suicidal. They might think, "Gee, I wish I were dead, things are going so badly," or "I don't know how I'll make it. I might just drive off the road if things don't get better." But things usually do get better. On the other hand, a clinical depression is characterized by a consistently low mood over a period of weeks, plus weight changes, sleep problems, and other physical symptoms. Pessimism is a part of the illness, just as fever is a part of the flu. Feelings of how bad things are are part of the depression. Depression, therefore, is bad enough alone, but combined with alcohol, it is a potent mix. "There is no way out." "I'm a bad person—the only way out is to kill myself."

Practical implications

The first is that alcohol, though it is a mood changer, cannot be counted on magically to brighten up someone who is feeling down. Therefore, if someone is really distraught or upset, going out and deliberating getting drunk is often the worst thing. Forget about the platitude that you can't drink problems away. The immediate danger is that drinking is going to accentuate the gloom, and that suicide will, in the drunken state, make sense. A tragic example comes to mind: An adolescent learned late in the final semester of her senior year that she had to attend summer school, and would not graduate with her class. You can imagine the shame, embarrassment, the "it's-the-end-of-the-world" feeling. The same afternoon she'd gotten that word, the traditional senior class party took place. There was lots of alcohol; she went and drank heavily. In her intoxicated state, the contrast between her own (in her mind) "desperate situation" and the light spirits of her friends was understandably painful. Following the party, she returned home and committed suicide. Without question, this was an alcohol-induced suicide.

Beyond these "passing crises" accentuated by alcohol, there are situations involving those who may be suffering a clinical depression. These people may even be in therapy. Anyone clearly already depressed is ill-advised to use any alcohol. Again, it is because it may well prove not to be the desired pick-me-up. In general, we might all reevaluate our almost automatic offer of a drink as soon as someone tells us they're in "the dumps." At the least we might stop and think whether the remark was as offhand as our virtually automatic responses. Sometimes a better response would be sitting down and being a good listener.

Probably the most difficult situation is being around someone who is in a depression. Often the whole situation creeps up on us unawares. What may easily happen to us if we are around someone in a depression is that we tend after a time to want to avoid them. Our own feelings when we are with them seem to mirror theirs, and we begin to feel unhappy ourselves. As a result, we begin to get impatient with their complaints, or tears, or silences, or lying in bed all the time, or pacing the floor half the night. Their view of the world is so pessimistic that it's natural to wish they'd pull themselves together, get busy, get out of the house, visit friends, *anything* but mope around. But that is just what they cannot do, unaided. This is why professional help is needed. We can all sympathize for a short time with someone who is having a case of the blues. If they persist and we notice impatience creeping in on our part, that is probably a good indication that we might try getting the person to seek help.

Whether offhandedly or very seriously, if anyone discusses taking his or her life, *take that seriously.* Do not be fooled by the myth that anyone who talks about suicide won't do it. What do you do if someone explicitly discusses suicide? If someone does speak of suicide, and especially if there's a plan in mind, this is very serious business. Try to set aside your worries about interfering. Assume that if someone has confided such information, it has been done with the hope that you will act. We are aware of the philosophical debates on whether someone has a right to commit suicide. Looking at it practically, anyone who thinks he does will just go ahead and do it! He wouldn't bother talking to others about it. Mental health professionals take the stance that persons who discuss suicide, are not doing so by chance. They are reaching out for help in settling the internal debate over life versus death. So the immediate step is to get professional help. Call a local mental health center or a suicide hot line. Most likely your friend or relative can be seen on an emergency basis. If for any reason you feel that you are being put off, given an appointment for another day, be insistent! In the meantime, if there is a plan worked out, do what you can to make the plan inoperable. If it involves stockpiled pills, ask that they be given to you. Alternatively, you can on your own, see that a gun is locked away with the key in your possession. Further, stay with your friend or relative, don't leave them alone. That, in and of itself, will probably undo the plan. Even if you are told you needn't hang around after you've made an appointment, stay or make sure someone else is present. Persons seriously contemplating suicide are all too likely to have the gloom redescend, and in a mixed-up emotional state, misinterpret your leaving as a sign of no one's caring, or as a signal the plan was the best thing.

The foregoing is the most dire situation with which anyone is likely to be faced. Even in less dramatic forms, when a possible suicide attempt is not immediately imminent, prompt action is still indicated. Even if someone has no plan worked out, take the steps necessary to get professional help. Keep in mind that depressed persons will seldom have the energy to resist your offer to help. Whereas alcoholics may become angry and try to fend off others' attempts to intervene, a depressed person will more likely acquiesce. Also be reassured that once the depression has been treated, previously suicidal persons will be very pleased that others prevented their action on suicidal plans.

In closing, we wish to address a few comments to those who may have lost a parent, a friend, a spouse, or a child to suicide. The suicide may have occurred recently or many years ago. The survivors of a suicide can experience a lot of pain and anguish, and at points, anger too. There are self-doubts, self-recriminations, the inevitable "if only I had . . ." Whether or not alcohol was involved, just reading this is likely to bring it all back. Unfortunately, as a society we have not been very sensitive to the survivors of suicide. Friends may avoid talking about it, which doesn't provide those left an opportunity to grieve, to express the sense of loss, or abandonment, or to voice out loud the haunting questions. Although the emphasis here has been on situations in which suicide may be preventable, the tragic fact is that many are not. Certainly, in the lives of those closest to the victim of suicide, after a suicide takes place the most pressing work is coming to terms with the loss. Though friends and family may assist this process, it may be aided too by professional help of a clergy member, a therapist, or a physician.

■ *Psychiatric illness*

In every area of medicine, there is distinctive terminology that can be confusing to the lay person. Also, with an increase in scientific knowledge about etiology of illnesses, the course of diseases, and effectiveness of various treatment approaches to them, there are corresponding changes in medical vocabulary. At times what was previously considered a single disease may come to be seen as different distinctive illnesses. Thus one can even witness the emergence of "new" illnesses—the most recent example being Legionnaire's disease. Though not "new" at all, it simply had not been distinguished before from other respiratory or pneumonia-like syndromes. All of this applies equally to psychiatric disorders, which cover disturbances of thought, emotion, and behavior.

The official classification of psychiatric disorders is set forth by the American Psychiatric Association in its diagnostic and statistical manual. The most recent manual (DSM III), adopted in 1980, represents a major departure from earlier diagnostic schemes. For one, it sets forth very specific diagnostic criteria, explicitly stating what signs and symptoms must be present to make each diagnosis. Also, it has significantly revised, reorganized, and in some instances renamed the major groupings of psychiatric problems. Accordingly for the first time, substance abuse disorders, into which alcohol dependence is placed, becomes a separate major category. (In earlier versions, alcoholism was under the heading of character disorders.) Similarly, another former category, neurosis, has been replaced by several separate diagnostic categories. Thus the layperson may be simultaneously faced with hearing of "new" psychiatric disorders while also discovering that many of the older labels still widely used by the lay population are no longer being applied medically.

The major categories of psychiatric illness are described in this section.

Organic mental disorders

This diagnosis is made when the disorder is caused by a known defect in brain function. The causes can vary, including traumatic or toxic insult to the central nervous system, the effects of a brain tumor, and the effects of a stroke. These impairments of brain function lead to a limitation of the ability to think and respond to the environment meaningfully. Usually there are significant changes in cognitive function. Hence there may commonly be problems with memory, loss of intellectual capacity, and an inability to concentrate.

These disorders can either represent permanent impairment or be largely reversible, largely dependent on whether the brain's function has been just temporarily interfered with (e.g., through ingestion of drugs or a blow to the head) or whether there has been permanent damage to brain tissue. Reversible organic mental disorders are referred to as delirium. Typically it is rapid in onset and usually resolved within days. Dementia generally refers to irreversible organic brain syndromes, which most typically have a more gradual onset with gradual deterioration of function over years.

In addition to the limitations these disorders create for an individual, an equally significant factor may be how the individual perceives them. If the symptoms appear slowly, the individual may be able to compensate and appear normal, especially if the environment is familiar, presenting no new problems to solve. On the other hand, if the symptoms appear rapidly, the person may be understandably panicked. As the individual experiences a reduction in thinking capacity, anxiety may be very prominent. Another not uncommon component can be visual hallucinations, especially at night, which can be particularly terrifying.

The treatment of organic mental disorders attempts, where possible, to correct the underlying cause. If it is a tumor, surgery may be the appropriate treatment; if drug-induced, withdrawal. If there are permanent impairments associated with mental disorders, rehabilitation measures will be initiated to assist the person in coping with limitations.

In relation to alcohol use, there are a variety of organic mental disorders, ranging from acute intoxication, which clearly impairs mental functioning; to withdrawal states, which can occur in the person physically dependent on alcohol; to permanent brain damage associated with long-standing, heavy alcohol use.

Affective disorders

Affect refers to mood and emotion; what you feel and how you show it. Here there are two extremes: people who are depressed, and those who are manic. People can fluctuate between these two extremes; this is called *bipolar illness.* People who are manic show characteristic behavior. Often they have grand schemes, which to others seem quite outlandish. Their conversation is very rapid, quick, pressured. Often they jump from topic to topic. If there were a conversation about the State of the Union, a manic person might say, "and, yes, New Hampshire is a very pretty

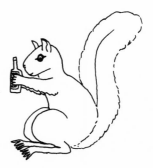

state. Governor Thompson was the governor of the state, and the governor of my car is out of kilter. The left tire is flat, out of air like a balloon Suzy got at the circus. . . .'' Although there is a logical connection between these thoughts, there's an inability to concentrate on one. Each thought is immediately crowded out by the next. Someone who is manic is often aggressive and irritable. They may feel themselves very attractive and sexually irresistible. Persons who are manic are perpetually in high gear and have difficulty sleeping. Simply being in their company might well make you feel exhausted.

Depression, which is the other side of the coin and is far more common, has all the opposite characteristics. Rather than being hyped up, these people grind to a halt. Depressed people feel *very* down. Speech is slow, movements are slow. Rather than a flood of things, they say nothing. Biological changes can accompany depression: disturbances of the normal sleep pattern, constipation, retarded motor activity, loss of appetite. In extremis, the depressed person stops eating, is unable to rest, experiences a complete depletion of energy, and expends available motor energy in repeated, purposeless motions such as hand-wringing and pacing. Such depression typically creates a sense of self-reproach, irrational guilt, hopelessness, and lack of interest in life. In full force these phenomena may culminate in suicidal thoughts, plans, or actions. Severe depression often involves disturbed biological function as well as guilt and is a life-threatening disorder. Available data increasingly point to a genetic component in the development of depression.

Both depression and mania are episodic disorders. Between episodes most persons return to a normal state. This is not to imply that one simply sits back and waits for the manic or depressive episode to pass. With the biologically seriously depressed individual, suicide is an ever-likely possibility. The manic individual can incur phenomenal problems that can wreak havoc in his or her life, as well as that of the family. These conditions are highly treatable, with medications. (See the following section on medications.) Talking therapies are of little use when someone's perception of reality and thought processes are so seriously altered.

Alcohol use and alcoholism can figure into affective disorders in several ways. As mentioned in the section on suicide, any alcohol use by someone in a depression is contraindicated. A depressant drug can with its drug-induced distortions of reality facilitate a suicide attempt. Clinicians have reported that persons with manic episodes, whose affective illness goes untreated, may tend to use alcohol as a self-medication. Also, though not yet understood, there does appear to be an increased incidence of affective disorder, namely depression, among family members of alcoholics and among female alcoholics.

Schizophrenic disorders

The schizophrenic disorders are a group of chronic remitting disturbances that are among the most incapacitating of the mental disorders. The term psychotic is often used to describe patients with schizophrenia. Psychosis refers to any disorder in which there is an observable disturbance of perception and function. Persons with a psychosis may be in significant disagreement with others as to what is reality. The psychotic individual has his own idiosyncratic notions of reality. Sitting in a room full of people, he might claim to be alone. Possibly, if we think of the statement in philosophical or poetic terms, it could make sense. However, as a statement of "fact" on which to base further interaction, it breaks down. Attempts to communicate are very difficult because the psychotic perceives reality very differently. This altered perception can be very subtle or very marked. The preference here is to think of it as a very gross disturbance. For example, suppose you were to see someone undressing in the parking lot outside your office, and then jumping on a car roof. Were you to ask why, a logical explanation might be given. But it wouldn't be an adequate explanation to get you to do it too. If the person is psychotic, the lingering question after the explanation would be, "But why are you doing *that?*" If only the perception of reality were disturbed, then such persons would rarely come to our attention. However, there is also a disturbance of function. It is because we observe strange behavior that we inquire about someone's perceptions and belief about the world. Ordinarily, we simply don't challenge one another. For someone to qualify as psychotic, you should expect there would be fairly uniform agreement among others that he's not on the same wavelength. Schizophrenic disorders are typically manifested by hallucinations (a sensory perception with no corresponding stimulus), delusions (a fixed, false belief), or incoherence of thought.

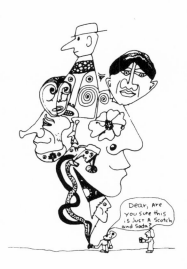

It has been estimated that 1% of the U.S. population suffers from schizophrenia. In years past, many of these persons lived in state hospitals, often located in rural settings. With the advent of psychotropic medications, which reduce the symptoms of schizophrenia, as well as the closing of state hospitals for financial reasons, the schizophrenic population has shifted into low-income urban areas.

The treatment of schizophrenic disorders involves medications (see following section) in addition to some ongoing supportive counseling.

Anxiety disorders

These disorders involve incapacitating anxiety. This symptom may appear episodically, as in panic attacks, or it may be unrelenting. Physical concomitants of arousal, such as diaphoresis, tremor, diarrhea, pallor, rapid pulse, shortness of breath, headache, and fatigue are common. The anxiety may be unattached to a particular situation, person, or thought (free-floating); or it may be associated with a specific object (phobia), a fear of being alone (agoraphobia), or a recurrent idea (obsession). In contrast to other mental disorders, which may show a significant amount of anxiety, the anxiety disorders do not involve major disturbances in mood, thought, or judgment.

Treatment of these can involve psychotherapy and/or behavioral modification approaches to provide the individual tools for coping with the anxiety. In terms of the appropriateness of medications for treatment of these, this is a topic on which there is lack of agreement. However, the thrust would seem to be that long-term use is both ineffective and invites drug dependence.

Somatoform disorders

The somatoform disorders (previously subsumed under neuroses) involve physical symptoms—such as pain, blindness, deafness, paralysis, anesthesia, and difficulty swallowing—which are considered to be a disguised expression of an emotional disturbance. The disguise may be so successful that no emotional distress is experienced by the patient at all. They may not even be anxious about the symptom, even though it appears serious. Inevitably, patients with these disorders have little insight into their emotions and are often quite skeptical when informed that their physical symptoms are related to the mental state. It is worth noting that a substantial number of persons, initially thought to have a somatoform disorder, do go on to develop a bona fide physical illness that went unrecognized, possibly because it was in the very early stages, at the time of the original examination. Clearly, for the diagnosis of somatoform disorder to be properly made, other possible physical causes have to be ruled out.

Treatment involves supportive counseling and "low-key" psychotherapy. It is also important that persons with somatoform disorders have a physician who can be supportive and provide continuity of medical care. One of the dangers is that such individuals may easily be "bounced" from specialist to specialist and receive at the least unwarranted diagnostic workups, or even nonessential surgery.

Substance abuse disorders

This is the category into which alcohol abuse and alcohol dependence fall, as do problems with other substances, be they narcotics, psychedelic drugs, licit or illicit drugs. In general, the feature that distinguishes abuse from dependence for this group is the presence of demonstrated tolerance and withdrawal syndromes with the latter. The alcohol-treatment field is not wholly satisfied with the diagnostic criteria set forth. Moreover, there has been nit-picking and various arguments for and against the criteria, which are not worth recounting here. On the whole nonetheless, we see this change in classification as a definite step in the right direction, simply because substance abuse is being treated as a distinct and separate entity, different and worth separating from other disorders. With that step taken, further refinements regarding proper definition of abuse versus dependence can occur. Moreover, the lively discussion engendered should stimulate necessary thinking and promote better understanding.

There are several other major categories that we will only mention. *Adjustment disorders* involve stressful life events, for example a death, divorce, job change. These are marked by poor adaptive responses so that the ability to function in the expected daily roles is impaired. *Psychosexual disorders* include disturbances in sexual functioning due to psychological factors, whether the disturbance is gender confusion or the inability to perform sexually in the absence of physiological problems. Homosexuality per se is no longer considered a psychiatric disorder, if it arouses no distress in the individual and the individual would not seek/wish for a heterosexual orientation. *Eating disorders* encompass abnormal eating patterns, and include two major conditions. One, anorexia nervosa, is predominantly a disorder affecting adolescent girls; it involves an intense fear of becoming obese, a disturbed body image, and a weight loss of at least 25% of original body weight. The other is bulimia, characterized by episodic binge eating, which is followed by dysphoric feelings. Patients with bulimia may induce vomiting after the gluttonous episodes. There is also a category, *psychological factors affecting physical condition.* It is characterized by a substantial interaction between the onset or course of a physical condition and psychological factors such as anxiety or depression. This category replaces the term psychosomatic disorders. The latter implied that only a limited number of diseases had important psychological determinants. However, it is current thinking that the importance of psychological factors in disease progression is not completely dependent on the specific disease involved, but on the individual and the environment as well. There are also *disorders first appearing in infancy, childhood, and adolescence,* which include mental retardation, attention-deficient disorders (hyperactivity), and developmental disorders (reading, language).

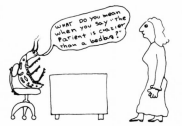

Finally, this diagnostic classification scheme also recognizes that there may be a variety of circumstances and occasions that would bring persons *without* psychiatric disorders into mental health services. Thus there is a category for conditions not attributable to a mental disorder that are a focus of attention or treatment. These include such things as bereavement, marital problems, occupational problems, academic problems.

■ *Medications*

Alcoholism does not exist in a vacuum. Alcoholics, as do other people, have a variety of other problems: some physical, some mental. They may be receiving treatment or treating themselves. The treatment probably involves drugs, prescribed or over the counter.

There may be tremendous confusion surrounding drugs. Often this arises from a communication gap. The doctor prescribes a certain medication intended to have a particular effect on a particular patient. The patient is unclear (and usually doesn't question) what the purpose is. He takes the drug without letting the physician know, in fact, what is occurring. Every drug has multiple simultaneous actions. Only a few of these effects are being sought when any drug is prescribed. These intended effects are called *therapeutic effects*. All other effects would be the side effects in that instance. In selecting a medication for a patient, the doctor seeks a drug with the maximum therapeutic impact and minimal side effects. Only feedback from the patient enables the doctor to make adjustments, if necessary. The regimen for taking a drug is as important as what is taken. There is a good reason for specifying before or after meals, for example. Often, as patients begin to feel better, they will stop or cut the dosage of prescribed drugs. One danger in this is that they have taken enough of a drug for relief of symptoms, but not enough to remove the underlying cause. People should be encouraged to consult with their physician *before* altering the way they take medications. Because treatment requires good communication, patients should be helped to ask any questions about their treatment and the drugs involved.

Psychotropic drugs

The group of medications of particular interest in relation to alcohol are the *psychotropic drugs*. Any drug that acts on the mind, thereby influencing behavior or mood, falls into this category. These drugs are likely to be among the most widely misunderstood. There is no denying that psychotropic drugs are widely prescribed. During 1974, 24% of the population took some form of psychotropic medication. Two years before that, 144 million prescriptions were written for minor tranquilizers alone, just one subgroup of the psychotropic drugs. Few persons would deny that such drugs are not only widely prescribed, but *over*prescribed. Because of their mood-altering properties, such medications may be candidates for abuse. However, all psychotropic medications are not alike. Each has its appropriate use. Not all are equally likely to present problems for the recovering alcoholic. However, in no instance should they be used in combination with alcohol (see Chapter 5).

A discussion of the three major categories of psychotropic drugs follows. Each has a different combination of actions and is properly prescribed for different reasons. These are the antipsychotic agents, antidepressant agents, and antianxiety agents.

The *antipsychotic* drugs are also called the *major tranquilizers.* This second name isn't really a very good way to describe their action. It has probably introduced confusion, but the phrase sticks. Antipsychotic agents, as the name implies, are drugs that relieve the symptoms of psychoses. In addition to the antipsychotic effect, these drugs also have a tranquilizing and a sedative action. They calm behavior and induce drowsiness. Different drugs in this group have differing balances of the three actions. The drug prescribed would be selected on the basis of the patient's constellation of symptoms. Thus a drug with greater sedative effects might well be selected for a person exhibiting psychotic and agitated behavior.

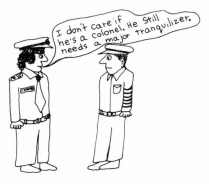

The antipsychotic medications most frequently encountered are listed below.

Brand name	Generic name	Daily dosage range (mg)
Thorazine	Chlorpromazine	100-1,000
Mellaril	Thioridazine	30-800
Stelazine	Trifluoperazine	2-30
Trilafon	Perphenazine	2-64
Navane	Thiothixene	6-60
Haldol	Haloperidol	3-50

These drugs interact with alcohol. Some possible effects include raising the seizure threshold and slowing the metabolism of alcohol.

On occasion, an antipsychotic agent will be prescribed, not to relieve psychotic symptoms, but for its sedative or tranquilizing properties. This is because these preparations are less likely to be abused than the usual sedatives or antianxiety agents. Generally their use is restricted to persons who have, or who have had, a serious psychiatric disorder. Medication may be prescribed not only during an acute phase, but afterward, to maintain an adequate level of functioning.

In working with alcoholics, a justified concern centers on the possible abuse of additional drugs. The abstinent alcoholic is less likely to abuse these medications than some other types of psychotropic drugs. These compounds are not chemically similar to alcohol and are therefore not subject to cross-tolerance or addiction.

The *antidepressants,* another major class of psychotropic drugs, do just what the name implies. They are used to treat the biological component of depression. They are not intended to help someone who is simply having a blue day. It takes a period of time of regular use for these medications to have their full action. Therefore, not an uncommon initial complaint of patients is that the medicine isn't helping. Commonly experienced side effects are sedation and tranquilization. These are most pronounced when the person first begins taking the drug. The physician may choose to have the patient take the drug at bedtime, so the sedation effect will not interfere with daytime function.

The most common antidepressants follow.

Brand name	Generic name	Daily dosage range (mg)
Tofranil	Imipramine	75-150
Elavil	Amitriptyline	75-150
Aventyl	Nortriptyline	75-200

There is no clear evidence that antidepressant agents are addicting. Again, in combination with alcohol, problems can rise with additive effects.

Lithium carbonate is worth special mention. Dissimilar to the antidepressants in chemical composition, it is nonetheless the mainstay of treatment in manic-depressive illness. Lithium has been invaluable in the control and leveling of wide mood swings associated with this illness. The dosage is geared to body weight, and the level of lithium is monitored periodically through blood samples. Any patient taking lithium should be seeing his physician regularly. An insufficient level of lithium will not help in control of symptoms. With too high a level, the patient may have a toxic reaction. Although it is unclear how lithium works, not only does it help during an acute episode, but just as importantly it reduces or prevents the intensity of subsequent episodes. Any patient taking lithium should be strongly advised to consult his physician if he is considering stopping this medication. Lithium is not a psychoactive drug that is at all likely to be abused by the patient.

The final group of psychotropic drugs are the *antianxiety agents.* Drugs in this class, along with barbiturates, are the ones most likely to be troublesome for alcoholics. The major action of these drugs is to promote tranquilization and sedation. Quite properly, alcohol can be included in any list of drugs in this class. The *antianxiety* agents are also called the *minor tranquilizers.* They have no antipsychotic or significant antidepressant properties. Two of the most widely prescribed drugs in the United States are antianxiety agents: Librium and Valium. Most of these prescriptions are *not* written by psychiatrists but by general practitioners, surgeons, internists, and orthopedists. The potential for abuse of these antianxiety agents is becoming far more broadly recognized. Accordingly, the total number of prescriptions written annually in the United States for Valium, for example, has tumbled from 61.5 million in 1975 to 39 million in 1979. Some estimates for 1980 are as low as 34 million, which would represent a 44% drop in a 6-year period.

Alcohol and the minor tranquilizers in combination potentiate one another. Because of their similar pharmacology, they are also virtually interchangeable. It's simply a matter of getting the correct dosage. This phenomenon is the basis of cross-addiction. Thus Librium is considered an excellent drug to manage withdrawal from alcohol and for detoxification. Essentially, the Librium is substituted for the alcohol, and then the patient tapered off the Librium. This interchangeability with alcohol is what makes Librium a very poor drug for alcoholics except for detoxification purposes. There is always the danger of creating an additional dependency.

The most common antianxiety agents follow.*

Brand name	Generic name	Daily dosage range (mg)
Librium	Chlordiazepoxide	10-100
Valium	Diazepam	6-40
Equanil, Miltown	Meprobamate	600-1,200
Atarax, Vistaril	Hydroxyzine	30-100

In the main, Americans are very casual about drugs. Too often, prescribed drugs are not taken as directed, are saved up for the "next" illness, or are shared with family and friends. If the attitude toward prescription drugs is so casual, over-the-counter preparations are treated as candy. Because a prescription is not required does not render these preparations harmless. Some possible ingredients of over-the-counter drugs are antihistamines, codeine, scopolamine, and of course alcohol. These can cause difficulty if taken in combination with alcohol. Or they may themselves be targets of abuse. For specific alcohol-drug interactions, see Chapter 5.

---

*We have lumped the antianxiety agents together for the purpose of this discussion. However, there are differences among them based on their chemical composition that have significance if abuse occurs. These will be elaborated on in the following section.

■ *Polydrug use*

There is increasing concern about polydrug use and abuse. This refers to simultaneous use of different mood-altering drugs, either one with another, or another drug in combination with that all-time favorite, alcohol. Different patterns of multiple drug use might be identified. One is most common among teenagers (or was several years ago). Naive drug users, they often took whatever was available, without particular regard for, or knowledge of, the specific effects. There were reports of teenage parties with "fruit salad." "Fruit salad" was a bowl of pills, with each guest contributing whatever he could glean from the family medicine cabinet. In what, to us, sounds like chemical roulette, the kids would take a handful of pills and supposedly "turn on" for the evening. From time to time, emergency rooms would be confronted with sick kids who had ingested unknown drugs in unknown quantities. This is one form of polydrug abuse, although admittedly not the most common variety.

Another form of polydrug abuse does not involve simultaneous use, but sequential use or abuse. Generally, people have their drug of choice, whether it is licit or a street drug. However, if what they want is unavailable, they will use something else that is—just like the cigarette smoker who is forced to settle for another brand when the vending machine is out of "his brand." It's only a temporary switch.

Then there are the folks who use multiple drugs in an attempt to achieve different particular moods or feeling states. You name the mood, and they have a formula of drugs in combination to achieve it. This may mean uppers in the morning, downers to unwind later in the day, drugs to counteract fatigue, drugs to promote sleep, drugs to feel "better." Those most likely to get into this drug-use pattern are persons with relatively easy access to drugs: nurses, physicians, pharmacists, and their spouses. This does not imply the medications are being stolen. Easy access can mean asking someone to write you a prescription as a favor. Anyone who works near the health care system or knows a physician is likely to make an informal request at some

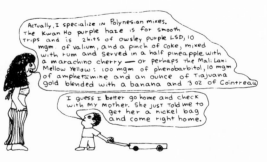

point. It may be for the birth control pills you didn't realize had run out, or poison ivy lotion, or just a few Librium because you are under a lot of stress now. Although the dynamics of this type of drug use have not been adequately described, in all probability it starts out innocently. The aim is not to get high, but to cope. Accustomed to the use of medications, often working at a pace beyond reasonable expectations for mere mortals, people may try a little chemical assistance to get by. Despite all their book knowledge of pharmacology, before they know it, they are in trouble. The drugs are no longer something to be used in special situations; they are essential for simply existing. Alcohol may well become a part of this picture.

It is our impression that the most frequent polydrug use does not involve illicit drugs or fit the patterns just described. Although alcohol workers all know of some horror story in which other drug use developed from injudicious use of medication prescribed as a part of identified alcohol treatment, this appears to be becoming increasingly less common. Yet polydrug use is reportedly on the rise. Among persons who have entered AA since 1977, 27% report a dual addiction. It is our suspicion that much polydrug use involving alcohol begins when people in the early stages of alcoholism start to ride the doctor circuit, in search of a physical answer to their problems. The complaint may be "nerves," "headaches," or "sensitive stomach," coupled with other vague complaints. These people do not go to their physicians deliberately trying to con them into a prescription. They truly want to be fixed up. Their drinking may not even look that different. Quite possibly the budding alcoholic may openly tout alcohol as a Godsend, given how he feels.

PHYSICIAN (dutifully taking the drinking history): How much do you drink?

PATIENT: Oh, not too much, mostly when I go out socially.

PHYSICIAN: How much is that, and how often?

PATIENT: Oh, not much, one or two drinks at a party, on occasion a cocktail before dinner. But I tell you, these headaches have been murder. And I've sometimes said, "I may not be a drinker, but I will be if they continue."

PHYSICIAN: They're that bad . . .

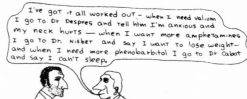

It all sounds straightforward. Our friend has tests done; nothing emerges to pin the headaches on. He is reporting stress at work, and eventually he walks out of the doctor's office with a prescription for a minor tranquilizer. This fellow may be headed for trouble. There is an ever-growing sensitivity of the medical community to prescribing minor tranquilizers for vague nonspecific problems. Nonetheless, a persistent patient will prevail.

Then there are those patients who have always been high-strung "nervous types," who are likely to get flapped easily. Somewhere along the line, they got some pills for their nerves. These pills just work wonders. They like to have a supply handy, "just in case." These patients often become quite skilled in reporting symptoms to ensure that the pill bottle in the medicine cabinet is always full. In this day of medical specialists, they might be seeing more than one doctor. And they may have each one writing the same prescription. As time goes on, the occasions warranting a pill become more numerous. Alcohol can come in here also. They simply may not be told of the dangers of mixing the medications with alcohol. Or they may dismiss the information if they are told. They are rarely informed of the time required to metabolize the drug from the system (or alcohol, for that matter) and simply think, "Oh, I took that 2 hours ago. A drink wouldn't hurt now!" This is a frequently seen phenomenon. After all, how many people do you know who believe alcohol is a terrific way to calm the nerves?

Withdrawal

Just as tolerance develops for alcohol, so too can tolerance develop for some other psychotropic medications, especially barbiturates, sedatives, and the minor tranquilizers. More are required to keep doing the same job. Add to this the all-American viewpoint that discomfort is pointless when chemical comfort is only a swallow away. With the development of tolerance, withdrawal syndromes may accompany abstinence. Several of these will be briefly described.

Barbiturates have been around since the beginning of this century. Central nervous system depressants, like alcohol, they have an abstinence syndrome very similar to alcohol's. At lower doses, withdrawal symptoms will most likely be limited to anxiety and tremulousness. At high levels, more serious withdrawal symptoms may develop. These can include convulsions and a "DT-like" syndrome of delirium, disorientation, hallucinations, and severe agitation. Barbiturate withdrawal presents a medical situation as serious, and potentially as life-threatening, as that accompanying alcohol withdrawal.

Drugs included within the category of minor tranquilizers can be subdivided into different groups depending on their chemical compositions. These differences are important when it comes to withdrawal and potential problems of abuse. Librium and Valium both belong to the subgroup known as the benzodiazepines. When drugs of this subgroup are abused, withdrawal symptoms may be present if use is abruptly stopped. Withdrawal symptoms can include tremulousness, sweating, and possibly convulsions. A full-blown "DT-like" picture generally is *not* associated with the benzodiazepines. However, it is increasingly recognized that physical dependence is not a casual issue. Clinically more and more persons are appearing for treatment following a long-standing use of Librium or Valium. Even if the symptoms of physical withdrawal associated with these substances are not as dramatic, getting off is no easy matter.

For other subgroups of drugs in the minor tranquilizers category, withdrawal can be much more serious. Be particularly alert to abuse of Miltown or Equanil, the brand names of meprobamate; Doriden (a glutethimide); and Quāālude (methaqualone). Withdrawal syndromes for these can be as dangerous as those associated with alcohol or barbiturates. (Doriden and Quāālude have hypnotic, sleep-inducing properties and may have been prescribed for sleep.)

Combine physical dependence on alcohol along with dependence on another drug, and the problems of detoxification are increased. Actually the task confronting the physician is to manage detoxification*s*. That is what is done, sequential detoxification, withdrawal of one drug at a time. Medical management can be a very delicate process in these situations. It is critical for multiple dependencies to be identified when someone first enters treatment. If alcohol detoxification is not going smoothly, the first question to be asked is: "Are there other drugs involved?"

Active alcoholics—other drug use

Multidrug use is important not only in terms of detoxification. It clearly has an impact on the drinking career. One observation is that the alcoholism process is accelerated when other drug use is present. This would not be unexpected, since the liver is the organ involved in the metabolism of many drugs. But more rapid physical deterioration is not the only problem. Depending on the drugs involved, there can be difficulties of a more acute nature on any drinking occasion. The effects may be additive, so there will be increased central nervous system depression. This can be a life-threatening situation.

In addition to physical problems that can occur with alcohol and other drug use, there are other difficulties for

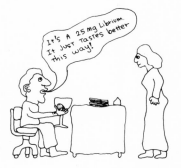

the active alcoholic. There are any number of ways the alcoholic can use other drugs. One way is to use other drugs to maintain and control the drinking. (Alcohol is the drug of choice.) Along the line, the alcoholic may have learned the warning signs of alcoholism. So by using pills, alcohol consumption may be maintained within what the drinker has decided are safe limits. What would *really* hit the spot would be a nice, stiff drink before a meeting. But instead the drinker settles for a capsule. He doesn't drink during the day, so he doesn't consider himself an alcoholic. So drug use can help the alcoholic keep alcohol use within "acceptable" limits. The drinking career can thereby, in his mind, be managed and extended.

Another pitfall is that other drug use can prevent the reality of the alcohol problem from sinking in. The minor tranquilizers are also known as the antianxiety agents. It might be said that anxiety is what will eventually move the alcoholic near treatment. This happens when the problems are such that one cannot explain them away or successfully drink them away, when the pain is no longer alcohol-soluble.

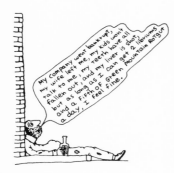

A little digression on anxiety. Anxiety, it seems to us, has been getting an unduly harsh press. Some anxiety is essential for normal, healthy functioning. It is an internal signal of potential danger and at times is essential for the preservation of life. The antianxiety agents, by turning off anxiety, may create a false sense of well-being. The individual using antianxiety agents will still intellectually know what is happening, but the emotional impact is blunted. The active alcoholic has plenty to be anxious about. Although pills may help turn it off, they will be unable to alter the source of the anxiety, which is the drinking and its consequences. Even if the alcoholic is at a point where the drinking is very troubling, when under the influence of pills, the drinking may not seem all that bad. So some anxiety seems necessary to produce change. We have a friend who says, "No one ever changes until it's too painful not to." This observation comes from long experience in a professional helping role. Removal of the alcoholic's pain can be a block to recovery. In the mildly mulled state of minor tranquilization, it may seem much easier to the alcoholic simply to continue the life pattern as before, including the drinking.

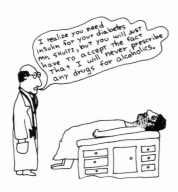

Polydrug use and abuse can take many forms, and there are great individual variations on these themes. It is not a subject that can be dismissed with any pat answers. As a nation of pill-poppers, we would all be well advised to be far less casual about our use of medications.

Chapter 10

Special populations: women, the elderly, adolescents, the employed

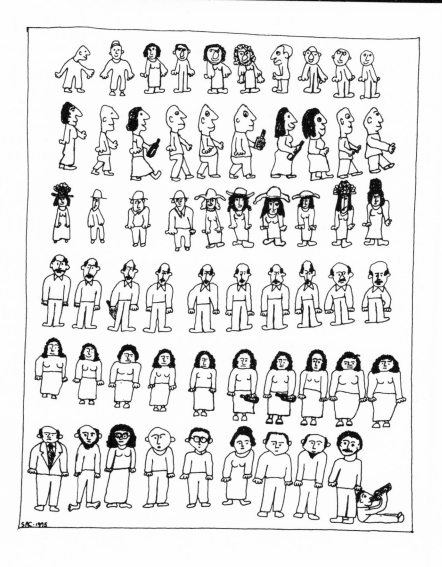

If there is a stereotype of the alcoholic or someone who has a drinking problem, that stereotypical individual is pictured as white, a male, in the 35- to 55-year age range, probably having a somewhat seedy appearance, and marginal work status. Say the word alcoholism and picture a woman? Never. A teenager? Of course not, they're too young. Getting loaded and feeling their oats is all it is. A white-haired grandmother who wears housedresses and oxford tie shoes? Really!

Although intellectually one may know that alcohol problems including alcoholism cross all age groups, occur in both sexes, and occur among persons of all ethnic backgrounds, the stereotype persists. It colors our thinking of what alcoholism looks like—that is, how it manifests itself—and how treatment should be organized. It undoubtedly influences the index of suspicion we have about who might have an alcohol problem.

For all these reasons, we wish to look specifically at alcohol problems and alcoholism in several groups—women, the elderly, adolescents, the employed—whose members collectively comprise the bulk of the alcoholic population. Aside from the insights you may glean about members of these groups, we hope to sensitize you as well to other differences that may exist. Clearly many other attributes are worthy of consideration that are not discussed here. Ethnicity, racial groups, religious affiliation, socioeconomic status, sexual orientation all have a bearing on alcohol problems and have been the subject of research. Persons seeking information about alcohol problems in any of these particular populations are referred to the End Papers (Chapter 11) for further sources of information.

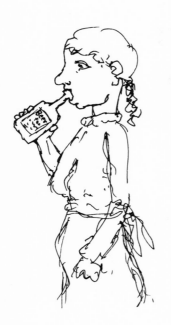

▪ *Women*

The alcohol problems of women is not a topic you will find much discussed until very recently. If you judged the presence of alcohol problems in women by the number of articles published on the subject, in either the scientific or popular press, you'd be forced to conclude there weren't any until the mid-1970s, when suddenly an epidemic struck! Alcoholism, heavy drinking, and problem drinking were long thought to be the concern principally of men. The reasons for this view are complex. Women's roles are changing, as will be discussed later. For centuries, however, women carried the burden of idealization. Women were "purer," objects to be loved and set on pedestals. There was—and still is to some extent—a virgin-prostitute dichotomy. Women fell clearly on one side or the other. Thus "ladies" didn't smoke, drink (never mind the Lydia Pinkhams), or swear. Although the picture has changed—

women do smoke, drink, and swear now in varying degrees —vestiges of the pedestal remain. "A woman drunk is worse than a drunk man." Therefore, not very many women drink too much. Therefore, if you encounter a woman alcoholic, pretend she isn't there. She is depressed, or suicidal, or mentally ill, or it will go away, or she is grieving the loss of her husband, and so on. The alcoholic woman was, and to an extent still is, ignored by all. Her family, if she had one, hid her from view as much as possible. She died, early and often. Even in the beginning years of AA (1935-1945) she was a rarity, a real minority.

For many years the estimates were that only one out of every seven alcoholics was a female; then the ratio cited was one out of four. More recently some authorities have claimed that there are almost as many female alcoholics as males. That the view of women and alcohol has changed little is evidenced by the title of an article in the September 1977, issue of *Good Housekeeping* magazine: "The *Shocking* Facts about Women and Alcohol." (The emphasis is ours.) To whom it was to be a shock wasn't clear—presumably, the readers. One of the shocks was that nearly half the estimated 10 million alcoholics are female. Another was "that the husbands of 9 out of 10 of these women will leave them." (Only one out of every ten women married to alcoholic men leave their husbands.) Also, the point was made that housewives make up the largest single category of women alcoholics. The article also mentioned the risk factor of alcohol use during pregnancy, which has been discussed earlier. These facts were certainly not news to anyone working in the alcohol field. That a major women's magazine calls these facts shocking says much about the avoidance of this issue by our society. If 5 million women were at risk because of some other illness, the hue and cry would be much greater.

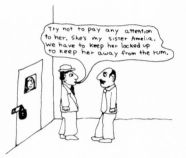

Paucity of research

What is really known about alcohol problems as they affect women is appallingly little. A review of the scientific literature found that between 1928 and 1970 there were only twenty-eight studies of women alcoholics published in the English language! Since then, many people have been industriously trying to fill the void. Previously, it was assumed that reported findings from studies of male alcoholics could just be extrapolated to females. There is a great deal of work currently under way to describe fully the characteristic manifestations of the disease in women, to pinpoint both the differences and similarities, to do studies on alcohol's physiological effects on women, to study the societal factors that influence the course of the disease and the treatment, and much more. The results to date are important, but tend mainly to point to additional areas of investigation that should be pursued. The most thoughtful writing on current research efforts generally ends with a statement that more information is required before firm statements can be made. We are at a stage where we are realizing how much we do not know. All that was thought to be known is rightfully being questioned and reexamined.

Women's roles and alcohol use

Women do not become alcoholics in a vacuum, any more than do other populations. Society plays a part as an influence. Women's roles in society now are less clearly defined than they once were. There are some hints and many questions as to how the changes taking place may affect the rates of alcoholism. As was seen in Chapter 4, cultural influences are only one of the three interwoven "causes" of alcoholism. One would suspect that the genetic factor, to date studied predominantly in men, will likewise play a part in the development of alcoholism in women as well. Any differences in women's psychological makeup that apply to alcohol's effects and distinguish them from men have yet to be explored adequately. However, research is going forth in this area, also. Culturally, several typical life-styles of today's women can be described and compared to those of the past. From this one can consider how these roles might influence women's use of alcohol.

There is first the now much denigrated role of full-time housewife. This role is subject to great variations on a theme, depending on social status, financial status, age, and area of the country in which one lives. Housewives range from those who enjoy the country club, fully electric kitchen, outside paid help, and volunteer work life-style to those women less financially advantaged who must do all their own work with little, if any, time-saving devices. One common thread for both, however, is that their schedules are built primarily around those of their families. They do whatever they have to do around and because of the husband's job and hours and children's school and extracurricular activities. Their activities may have a fractured quality. Interruptions, minor crises, and unfinished business seem to be constant. There is also a sameness to their routine, which varies only with the seasons—school, vacation, holidays. Boredom, too much to do, and too little reward are fairly common complaints. Today's housewife may have some advantages, such as wash-and-wear clothing, convenience foods, and electric appliances; but there were some things about the "good old days" that really were! One of those positive things was support—extended families nearby. People tended to be less mobile. They grew up, married, and remained living in the same area.

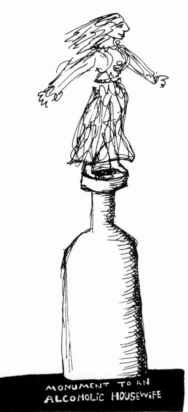

MONUMENT TO AN
ALCOHOLIC HOUSEWIFE

Grandparents, aunts, sisters, and cousins were around for help with children, during illnesses, or when canning time came around. Certainly an "all for one and one for all" feeling wasn't always present, but there were usually at least some family members close by to call on for aid. For many women today, their families are far away, with visits only once or twice a year. Supports are either friends or, when there aren't many of these, agencies of one kind or another. When daily life got to be too much in the past, women had the option of a grandmother or two or other women in the family to help out. Today women have to pay sitters or housekeepers.

We suspect that one outlet no longer available was "the vapors." Women in the old stereotypical view were "weaker," more "emotional," and "delicate." It was accepted practice to take to their beds under stress. This was possible because there was usually someone to take over for a brief period, to allow for the temporary collapse. It could well be that this acted as a safety valve and actually was beneficial. In order to justify the expense of temporary household help today, the woman *really* has to be sick in a big way. Who knows how many tranquilizers and drinks are used to ward off what was previously taken care of by a day or two in bed!

Today's increased pace also enhances the use of alcohol. Children don't just go to school, come home, study, and help with chores. There are Boy Scouts, play rehearsals, dancing and music classes, riding lessons, Little League, baby-sitting jobs, and most of these trips require a chauffeur. And they are often in conflict with the things the other children have scheduled. Add to this the vicissitudes of life, minor accidents, pets, and so on. After a fractured, harried day, a drink may be a very welcome way to unwind enough to get dinner on the table and relax or do the laundry, or entertain business associates of the husband. . . . There is also the psychological impact created by the self-questioning most housewives now are subject to, with the implication often that such a role is unrewarding, unnecessary, and behind the times. Whether this is true or not, the question is being raised.

Figures now show that over half of adult women work outside the home. Many do so because of financial necessity. Most of this group are not trained professionally and must take the jobs available to them. The magazine articles of late have focused primarily on women who like their work and have some skills and/or training that allow them a choice. This has glamorized the working woman and distorted the picture. Many women are forced by need to support themselves and their children or add to the family income to survive. And many of these women are in low-

paying, highly unsatisfying jobs. They are not working outside the home because they want to. Usually these women
fill the homemaker role as well. Therefore, they carry the
burden at home and in essence hold two full-time jobs.

Others work out of a need to have more in life than un-
made beds, dishes, and cleaning something all the time.
With more options open, women are no longer forced to
stay at home if they find that unrewarding. For these
women, work outside the home is something they are glad
to be able to do. More younger women are choosing careers
they plan to pursue whether they marry or not. They are
more aware of the financial realities and the probability
that they will be spending at least a portion of their adult
life working outside the home. They are more aware of the
desirability of being more self-reliant. As a consequence,
they are more realistic in preparing themselves to do something that will be financially and personally rewarding.

There have always been some, and will be more and
more, women who wish to pursue a professional career.
Whether it is the law, medicine, the arts, education, or the
business world, these women are pursuing something they
really wish to do. Their careers are very important to them;
they don't wish to put them in second place. The times may
be changing sufficiently to make this easier for women to
do. If changes are coming in the professional world, it
seems they come at the rate of the proverbial snail. It still is
harder for a woman to advance professionally or at a rate
financially equal to that of her male counterpart. A survey
of colleges and universities showed women still not holding
positions of real power and being paid less than men in
comparable positions. It is doubtful the picture is much
different in other segments of society.

What happens to working women back in the home? A
survey of working women with families showed that they
had reduced the amount of housework they did by only
about 35% when they began full-time employment. Thus
they will have many of the same pressures of women who
work at home plus whatever other pressures are incurred
on their jobs. Alcohol has always been an accepted way to
"relax" after a hard day at work for men. It is rather
natural to assume that women would find the same to be
true for them. They can also add all the other reasons men
give for drinking: entertaining clients, to be one of the
"crowd." Equal opportunities for women have not totally
arrived and society still holds the view generally that most
household chores "belong" to women, hence the situation
for most working women is far from ideal. They are faced
with many compromises that are unsatisfactory to them.
And dissatisfaction and alcohol have long been compan-
ions.

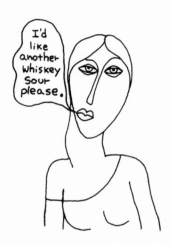

The foregoing may imply that virtually all women are married and the only variations are working outside the home versus being full-time homemakers and having children or not. The reality is far more complex. Women are marrying later. More and more marriages are ending in divorce. Despite changing patterns in child custody, the odds are on the rise that a woman will head up a single-parent family. And with remarriage, the woman may well be in a new ready-made "blended family": she, her new spouse, and the children of their previous marriages. "And they lived happily ever after" is no longer the norm.

Some suggestions

With this background on the changing roles of women and how these might prompt the use of alcohol, and in light of what was first discussed on how little is definitively known about women and alcohol, what should women be aware of as possible problem areas?

Often mentioned in discussion of female alcoholism is the fact that many more women than men can point to a specific trigger for the onset of their drinking. This might be a divorce, death of a spouse, children leaving home, a depression, or some other significant event. If a woman is experiencing a stressful time in her life, she needs to be aware of the dangers of using alcohol or drugs, including prescription drugs, to cope. She runs a higher risk of addiction at such times. If drinking does increase, or alternately, she uses pills to "get through," it should not be assumed that the drinking and/or pill-taking is "only" temporary and will end when the crisis is over. Too many crises seem to take on a long-term life of their own, or lead to others, "justifying" the continued use of alcohol and/or pills long after the original event. The problem for those around a woman caught in this trap is usually an overabundance of sympathy. We agree that whatever happened to her is truly awful and, overtly or covertly, imply that we'd probably do the same if something that bad happened to us. It is almost impossible to face the fact that the alcohol and/or pill use is now a severe problem itself if the focus remains on the original crisis.

This brings us to the much-publicized fact that mood-altering drugs are prescribed much more frequently for women than for men. Cross-addiction is therefore a real possibility. If there is no recognition of this possibility, a woman might use a "spice rack" approach to her problems and come up with a real witches' brew. Women need to be much more cautious in their acceptance of medications and to ask for clear and complete instructions regarding any hazards associated with them.

It has also been suggested that women's alcoholism progresses somewhat differently from men's. The whole disease process appears to be telescoped; it starts later and gets worse faster. Many may show the same characteristic developments that men do, but the order in which they appear can be different. Thus it cannot be automatically assumed that a woman is or is not in a particular phase because she does or does not manifest the symptoms associated with that phase. (It should be recalled from Chapter 3 that the Jellinek phases were based on the typical progression seen in male alcoholics. One can never expect the symptoms always to show up in order: one, two, three, and so on.) As the course of alcoholism in women is studied more fully, a similar model may be constructed to depict the typical progression of alcoholism in females. In the meantime, anyone concerned about a woman's drinking shouldn't be lulled into a false sense of security based on any description of symptoms in males. If you were concerned in the first place, stay concerned until she's been checked out by a knowledgeable professional.

Women are not, in general, free from society's biases toward them. A great problem in the identification and treatment of women with alcohol problems is the general view that it is "worse" for a woman to drink to excess. This view is widely held, and held equally by women. Several possible results follow from this. One is that a women will delay coming for treatment and deny her problem until no other course is open to her. Her family will also make more effort to deny and/or cover up the possibility of an alcohol problem. If she does appear for treatment, her self-respect is likely to be very low or nonexistent. She holds a very low estimate of herself. She may be so guilt-ridden that she is unable to see any acceptable way out of her dilemma. Because she has delayed seeking treatment, she may be physically and emotionally in worse shape than her male counterpart. Unfortunately, she may also be led astray in her first attempts to gain help. One cannot expect that all caregivers are completely untouched by society's views. Professionals too may be reluctant to see an obvious alcohol problem, focusing instead on some secondary issue.

In some circles there has been concern about professionals' insensitivity to women's issues. Correspondingly, there has been an emphasis on seeking a therapist, counselor, or agency primarily serving women. While recognizing the history behind this and the merits, we have one caution. We believe the greater danger to an alcoholic woman is an insensitivity to alcoholism. The primary goal is to have the alcoholic woman seen by someone knowledgeable about alcohol problems. whether that worker be affiliated with an alcohol-treatment agency or a feminist health service.

Mothering and female sexuality are two aspects of self-esteem unique to women. If the woman alcoholic now trying to stay sober has children, some of the questions she may well be asking herself are: "Am I a good mother?" "Can I be a good mother?" "Can I ever cope with my children if I don't drink?" These may not be explicitly stated, but they do cross her mind. They can begin to be answered hopefully positively, as she gains sober time. However, in some cases where there has been child abuse or a child is having special difficulties, a children's agency, a family-service agency, or a mental health clinic may be helpful in dealing with this type of problem. One of the things any recovering alcoholic mother will need to learn to regain her self-esteem as a mother is a sense of what the "normal" difficulties are in raising children. Support groups, AA, counseling, or all of these can help her to achieve a more balanced sense of her role as a mother. She needs to realize that getting sober and staying that way are the first big steps in fulfilling her responsibilities as a mother.

In terms of her *sexuality,* there may be a number of potential questions. If there has been a divorce or an affair, she may well be wondering about her worth and attractiveness as a woman. Even if the marriage is intact, there may be sexual problems. On the one hand, the sexual relationship may have almost disappeared as the drinking progressed. On the other, it may have been years since she's had sexual intercourse without benefit of a glass of wine or a couple of beers to get her "in the mood." Again, sober time may well be the major therapeutic element. However, couples' therapy and/or sexual counseling may be needed if marital problems are not resolved. In cases where the sexual problems *preceded* the active drinking, professional help is certainly recommended. Sobering up is not likely to take away the existing problem in some miraculous fashion. To let it fester is to invite even more problems.

An uncomfortable reality is the *lack of a supportive family* for the woman in many cases. Even in the one out of ten situations in which the family is still intact, husbands of alcoholic women seem less willing to become involved in family treatment than are wives of alcoholic husbands. The effects of alcoholism on the family have been discussed. It is clear that the most desirable and effective treatment includes family members. But it is also clear that recovery from alcoholism can and does take place under less than optimal conditions. Women need not use this as an excuse to stay sick themselves.

One note on *women and AA*. The latest figures from the General Services Board of AA indicate that over a third of the members coming into AA are women. It appears that whatever the differences between male and female alcoholics, AA manages to achieve the same rate of success with both. A few trips to local AA meetings should assure a woman that it is no longer the male stronghold it once was.

Though we have noted the paucity of generally available research material on women, the subjective viewpoint is receiving attention. Several women have recently written books about their personal troubles with alcohol and the subsequent recovery. There are also several books that survey the themes of women and addiction.

Being aware that alcoholism, alcohol problems, and treatment issues are not identical for men and women is most of the battle. We can all look forward to the developments to come as more research on alcohol and women is conducted and reported.

■ *The elderly*

*Dishonor not the old: we
shall all be numbered among
them.*

APOCRYPHA: BENSIRA 8:6

On Art Linkletter's show several years ago, he was interviewing children, and they came up with the following answers to a question he posed: "You can't play with toys anymore . . . the government pays for everything . . . you don't go to work . . . you wrinkle and shrink." The question was "What does it mean to grow old?" The responses of the children contain many of the stereotypes our society attributes to the elderly. They also show that this negative picture develops from a very early age. There is a stigma to growing old. The notion is that the elderly have no fun, no money, no usefulness, and no attractiveness.

It is important to recognize that in considering the elderly, we all really are talking about ourselves. It's inevitable. We will all age; we will all become the elderly. A participant at a recent geriatric conference reported being asked by a friend, "Give me the inside scoop . . . what can I do to keep from getting older?" The response the person received was simple: "Die now!" There is no other way to avoid aging. So, for those not themselves among the elderly, in thinking about older prsons, imagine yourself years in the future, since many of the circumstances will probably be the same.

Of the approximately 250 million persons in the United States, 20 million are over age 65. This is the group arbitrarily defined as the "elderly," or "aged." Each day, 3000 die and 4000 reach their sixty-fifth birthday, so there's a net gain of 1000. By the year 1990, it is estimated that over 35 million persons will be over age 65; this will represent a larger percentage of the population than ever before. Consequently, the problems of the elderly, including alcoholism, that will be discussed are going to become a growing concern for our society.

Coping styles

Despite the inevitability of aging and despite the inevitability of physical problems arising as the years pass, there's an important thing to keep in mind. It has been said many times and in many different ways that you are as young as you want to be. But this is only possible if the person has some strengths going for him. The best predictor of the future, specifically how someone will handle growing old, is how the individual has handled the previous years. Individuals who have demonstrated flexibility as they have gone through life will adapt best to the inevitable stresses that come with getting older. These are the people who will be able to feel young, regardless of the number of birthdays they have celebrated.

Interestingly, as people get older, they become less similar and more individual. The only thing that remains alike for this group is the problems they face. There's a reason for this. Everyone going through life relies most heavily on the coping styles that seem to have served them well previously. With years and years of living, individuals gradually narrow down their responses. What looks, at first glance, like an egocentricity or eccentricity of old age is more likely a lifelong behavior that has become one of the person's exclusive methods for dealing with stress. An example illustrating this point arose in the case of an elderly surgical patient for whom psychiatric consultation was requested. This man had a constant smile. In response to any question or statement by the nurses or doctors, he smiled, which was often felt to be wholly inappropriate. The treatment staff requested help in comprehending the patient's behavior. In the process of the psychiatric consultation, it became quite understandable. Friends, neighbors, and family of the man consistently described him as "good ole Joe, who always had a friendly word and a smile for everyone, the nicest man you'd ever want to meet." Now under the most fearful of situations, with many cognitive processes depleted, he was instinctively using his faithful, basic coping style. Very similarly, the person who goes through life with a pessimistic streak may become angry and sad in old age. Or the people who have been fearful under stress may be timid and withdrawn in old age. Or the people who have been very organized and always reliant on a definite schedule may try to handle everything by making lists in old age. What is true in each case is that the person has settled into a style that was present and successful in earlier life.

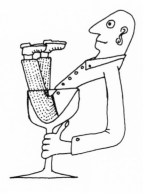

Main stresses

In understanding the elderly, four areas of stress need to be considered: stresses that arise from social factors; biological or physical problems; psychological factors; and, unfortunately, iatrogenic stresses due to the helping professions as they serve (or inadequately serve) the elderly.

Social stresses. These can be summarized under the phenomenon of the national addiction to youth. Television commercials highlight all types of products that can be used to disguise the process of aging. There's everything from hair colorings to dish detergents, which if used will make a mother's hands indistinguishable from her daughter's. Look around you. Who's being hired and who's being retired? Aging is equated with obsolescence and worthlessness. People who have been vital, contributing members of an organization suddenly find themselves with the title "honorary." It is often not an honor at all! It means these people have become figureheads, they have been replaced. The real work has been taken over by someone else, someone of younger age.

Consider for a moment the social stresses due to the biases of the helping professions. The National Institute of Mental Health only a decade ago spent a mere 1.1% of its budget for research on problems of the elderly. Only 1% of its budget for services went to provide for care of the elderly. This is now changing, but it gives a graphic picture of the relative importance placed on this group of people in the recent past. The real issue is one of *attitude.* If one examines the dynamics behind this attitude, then one can see why there has been "disinterest" and "avoidance." Generally, the medical profession and other helping people, as well as family and friends, are overwhelmed by the multiplicity, chronicity, and confusing nature of the disorders of aging. Caregivers often feel helpless with the elderly and harbor self-doubts about whether they can contribute, both in a satisfactory manner and in a manner that is personally gratifying. To put it another way, most of us like to see results, to see things happen, to believe there is a "before" and "after" picture, in which the difference is clear. Also, it is important for caregivers as well as others to feel that the part they have played, however big or small, has influenced this difference.

Often the elderly are seen as complainers, by both family and helpers. We all like it when someone puts out his hand and says "Thank you," but the elderly often say, "Don't bug me . . . I don't want help." If you check who voluntarily comes into most clinical agencies, it's not the elderly. Those who do come are usually coerced into it. Helpers do not like complainers. What do the elderly say? "This hurts, that hurts . . . you're not nice enough . . . you don't come soon enough . . . my old doctor was much better . . . do this, do that." Helpers like patients who receive maximum cures in the minimum of time. This certainly is not the elderly. There are more visits, more problems, more time. Helpers like patients who get well. How many of the elderly are cured? How can anyone take away their diabetes, their arthritis, the pain from the memory of a lost spouse? Helpers like patients who take their advice. With the elderly, suggest A, and they'll often do B.

The family may experience this frustration too. They may have their offers of assistance refused, only to hear their elderly relative later say how hard things are when you are alone with no one to help out. These interactional dynamics are understandable but they only aggravate the problem. They rub others the wrong way, the result being that many potential caregivers or family decide they don't like being with the elderly, and it shows. Very few clinicians volunteer to take on elderly clients. If an elderly client comes into a helping agency, the chances are good that the person who sees the client may soon decide to transfer the case to someone more "appropriate" or refer the patient to another agency. Family members may feel alternately frustrated, angry, guilty, and generally helpless. Also, the older person may feel like a nuisance, and may be very lonely.

Another factor that can impede relationships with the elderly is that the elderly *may resent others' youth, just as the others fear their elderliness.* Also, the elderly generally dislike the dependent status that comes from relying on children, or that goes along with being a client or patient. It is the opposite of what they want, which is to be independent and secure and feel a sense of worth. Being dependent implies that something is wrong with them. It also means that someone else is partially in charge and telling them how to run their lives.

Psychological stresses. The common denominator is loss. No matter how you slice it, the elderly must constantly deal with loss. The elderly may try to handle loss in a number of ways. One is the widely used defense of *denial*. In response to an observation that a client's hand is more swollen, he may well say, "Oh no, it's no different than it's always been." If a close friend is in the hospital and very seriously ill, she may dismiss the seriousness and claim it is "just another of her spells, she'll be out, perky as ever in a day or two." Another common way of handling loss is by *somatization*. This means bringing the emotional content out in the open, but "saying" it in terms of the body hurts. This is why so many of the elderly are labeled hypochondriacal. When he says his knee hurts and he really cannot get up that day, what he also may be saying is that he hurts inside, emotionally. Because he may not get attention for emotional pains, having something wrong physically or "mechanically" is socially more acceptable.

Another way of handling loss is *restricting affect.* Instead of saying it does not exist, as with denial, there is a withdrawing. They become less involved, so they don't hear about the bad things happening. By being less a part of the world, they are less vulnerable. Unfortunately, all these defenses boomerang and work against the elderly. How are love, affection, and concern expressed? Through words, behavior, and many nonverbal cues—a smile, a nod, a touch. After so many years of living, the elderly certainly know the signs of affection and caring or of distancing and detachment. By withdrawing when they are fearful, they may well see others reciprocally withdrawing. The elderly may then be left without any source of affection, interest, and caring. This they in turn read as dislike, and they may then feel their initial withdrawing was justified. Therefore, one of the prime techniques in dealing with the elderly is to reach out to them, literally. Smile, touch them, sit close to them. Attempt to reach through the barrier they may have erected with the "protective" psychological defenses mentioned.

The elderly frequently overinterpret what helping people instinctively say when reaching out to the aged. There are often statements like "you're lucky to be alive . . . quit worrying about things . . . grow old gracefully." What the elderly hear is someone telling them to ignore their losses, or that the person making such statements does not want to get close to them. The elderly's response is that they do not want to grow old gracefully, they do not want to be "easy to manage," they want to go out with a band, leave a mark—they want to be individuals to the last day.

In the geriatric population losses are steady, predictable, and often come in bunches. And even if they do not, they are still numerous. What are the specific losses?

There is the loss that comes from the *illnesses* and *deaths* of family and friends. The older you get, statistically the more likely that those about you will begin to falter. So there are the obvious losses of supports and companionship. Not necessarily as obvious is that the deaths of others also leads to questioning about loss of self, anticipation of one's own death. This may sometimes be the source of anxiety attacks among the elderly.

There is the loss that comes from the geographical *separations of family*. This begins earlier in life, as children go to school and later leave home for college, the service, and eventually to marry. For the elderly, this may be especially difficult, since 50% of all grandparents do not have their grandchildren living close by. As new generations are being born, they are not accessible to the older generation whose lives are coming to a close.

There is the loss of *money* through earned income. Whether income is supplemented through pensions, social security, or savings, the elderly do not have as much money as earlier in their lives. Dollars not only represent buying power, they also have symbolic values. Money represents power, stature, value, and independence. Lack of money has obvious implications in vital areas of self-esteem.

There are the losses that accompany *retirement:* loss of status, gratification, and often most important, identity. With retirement, you lose who you've been. This refers not only to retirement from a job. It includes retirement from anything, from being a mother, or a grandmother, or from being a person who walked around the block. Often accompanying retirement is a loss of privacy. For married couples, retirement may mean more togetherness than they have had for years. Both will have to change routines and habits and be forced to accommodate the presence of the other. The expectations may also be tremendous. Retirement, in most people's fantasies, is thought to usher in the ''golden years,'' provide the opportunity to do the things that have been put off. There may well be a letdown.

There is also the loss of *body functions and skills,* which may include a loss of attractiveness. Older people may develop body odors. They lose their teeth. They are more prone to infection. For women, the skin may become dry, including the skin of the vagina, which can lead to vaginal discharges and dyspareunia (painful intercourse). For men, there is a general loss of muscle tone. Everything begins to stick out where it shouldn't. As physical problems arise, this may lead to loss of skills. The carpenter with arthritis or the tremors of Parkinson's disease will be unable to do the things that were formerly possible and rewarding.

How about sex and the elderly? The most prevalent lay myth is that the elderly have no interest in sex. Physiologically, aging of itself need not greatly affect sexual functioning. With advancing years, it takes a little longer to achieve an erection, a little more time to the point of ejaculation, orgasm is a little less intense, and a little more time is required before orgasms can be reexperienced. But if physically healthy, there is no reason the elderly should not be sexually active. The biggest factor influencing sexual activity in the elderly are the availability of a partner and social pressures. Among the elderly, when a partner dies, the survivor is often not encouraged to date or remarry. What is considered virility at age 25 is seen as lechery after age 65. Even when both partners are alive, if they are living in an institution or in the home of children, sexual activity may well be frowned on, or ''not allowed.''

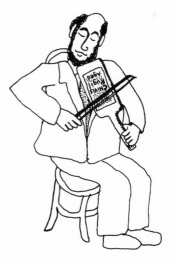

Another loss is of *sensation.* With aging, the senses become less acute. What this means is that the elderly are then deprived of accurate cues from their environment. This may be a big factor in the development of suspiciousness in older persons. Any paranoid elderly person should have hearing and vision evaluated.

The most powerful loss, the loss no elderly person is pre-

pared to understand or accept, is the loss of *thinking ability*. This may happen imperceptibly over a period of time.
It comes from the loss of cortical brain function. Suddenly
a person who has been an accountant or a schoolteacher,
for example, is adding 2 + 2 and it doesn't equal 4 every
time. This is embarrassing and scarey and though maybe
able to stand losing other things, to "lose one's mind" is
the ultimate indignity.

The result of all or any of these losses is that self-respect,
integrity, dignity, and self-esteem are threatened. The implication can be that usefulness is questioned and life is
ebbing away. The feeling may well be that "my work is
over."

Biological stresses. Of the elderly, only 5% are institu-
tionalized in nursing homes, convalescent centers, or similar facilities. However, 45% of the elderly have some serious physical disability such as heart disease, diabetes, lung
disease, or arthritis. About 25% also have a significant
functional psychological problem, with depression the
most prevalent. Understandably, as life expectancy increases and we live longer, there is more vulnerability to
the natural course of disease. For this part of the population, receiving medical care and paying medical bills can
mean additional big problems. The elderly have twice as
many visits to a physician, their average hospital stay is
three and one-half times longer than for persons under age
65, and the hospital stay costs five times more than for the
under-65 group. Ironically, for this medically fragile
group, insurance coverage (including Medicare) is often
less adequate than is coverage for younger persons. Thus
those with the greatest need for medical care, the highest
medical expenses, and the least ability to pay have the
poorest insurance coverage of any group.

Alcoholism is also a big problem for the elderly. Dr.
Robert Butler of the National Institutes of Aging,
estimates that 20% have a significant alcohol problem.
These problems are also ignored for many of the same
reasons that sex in the elderly is dismissed without a further thought. "That nice old lady drinks too much (or is
interested in sex)!" "Never!" Some of these elderly have
had a long history of alcohol use and abuse; they may have
been alcoholic for a good long time, but with adequate
medical care have somehow lived to old age. However,
with the overall deterioration of physical functioning, the
alcohol use may begin to take a heavier toll and become an
increasingly difficult problem. Also among the elderly are
persons who do not have a prior history of alcohol abuse;
their alcoholism may be described as late onset. The stresses
of aging may have been too great or come too fast and at
the wrong time. They have turned to alcohol as a coping

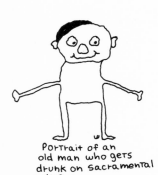

Portrait of an
old man who gets
drunk on sacramental
wine

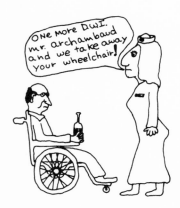

One more DWI.
Mr. Archambaud
and we take away
your wheelchair!

mechanism. The subgroup of the total population with the highest risk for alcoholism is widowers over age 65. Whatever the variety of alcoholism present, intervention is important. All too often we are likely to dismiss the elderly with ''what do they have to live for anyway . . . they have been drinking all these years, they'll never stop now . . . I don't want to be the one who asks them to give up the bottle.'' The *quality* of any amount of life left to any of us would better be the paramount concern. We wouldn't hesitate to assume that a 35-year-old man ought to get treated for his problem even though he could easily be killed in an auto accident next year. The elderly deserve just as much, if not more, consideration.

Depressive illness is very prevalent among the elderly. There may well be a physiological basis for this. The levels of neurochemicals (serotonin and norepinephrine) thought to be associated with depression change in the brain as people get older. These depressions, then, are not necessarily tied solely to situational events. But because so many things are likely to be going on in the surrounding environment for the elderly, it is too easy to forget the potential benefits of judiciously prescribed antidepressants. Malnourishment is all too common in the elderly. This can cause several syndromes that may look like depressions. Many physical ailments, due to disease processes themselves, manifest as depression.

Let us eat and drink; for tomorrow we die.

I CORINTHIANS 15:32

Depression in the elderly may not present like depression in younger persons, with tearfulness, inability to sleep, or loss of appetite. Some of the tips for recognizing depression in the elderly are an increased sensitivity to pain, refusing to get out of bed when physical problems don't require bed rest, poor concentration, a marked narrowing of coping style, and an upsurge of physical complaints. Often, the poor concentration leads to absent-mindedness and inattentiveness, which is misdiagnosed as defective memory and ultimately as ''senility'' with the depression unrecognized and untreated. Senility is really a useless clinical term. The proper phrase should be dementia, which means irreversible cognitive impairment. However, all cognitive impairment should be considered reversible (delirium) until proven otherwise. The elderly deserve an aggressive search for potentially treatable, reversible causes of organic brain syndromes by qualified medical personnel.

Suicide among the elderly is a very big problem. Twenty-five percent of all persons who commit suicide are over age 65. The rate of suicide for persons over 65 is five times that of the general population. After age 75, the rate is eight times higher.

Iatrogenic stresses. Unfortunately, the medical problems

of the elderly may be aggravated by the medical profession's insensitivities to the psychological and basic physiological changes in the elderly. All too often there is overprescription of medication in attempts to keep behavior controlled rather than diagnosed. Too few clinicians take into account the dramatically altered way the elderly metabolize medications, which means that fewer medicines in combination and lowered doses of any drug are required. Rarely is there any thought of whether the patient can afford the medicine prescribed. Also there is an overestimation of the patient's ability to comply with directions for taking medications. A poignant example of this was the case of an elderly woman who was discharged from the hospital with a number of medications. She had been admitted in severe congestive heart failure but had responded well to chemical treatment of hypertension and fluid retention. Within 2 weeks of returning to her home, her condition began to deteriorate, which was a source of dismay and consternation to her physicians. The patient was thought surely to be purposefully causing her ailments, and a psychiatrist, who was asked to consult on the case, decided to make a home visit. The woman knew which medications to take, when, and for what conditions. However, there was one problem. As she handed the bottle of capsules to the psychiatrist, with her crippled arthritic fingers, the "diagnosis" became obvious: the childproof cap! She had been unable to open the bottles and therefore unable to take the medicine. This is a vivid reminder of the need to consider *all* the available information in dealing with the problems of the elderly.

Practical suggestions

If the elderly have some symptoms of psychological problems or physical problems, including a problem with alcohol, the same treatment should be sought as would be for someone younger. Too often, problems of the elderly are dismissed under the assumption the elderly are just complainers, "senile," unlikely to benefit, likely to die soon, or incapable of appreciating help.

Because many elderly persons are reluctant to seek or receive professional help, a family member is often the person to make the first contact. The family's views of the situation, their ideas and fears, need to be aired. Whatever the problem, the chances are good that something can be done to improve the picture if the advice of a concerned caregiver is sought and followed. It often comes as a surprise to families that their elderly relative may get better. Professionals can help the family too, as it copes with a possibly difficult situation, by arranging for homeworker service or for Meals-on-Wheels, or making simple suggestions about routines that can make a difference.

In dealing with the elderly, remind yourself they are persons who are survivors. The fact that they have made it even this far means they have some strengths. These peole have stuck their necks out in the past and taken risks. Find out how they have done it, and see if you can help them do it again. Also, raise their expectations that indeed they *can* "make it" again, just as they have before.

Use all the possible resources at your disposal. In many instances the elderly need to become reinvolved in the world around them. Meaningful contacts can come from a variety of people, not just from professional helpers. The janitor in the client's apartment building, a neighbor, or a crossing guard at the street corner may all be potential allies. If the person was once active in a church group, civic organization, or other community group, but has lost contact, get in touch with the organization. There is often a member who will visit or be able to assist in other ways. Many communities have senior citizen centers. They offer a wide range of resources: everything from a social program, to Meals-on-Wheels, to counseling on Social Security and Medicare, to transportation. If there is a single agency to cultivate, this is the one.

The importance of reaching out, showing interest, and having physical contact has already been mentioned. Another very important thing to do is to provide cues to orient the elderly. Mention dates, day of the week, current events. For anyone who has had any cognitive slippage, good cues from the environment are very helpful. In conversation with the elderly, don't stick with neutral topics like the weather all the time. Try to engage them in some topics of common interest to you both (gardening, baseball, etc.) as well as some controversial topic, something with some zip. This stimulates their egos, since it implies you not only want *their* opinions, but you want *them* to listen to yours.

Try not to suggest offhandedly to elderly friends or relations that they "go see someone" about a problem. Think about what it means for an elderly person to go for help. Are there long waits at several different offices on several different floors? Does it require navigating difficult stairs, elevators, and hallways in the process? Are there times of day that make the use of public transportation easier? Consider such factors, and make adjustments to make it much easier for your elderly relatives or friends to receive help in as uncomplicated, convenient, nonembarrassing, and economical a fashion as possible.

Separate sympathy and empathy. Sympathy is feeling sorry for someone. The elderly don't want that; it makes them feel like children. Empathy means you understand, or want to understand. This is what they would like.

Display integrity with the elderly. Do not try to mislead them or lie to them. They are too experienced with all the con games in life. If they ask you questions, give them straight answers. This, however, does not mean being brutal in the name of "honesty."

Beware of arranging things for the elderly that will be seen as something trivial to occupy their time. If there is a crafts class, the point ought to be to teach them a skill, an art, not to keep them busy. Many of the elderly also have something they can teach others. The carpenter who is no longer steady enough to swing a hammer and drive a nail will be able to provide consultation to do-it-yourselfers who want to remodel their homes. The elderly have a richness of life experiences and much to contribute. Growing recognition of this fact and encouragement of sharing by the elderly can enrich the lives of us all.

■ *Adolescents*

Adolescence is indeed a special period of life. It lies at the back door of childhood yet at the very doorstep of adulthood. There is no comparable time in life when more physical and emotional changes take place in such a narrow span of time.

Adolescence as a term is less than 150 years old. Before that time, one grew straight from childhood into adulthood. The needs of family and culture demanded earlier work and community responsibilities. Survival depended on it. With increasing industrialization, children left the factories and fields to spend more time in school, play, and idle time. Society became increasingly aware of the presence of teenagers as a group who had and still have as yet fairly indefinable roles and rights. Most texts define adolescence as the time span from 12 to 21. Physical and legal determinants would suggest otherwise. Physical changes indicative of the beginning of adolescence may begin as early as age 7 and not end until the mid 20s. Legal age has fluctuated within state and federal differences. Varied drinking ages, youthful draft requirements, and reduced voting age have clouded the definition.

Physical changes

The most striking aspect of adolescence is the rapid physical growth. These changes are mediated by the sex hormones. The rough charts above indicate that the first recognizable change in the male is due to fat increase dictated by a small but gradual increase in estrogen. Every boy gains weight at the expense of height during these years. Some boys due to become tall and muscular men are actually chubby and effeminate looking during these early

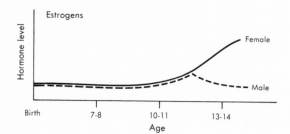

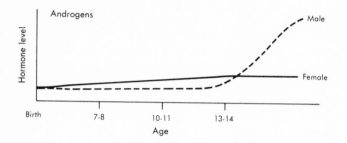

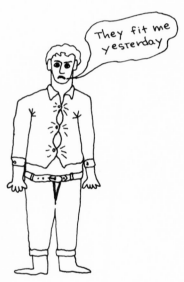

adolescent years. To add insult to injury, the next body part to grow is his feet, then thighs, which make him appear short waisted and gawky. This slows, allowing the rest of his body to catch up. Androgen influence may not come for a few years, with often unrecognizable pigment changes in the scrotal sac, then enlargement of the penis, testes, the beginning of pubic hair, and early voice changes. His first nocturnal emission or "wet dream" may occur as early as age 10 or as late as age 15. Even so, the majority of boys remain "relatively sterile" till age 15. The major male growth spurt appears at age 14½ and is due to growth in the backbone. This averages 4 to 4½ inches over an 18-month period. Some boys will shoot up 8 to 10 more inches during this time. Axillary and facial hair soon follow. Facial hair may develop entirely in one year. Other boys, equally normal but with different genes, may not complete the facial and body hair growth till the mid to late 20s.

We are indeed taller than our ancestors, which can be shown from historical evidence. Clothing, doorways, and furniture were made for shorter men and women. Better nutrition is mainly responsible for the changes seen.

A girl's first hormonal response is around age 7 or 8 with a normal vaginal discharge called *leukorrhea*. Her feet then grow, but this is rarely as noticeable a change as in the male. A breast "button" begins about age 11 under the skin of one breast first, to be followed in weeks or months under the remaining breast.The breasts develop into adult breasts over a span of 4 to 5 years. Pubic hair begins approximately 6 months after breast button stage. Her hips

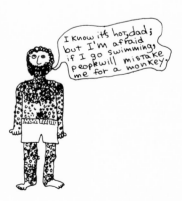

widen, and the backbone gains 3 to 4 inches before she is ready for her menses. Although a critical body weight is not the only initiator, the body is influenced by this. If other criteria are met, such as developing breasts, pubic hair, widened hips, and growth spurt, a sample of American girls will begin their menses weighing from 100 to 105 pounds. Nutrition has a great deal to do with the menarche (first menses); girls in countries with poor nutritional standards begin their menses 2 to 3 years later. The mean age for menarche in America is 12. (Pilgrim girls, who suffered from many nutritional deprivations, often had menarche delayed until age 17.) A regular menstrual cycle is not established immediately. Quite commonly a girl will have anovulatory (no egg) periods for 6 to 18 months before having ovulatory periods. This change may bring an increased weight gain, breast tenderness, occasional emotional lability, and cramps at the midcycle. These are consequences of progesterone, a hormone now secreted by the ovary at the time of ovulation. An adult pattern in ovulation will not be completed till the early 20s.

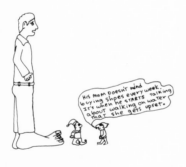

Until puberty, boys and girls are equally strong in muscle strength (if corrected for height and weight). Total body fat increases in girls by 50% from ages 12 to 18, whereas a similar decrease of 50% occurs in boys. Muscle cell size and number increase in boys, muscle cell size alone increases in girls. Internal organs such as the heart double in size. Blood pressure increases with demands of growth. Pulse rate decreases, and the ability to break down fatigue metabolites in muscle prepares the male, especially, for the role of hunter and runner that was so important for survival centuries ago.

Marked fatigue coupled with overwhelming strength is often difficult to appreciate fully. An adolescent may wolf down several quarts of milk, a full meal or two, play many hours of active sports, and yet complain bitterly of severe fatigue at all times! This human metabolic furnace needs the food and rest as well as the drive to have the machine function and test itself out. These bodily inconsistencies often show in mood swings and unpredictable demands for self-satisfaction and physical expression.

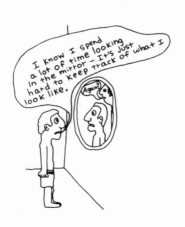

The rapidity of these changes tends to produce almost a physiological confusion in many adolescents. Quite commonly, they become preoccupied with themselves. This can lead to an overconcern with their health. In some instances, it is almost hypochondriacal. Adolescents may complain of things that to an adult appear very minor. The thing to remember is that their concern is very real and deep. Attention should be paid to their concerns. Remembering the rapid rate of physical changes that confronts the adolescent makes their preoccupation with their bodies understandable.

Characteristics

Adolescence characteristically is an extremely healthy time of life. In general, adolescents don't die off from the kinds of things that strike the rest of us, such as heart disease. The major causes of adolescent deaths are accidents and suicide. The result of this healthiness is that adults tend to assume that adolescents with problems are not really sick and do not give their complaints the hearing they deserve.

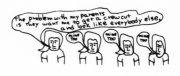

Another characteristic of adolescence is a truly tremendous need to conform to their peers. There's the need to dress alike, wear the same hairstyle, listen to the same music, and even think alike. A perpetual concern of the adolescent is that he or she is different. Although the sequence of physical development is the same, there is still variation in the age of onset and the rate of development. This can be a big concern for adolescents, whether the teenager is ahead, behind, or just on the norm. Worry about being different is a particular concern for the adolescent who may want or need professional help. the adolescent won't go unless it is "peer acceptable." Kids often stay away from caregivers out of fear. A big fear is that if they go, sure enough something really wrong will be found. This, to their minds, would officially certify them as *different*. They can't tolerate that.

Also characteristic of adolescence is wildly fluctuating behavior. It frequently alternates between wild, turmoiled periods and times of quiescence. A flurry of even psychotic-type thinking is not uncommon. This doesn't mean adolescents are psychotic for a time and then get over it. There are just some periods when their thinking really only makes sense to themselves and possibly to their friends. For example, if not selected for the play cast, he may be sure that "proves" he will be a failure his entire life. Or, if she is denied the use of the family car on Friday, she may overreact. With a perfectly straight face, she may accuse her parents of *never* letting her have the car, even as she stands there with the car keys ready to drive off.

Adolescence is very much a time of two steps forward and one back, with an occasional jog to one side or the other. Despite the ups and downs, it is usually a continuing, if uneven, upward trip to maturity.

Another point of importance: in early adolescence, the girls are developmentally ahead of the boys. At the onset of puberty, girls are physically about 2 years ahead. This makes a difference in social functioning because social development takes place in tandem with physical development. This can cause problems in social interactions for boys and girls of the same age. Their ideas of what makes a good party or what is appropriate behavior may differ con-

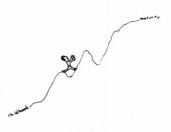

siderably. The girls may consider their male peers dumbos. The boys, aware of the girls' assessments, may be shaken up, while the girls feel dislocated too. With the uneven development of boys and girls during early adolescence, girls have an edge in school. In reading skills, for example, the girls may be a year ahead of the boys. There is a catching up period later, but in dealing with younger adolescents, keep this disparity in mind.

Four tasks

When does adolescence end? There are fairly clear-cut signs that mark the beginnings of the process. There is more to adolescence than just physical maturation. Defining the end can lead to philosophical discussions of "maturity." Doesn't everyone know a 45- or 65-year-old "adolescent?" There's more to assigning an end point than just considering a numerical age.

One way of thinking about the adolescent period is to assign to it four tasks. From this point of view, once the tasks have been reasonably accomplished, the person is launched into adulthood. These tasks are not tackled in any neat order or sequence. It is not like the consistent pattern of physical development. They are more like four themes that are interwoven, the dominant issues of adolescence.

One task of adolescence is *acceptance of the biological role*. This means acquiring some degree of comfort with your identity as either male or female. This is an intellectual effort. It has nothing to do with sexuality or experimentation with sexuality.

A second task is *the struggle to become comfortable with heterosexuality*. This doesn't mean struggling with the question of "how to make out at the drive-in!" It's the much larger question of "How do you get along with the opposite sex at all, ever?" Prior to adolescence, boys and girls are far more casual with one another. With adolescence, those days are over. Simply to walk by a member of the opposite sex and say "Hi" without blushing, giggling, or throwing up can be a problem. To become a heterosexual person—able to carry on all manner of social and eventually sexual activities with a member of the opposite sex—does not come easily. It is fraught with insecurity and considerable self-consciousness. If you force yourself to remember your own adolescence, some memories of awkwardness and uncertainty come to the fore. Thus there is the adolescent who doesn't ask for a date because of the anticipated *no*. Being dateless is much more tolerable than hearing a no.

Another task is *the choice of an occupational identity*. It becomes important to find an answer to "What am I going to do (be)?'' There are usually several false starts to this one. Think of the 5-year-old who wants to be a fireman. He probably never will be, but he gets a lot of mileage for awhile just thinking he is. It is not so different for adolescents. It is not helpful to pooh-pooh the first ideas they come up with. Nor is handing over an inheritance and saying ''Go ahead'' recommended. They need some time to work it out in their heads. A fair amount of indecision, plus some real lulu ideas, are to be expected.

The fourth task is *the struggle toward independence.* This is a real conflict. There is the internal push to break away from home and parents, and, at the same time, the desire to remain comfortably cared for. The conflict shows up in rebellion, since there aren't many ways to feel independent when living at home, being fed, checked on, prodded, and examined by parents. Rebellion of some type is so common to this period of life that an adolescent who does not rebel in some fashion should be suspect.

Rebellion. Rebellion can be seen in such things as manner of dress and appearance. It is usually the opposite of what the parents' generation accepts. Little ways of testing out crop up in being late from a date, buying something without permission, arguing with the parents over just anything. The kids are aware of their dependency, and they don't like it. There is even some shame over being in such a position. It is important that the parents recognize the rebellion and respond to it. In this era of Dr. Spock and ''Be friends with your kids,'' a lot of well-meaning parents have accepted *any* behavior from their kids. For example, if the kids, for the sake of rebellion, brought home some grass to smoke, their parents might light up, too. Often the kids will do whatever they can, just to get their parents angry. They are so often reminded by others of how much they look or act like their father or mother. And they don't want that. *Adolescents want to be themselves.* They don't want to be carbon copies of their parents, whom they probably don't much like at the moment. Going out and doing some drinking with the gang, doing something weird to their hair that Mom and Dad will hate, not cleaning their rooms, helping the neighbors but not their parents are all fairly usual ways of testing out and attempting to assert independence.

Destructive rebellion can occur when the parents either don't recognize the rebellion or don't respond to it. It can take many forms, such as running out of the house after an argument and driving off at 80 or 90 miles per hour, getting really drunk, running away, or, for girls, getting pregnant despite frequent warnings from their overrestrictive parents to avoid all sexual activities.

There are many roadblocks to completion of these four

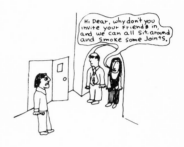

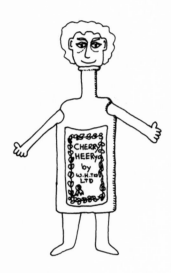

basic tasks. One results from a social paradox. Adolescents are physically ready for adult roles long before our society allows it. Studies of other societies and cultures point this out. In some societies adolescence doesn't cover a decade or more. It is about a one-hour trip! Light a fire, bat a gong, send the boy into the woods to pray to the moon; when he returns, hand him a spear and a wife, and he's in business. Our society dictates instead that people stay in an adolescent position for a frightfully long time: junior high school, senior high school, college, graduate school. . . . Another social paradox comes from the mixed messages. On the one hand, it's "be heterosexual, get a date" . . . "get a job" . . . "be grown up." On the other, it's "be back by 1 AM" . . . "save the money for college" . . . "don't argue with me." The mixed-upness of "grow up, but stay under my control" can introduce tensions.

The above is a very brief overview of adolescence. There are many excellent books on the subject should you want a more in-depth study. For our purposes here, it will suffice as a context in which to consider alcohol use.

Alcohol use

Adolescents do use alcohol, and in many different ways. Some of these ways are a normal part of the whole process. The "try it on" thread runs throughout adolescence. Alcohol is just one of the things to be tried. It is, after all, a massive part of adult society. So it's natural that the adolescent struggling toward adulthood will try it. Drinking is also attractive for either rebellious or risk-taking behavior. It is most usually introduced in a peer group. At present, it is not very acceptable to say, "No, thank you." Here again, the need to conform comes into play. Alcohol use to some degree is a part of the adolescent experience. Statistics now show that by age 18 the number of drinkers is the same as for the adult population. In a recent survey of high school youth, at least one half said they are in social situations where alcohol is served once a month or more. Of this group, one half said they drink "once a week, twice a week or more." Beer is the beverage most often drunk by both the frequent drinkers and those who had only tried drinking a few times. Many adolescents do not know that beer is as intoxicating as distilled spirits. Forty-two percent thought five to seven cans of beer could be drunk in 2 hours without risk of intoxication. They are short on facts and tend more than adults to rely on myths. Seventy percent believed cold showers could sober someone up, and 62% thought coffee would do it. Very few realized that only time takes care of it.

They also minimize the consequences of drinking. Only 8% thought their driving ability would be "much worse"

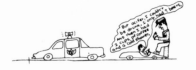

under the influence. They don't feel they are likely to get stopped by the police for drinking, or that the consequences could be severe if they are. They also don't consider their being in an accident a real possibility, much less one that might result in serious injury or death.

The children of alcoholics might use alcohol for other reasons, as well. They are dreadfully ashamed of their parents' alcoholism. They really hate it. They might deliberately, and very openly, come in drunk as a way of saying, "See what you're doing!" They are also quite likely testing out. They are very worried that they might turn out like Mom or Dad. Although they have grown up with alcoholism, their knowledge of it is quite superficial, spotty, and filled with fantasy.

This is why Al-Anon, Al-Ateen, or educational support groups are so important for them at this time. They try alcohol, and their logic goes, "I can go out and drink on Friday or Saturday, but on Monday I don't have to. I can leave it alone. See, I am different; I can handle it." Even explaining that alcoholism doesn't usually show up instantly, that almost everyone can handle it at first, isn't very convincing. They have a hard time accepting this. Adolescents are very oriented to the present. There is just this day. If they think about the future at all, they base it on how they feel *right now*. They sincerely feel they have proved their immunity from alcoholism forever if they don't show all the problems from the time of their first drinking experiences.

Alcohol problems and alcoholism

Since drinking is so prevalent during adolescence, it should not be a surprise to discover that alcohol problems and even alcoholism show up in this age group. Much press coverage has been given lately to "teenage alcoholism." Whether it is indeed more prevalent or simply being detected earlier is not easily answered. Some of both is probably true. That it exists is no longer arguable. The whole range of alcohol problems besides alcoholism are also happening to adolescents: driving while intoxicated, accidents, fights, arrests, injuries. Driving while intoxicated, in fact, may be quite prevalent, because the young person lacks experience in both driving and drinking. Education about alcohol use or early intervention when a problem is detected is vital, more so than in almost any other age group. It is very important to question the role alcohol plays in their lives. How to do this effectively is the real problem.

Practical suggestions

Most of us feel ill-equipped to deal with alcoholics of any age. Because most of us feel inadequate in our encounters with adolescents as well, to approach an adolescent about a drinking problem seems an impossible task. Unfortunately, there aren't any easy answers. The problem can't be ignored in the hope they will outgrow it. As parents or teachers or doctors or friends, we can't afford to look the other way. Too many of them die in alcohol-related incidents or traffic accidents. The risk is too great. We need to take their use of alcohol as seriously as we would their use of an illegal drug. They need help. They need a professional who is a specialist in both adolescence and alcohol problems. Because of the very task of establishing independence that is part of their development, they are unlikely simply to accept parental injunctions related to the use of alcohol. If we are parents of a young person in trouble, we need help as well. As discussed in Chapter 7, families are affected by a problem that any member of the family has. The dynamics that exist between adolescents and their families may render even more important the seeking of professional help by parents for themselves as soon as they suspect an alcohol problem developing in their child. Attempting to institute disciplinary measures may only drive the problem underground, cut off communications with the child, and indeed cause the problems to multiply. If we try to educate them at this point, we run the risk of being accused of using "scare tactics." Education about alcohol is important, but it should take place long before they are using it with any regularity. (As an aside, another point to remember is not to give a child inaccurate information about alcohol, or anything else for that matter. It is far safer to suggest they read a book on the subject or talk to an expert than to have them distrust you on all counts because of one incorrect statement.)

It is difficult at best as parents to admit that we are unsure about what to do in raising our children. We seem to operate under the misapprehension that we "ought" to be able to manage better, to handle it ourselves. A helpful thought to keep in mind is that most of us are as inexperienced at being parents as our children are at growing up. We're all in it together. Each child and each stage of development is a whole new experience for each one of us. We can't expect them to be just like we were when we were that age, even if we could remember that accurately. When we take on a new job we expect to receive some training even if we have spent years in school preparing for just such a job. Each business, or office, or what-have-you, has its own particular set of expectations, and we readily accept all the help we can get from more experienced workers in order to do a good job. To walk in smugly assuming we knew all there was to know would most likely set us up to fail. It would seem that we might begin to view the difficult and important job of parenting in the same light.

In seeking professional help, it goes without saying that locating someone knowledgeable about alcohol is important. Beyond that, in seeking assistance for an adolescent, look for someone who has a reputation for doing well with adolescents; a school counselor might be able to provide a good lead. You don't want an austere authority figure, the doctor in a white coat whose diplomas are dripping off the walls and who has a remote and cold clinical matter. Teenagers probably are having some degree of difficulty with authority figures, and they don't need that barrier set in place. On the other hand, beware of the guru type with gold chains, playing records, sitting on a floor cushion sucking a "roach" when they arrive. Adolescents spot phonies a long way off and they place a premium on honesty. Though they like to feel that a counselor isn't out of touch with what is going on in their world, they don't expect the counselor to be living there too.

Once professional treatment is sought, an issue to be faced is confidentiality. Parents naturally are concerned about their children's welfare, and they do have legal rights as regards being informed. This is something that probably ought to be addressed openly at the outset, so that the parents and adolescent both know how this will be handled. Dr. MacNamee, whose contributions help form this chapter, tells whomever he sees that though most of what they say will be held in confidence, if they tell him anything that scares him about what they might do, that would be harmful to themselves or others, he is going to blow the whistle. He makes it clear he won't do it without telling them. Nonetheless, however, he will do it. Adolescents will usually accept this. It may even be a relief. It may help to know that someone else is going to exert some control, especially if they are none too sure about their own inner controls at the moment. In a similar vein, Dr. MacNamee suggests keeping the adolescent posted on any contact he has with others. If a parent calls, he will start off the next session by informing the adolescent, "Hey, your Dad called me, and he wanted . . ." If a letter has to be written to a school probation officer or other contact, he shares what has been written with the adolescent. The chances are fairly good that the teenager's fantasy about what might be said is far worse than anything he would actually say, no matter what the problem. Since trust is such an issue with adolescents, it is important that others be willing to say *to* them what they say *about* them behind their backs.

Also, once professional help has been sought, it is important to follow through with all the recommendations. It is also important to let the adolescent take reasonable responsibility for his or her own treatment program, whether it consists of weekly sessions with a therapist, family meetings, AA meetings, or any other treatment approaches.

One area to be particularly aware of is that because being alcoholic is still stigmatized, parents and friends may be more uncomfortable than the child about AA attendance for adolescents. It is important to know how AA might be of use to adolescents with alcohol problems and not to discourage their attendance. The first thought might be that the adolescent would never identify with a group of predominantly 35- to 55-year-olds. In many areas that stereotype of the AA group doesn't necessarily hold true; there are now in some locales what are called "young people's groups." There the average age is early to mid 20s. Even if there are not any young people's groups in your vicinity, age need not be a barrier to an adolescent's affiliating with AA. On the contrary, there are several features of AA that might attract and intrigue the adolescent. It is a group of adults who will definitely not preach at him. Furthermore, given the collective life experiences wihin AA, the members are not likely to be shocked, outraged, or, for that matter, impressed by any of the adolescent's behavior. The members will generally treat the adolescent as an adult, presumably capable of making responsible choices, although cognizant that to do so isn't easy for anyone. There is within AA a ready assortment of potential surrogate parents, aunts, uncles, and grandparents. The intergenerational contact, possibly not available elsewhere to the adolescent, can be a plus. Also, AA remains sufficiently "unacceptable" so as not to automatically be written off by the adolescent wary of what he considers traditional, staid, "establishment," and out-of-it adult groups. The adolescent is full of surprises; his receptivity to AA may well be another one.

Changing times

In closing, some comments on the changing times and some speculation on its impact on adolescence seems in order. Much of adolescence is concerned with sexual maturation, acceptance of biological roles, adaptation to a heterosexual world, and selection of an occupational identity. What impact does the sexual revolution, the women's movement, gay liberation, or the counterculture have on these tasks? Adolescents appear to be faced with a wider range of choices than previous generations were in the struggle to answer the question "Who/what will I be when I grow up?" How many adolescents' parents had to seriously consider whether they'd marry or just live with someone? Whether to finish school or hitchhike across the country? Whether they were straight, gay, or bisexual? Whether they'd go to graduate school or become a potter?

Having to deal with such questions conceivably leads to healthier adults. But it would also seem to make accomplishing the tasks of adolescence more complicated. Moreover, it conceivably leads to more casualties along the way. Adolescents do not have culturally agreed-on stereotypes to rely on and provide guidance as they attempt to navigate this period of life. Potentially, part of the role of those in contact with the adolescent is to help him discover which of the many possibilities fits him. Relationships with people who care and can communicate effectively with them— whether parents, teachers, or older brothers, sisters, friends —can be an important point of reference as adolescents attempt to chart a course.

The questions the adolescent is grappling with are heavy ones. It will not be helpful if those who wish to help find them gut-wrenching. In no other area is it more necessary to be aware of personal biases and hang-ups. If the person is not comfortable in dealing with some of the issues the adolescent raises, the only course open is to send the adolescent to a professional better equipped to deal with the issues.

▪ *The employed*

The majority of alcoholics are members of the work force. One estimate, probably a conservative one, is that 8% of the nation's work force is adversely affected by the use of alcohol. Business and industry are beginning to recognize the costs to them of employees with alcohol problems. As a result, there has been a rapid development of special programs by employers to identify problems and initiate alcohol treatment. These programs, generally called either *employee assistance programs* (EAPs) or *occupational alcohol programs*, will be discussed later in this section. What is much less often discussed is how being a worker may influence the development of alcohol problems and the course of treatment.

Although not often mentioned, drinking is interwoven into work. And why not? As noted in Chapter 1, drinking is tied to all other parts of life. For some concrete examples of its intrusion into work, consider the office party, the company picnic, and the wine and cheese reception. There are martini lunches, the "drink date" to "review business," and the bar car on the commuter train. What is the good old stanby gift for a business associate? A fifth of good liquor. A round of drinks celebrates the close of a business deal. The construction crew stops off for beers after work. T.G.I.F. has become a catch phrase and an occasion for a drink. The company bowling team is cheered by beer. The list could be extended.

Abstaining is favorable both to the head and the pocket.

HORACE GREELEY

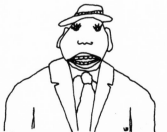

.Portrait of a man who stops in a bar for 3 drinks on his way home from work every night.

How might the almost universal presence of alcohol around the work setting be explained? To our knowledge, this has not been systematically, or even haphazardly, investigated. Based on observation, there does seem to be one common denominator to any drinking connected with work. The Kinney-Leaton Law states that alcohol will be conspicuously present at any social gathering composed of people who know one another primarily from work. As a corollary, people who may not associate drinking with social gatherings of friends, family, or neighborhood folk will choose to drink at a social function that is tied to work. It would seem that being initially ill at ease at social gatherings, which is a common feeling, might be more threatening if the function consists of co-workers. Alcohol is often used to lessen anxiety. On the other hand, drinking with co-workers may be considered "time out"; co-workers may be far more tolerant of one another's getting a little "tanked" than they would be if the drinking were being done with spouse, family, or close friends.

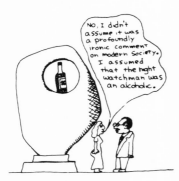

What is common to many work situations is that drinking is not only accepted; it is expected. This is not to imply that nondrinking is frowned upon, but it is considered unusual. The only perceived reason for supplying a nonalcoholic alternative is for the few who never drink. The assumption is that if you drink at all, you'll certainly want to take advantage of the opportunity!

If the use of alcohol is tolerated, the potential for alcohol problems among susceptible individuals rises, and more so if drinking is subtly encouraged. Employers have generally not been considered responsible for their employees' drinking practices. After all, employers are not making employees drink. Or are they? Several recent court rulings have held that an employer, in certain situations, is responsible. The following two cases demonstrate this. From the *New York Times:*

Douglas M. Jolly, A District of Columbia policeman, proved overqualified for an undercover assignment that required him to spend a lot of time in bars, a civil service board ruled Thursday, so he will get a tax-free pension of two-thirds of his $13,000 annual salary. Testimony showed that although Mr. Jolly had been a "health fiend" who seldom touched alcohol, his assignment as a narcotics and liquor-law investigator produced such a case of alcoholism and resulting medical conditions that he had been retired on full disability. He has also stopped drinking.

Laurie Johnston

Also from the *New York Times:*

Office Party Blamed in Death of Employee

San Francisco, Oct. 31 (UPI)—The widow of a man killed in an auto accident after he became intoxicated at an office party is entitled to receive workmen's compensation, the California Supreme Court ruled yesterday.

The court said the "proximate cause" of death of Daniel Mc-Carty originated with his employment at a plumbing concern, which gave a party on company time during the 1971 holiday season.

"An employer who tolerates and encourages employee drinking in connection with the job may not later assert that the injury was caused by the intoxication of the employee," the court ruled.

Although a job cannot be said to cause alcoholism, it can contribute to its development. Some of the factors in a job that may be conducive to the development of alcohol problems are noted in the following discussion.

High-risk factors

Certain types of work and work situations appear to aggravate and reinforce alcohol abuse. This statement is substantiated by the high percentage of managerial, white collar, and professional people reported to have alcohol problems. Alcoholism is also a serious problem for, among others, the military, physicians, executives, and airline employees. What do all these diverse occupations have in common? According to one view, they have "job-based risk factors." The two major categories of these are absence of supervision and low visibility of performance. It might be useful to review these twelve risk factors:

- Absence of clear goals (and absence of supervision)
- Freedom to set work hours (isolation and low visibility)
- Low structural visibility (e.g., salespeople away from the business place)
- Work addiction
- Occupational obsolescence (especially common in scientific and technical fields)
- New work status
- Required on-the-job drinking (e.g., salespeople drinking with clients)
- Mutual benefits (informal power struggles in upper organizational levels may lead to heavier drinking)
- Reduction of social controls (occurs on college campuses and other less-structured settings)
- Severe role stress
- Competitive pressure
- Presence of illegal drug users (less an issue for alcohol abusers)

An interesting conclusion from this research is that deviant drinking is not concentrated in any one social class or occupational group.

The workplace cover-up

If bringing up the drinking practices and potential problems of a family member or close friend makes someone

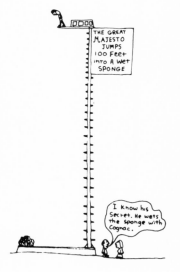

The contract of the National Brewery Workers of America specifies that union members may drink beer in unlimited quantity during breaks. (Do they have an industrial alcoholism program?)

squirm with discomfort, the idea of saying something to a co-worker is virtually unthinkable. There is a separation that almost everyone accepts between work and home or professional and private life. The reticence people feel about butting into someone else's life, especially around drinking, is as true in the work setting as anywhere else. What happens on the job is the legitimate concern of the business and co-workers. Anything outside the job setting is considered someone's own private affair. So until the alcohol problem flows into the work world, the worker's use of alcohol is considered no one else's business. That doesn't mean that no one sees a problem developing. It is our suspicion that someone with just a little savvy can spot potentially dangerous drinking practices. The office scuttlebutt or work crew's bull sessions plus simple observation make it common knowledge who "really put it away this weekend" or the "poor devil who just got picked up DWI" or "you can always count on Sue to join in whenever anyone wants to stop for a drink after work."

Even if an employee does show some problems on the job, whether marginal to or directly related to alcohol use, co-workers may try to "help out." This may mean covering up any work difficulties so that supervisors or management don't find out, by doing extra work, or not blowing the whistle. Co-workers are also not immune to the alcoholic's deceptions. Out of misguided sympathy, they may well feel they are helping the alcoholic" until the pressure's off about _____." Because employee-assistance programs, if they are present, are based on identifying work deterioration, any attempt by co-workers to help cover up job problems makes spotting the alcohol problem all the more difficult. If a company does not have a program to help alcoholics, odds for a cover-up by co-workers are greater. It may well be true that if management does spot a problem, the worker will be fired. Co-workers, knowing how important that paycheck is, believing promises by the alcoholic to shape up, and fearful of what dire things may follow the loss of the job, are likely to minimize and conceal the problem.

Another important party in this concealment strategy is the spouse. With the predictable strains in the emotional realm, parental roles, and sexual relationship, the last straw is the potential loss of financial support. The spouse usually doesn't want to do anything to threaten the paycheck. So spouses will do whatever they can to get the alcoholic to work. On the other side of the coin, they'll make excuses whenever possible for those occasions when work is missed. The spouse may buy the alcoholic's rationalization that the drinking is a product of stress at work. Therefore the spouse may support job changes in the hope that they will relieve the drinking and consequent problems.

Eventually the problems become too diffuse for the cover-ups to work anymore. Or the spouse leaves, or the co-workers get sick of the whole thing, or the alcoholic comes in drunk or has an on-the-job accident. At this point, in the past the alcoholic usually got fired. It can be assumed that this still happens in many companies. The employee is out, and the company may have lost a formerly valuable and well-trained worker. Statistically, this is a costly problem for companies all over the country. There are, however, other solutions to this dilemma. Nationally, it is estimated that 5000 work organizations have employee-assitance or occupational alcohol programs. Of the Fortune 500 companies in 1978, 57% had programs, a 25% increase over the proportion in 1972. Basically, the thinking behind these programs is that it is cheaper for the companies to identify problems earlier and then use the job as leverage to get the employee into treatment and back to work at an efficient level.

Cost effectiveness

In a study conducted by an economist at the School of Hygiene and Public Health at Johns Hopkins University, employee programs were found to be cost effective. The 3-year study, begun in 1972, involved unions and management in twelve companies employing 134,000 people. In the Baltimore project, where the cost for 206 referred patients was $230,000, the twelve employers saved $454,000 in reduced absenteeism the first year of the program and $600,000 the second year. Savings are expected to be $1 million in the third year and to grow geometrically. Absenteeism was the only factor analyzed in this particular study because it is the most easily measured. But there are a number of other areas that have been identified as potentially beneficial to the employer, including reduction of on-the-job accidents, less equipment damage, and improved morale, leading to increased productivity.

Why so few programs?

If all this cost effectiveness is for real, why do not more businesses have programs? There is no single clear-cut reason, but several possibilities can be mentioned. One is company size. Small companies may be quite informal and have a more personal approach. They may also not have funds or the need to hire a professional to set up and run a program just for them. Consortiums are one emerging answer to this one.

Another frequently mentioned roadblock is the executive or "president alcoholic," who is certainly less likely to insitute a program that is personally threatening. It is often said that programs are designed to identify alcoholics at all levels *lower* than that of the person approving the program. It would clearly be difficult for the personnel manager to set up or OK a program when he feels sure that his immediate superior already has a problem. One way out of this bind would be to apply the program to all levels below this.

And, of course, the pervasive American idea that alcoholism is a choice and those who choose it deserve what they get is just as influential in business as elsewhere. There is surely a host of other reasons for the paucity of programs, but with slowly changing attitudes, publicity above successful programs, and better available insurance coverage, there is hope that the future will be brighter for the employed alcoholic.

Now on to a bit about identification of troubled employees, types of programs, and so on.

Philosophy, "the bottom line," or toward a more productive work force

Facts and experience suggest that the occupational environment may be one of the most efficient and economical means of providing an opportunity for early identification and treatment of alcoholism and alcohol-related problems. The problem drinker's daily contact with other employees, supervisors, union stewards, medical department, and personnel staff increases the possibility of others noticing the behavioral changes and impaired job performance that accompany a developing alcohol problem. This early recognition and confrontation is critical; otherwise, the problem drinker tends to use employment as the indicator that he's still OK. After all, he can still go to work!

Chances for recovery are also increased by reaching the alcoholic at an earlier stage, for the following reasons:

1. Physical health has not deteriorated significantly.
2. Financial resources are not as depleted.
3. Emotional supports still exist in the family and community.
4. Threat of job loss is present as a motivator.

Program approaches

The two major approaches to occupational programming are the *broad brush* and the *alcohol-only*. The former *(troubled employee or employee assistance)* is directed at all employees, regardless of the type of problem affecting work performance, which may include personal, family, financial, legal, drug, or alcohol problems. The alcohol-only approach is limited to employees with alcohol problems that inhibit their productivity.

An advantage of the broad brush approach is that alcoholism is not the only factor that affects employee behavior or work performance. And the moral stigma that is still attached to alcoholism inhibits many people from seeking help or referring others. Thus the neutrality of Employee Assistance Program on the door allows certain workers to enter without fearing others will know the particular problem that they might have.

The argument for the straight alcoholism approach is that such directness cuts through the denial and manipulation of the alcoholic and is thus more effective.

Program components

Regardless of approach, staff, or program model, any organization that determines a need exists for developing a program will find there are certain components critical to all.

1. A *written policy* must be issued, one that is supported by management and labor. If there are unions at the facility, these groups should be represented at every level of planning, implementation, and review. As many companies have sorrowfully discovered, without the cooperation and representation of all elements of the work force, a program cannot succeed because there will be competition and distrust.

2. A trained and qualified *Program Coordinator* should be hired. This individual will be responsible for determining the program approach and developing and implementing program, policy, and procedures. This person might function under the umbrella of a medical department, personnel department, a separate department, or at an outside service agency.

3. *Training sessions* should be offered to supervisors, managers, and union stewards to help them recognize problems and also to teach them the referral process.

4. *Information* and *education* should be available to all employees on a continuing basis to ensure proper and full utilization of the program.

5. *Total confidentiality* must be guaranteed to the employee/client. The Federal Privacy Act of 1975 provides strict guidelines regarding client information sharing and record keeping.

6. A *program description*, via a brochure or handbook, is important so that employees will know what services are being offered. Also, information should be given about referral procedures, employ*ee* responsibility, and employ*er* responsibility.

7. *Payment options* must be determined and then clearly stated, so that the employee/client will be prepared. Some companies include this service with employee

There are two things that will be believed of any man whosoever, and one of them is that he has taken to drink.

BOOTH TARKINGTON

health benefits. Others prefer a different arrangement, and the employee might then be asked to assume responsibility for some part of the payment.

8. An *evaluation* or *review* component is critical. It
might be administered by the program coordinator,
an advisory board, or a joint labor-management committee. The purposes would be to provide for account-
ability, monitor program implementation, review
and advise, disseminate information, and conduct a
cost-benefit analysis.

Special features

An important technique in dealing with the alcoholic
employee is sometimes called *intervention, constructive
coercion,* or *confrontation.* The technique is used in the
work setting to motivate the individual to seek help to improve job performance and retain the job. The use of "job
leverage" can also be an excellent tool to use to keep the
employee motivated and involved in treatment.

Confrontation is actually a process that occurs within
the company's normal evaluation and disciplinary procedures. A supervisor, manager, or union steward who notes
certain behaviors and signs of deteriorating job performance documents them. Some of the most common signs
and symptoms used to identify the problem drinker are the
following:

- Chronic absenteeism
- Change in behavior
- Physical signs
- Spasmodic work pace
- Lower quantity and quality of work
- Partial absences
- Lying
- Avoiding supervisors and co-workers
- On-the-job drinking
- On-the-job accidents and lost time from off-the-job ac-
cidents

One can see the importance of training supervisors and
others in recognizing these signs, so that early detection
can occur. Training is also critical to helping employers to
document and not diagnose. In organizations where there
has been no such training or education, the common response to the problem drinker is to "kill him with kind-
ness." His co-workers and supervisors cover up, advise,
threaten, and finally give up.

If there is a company program, the procedure would be
to identify, document, and then confront the employee
with the facts and an informal offer of referral for help. If
unsuccessful, the next phase would be a stepped-up disciplinary procedure, including a time limit and a formal re-

ferral with the "threat" of job loss if performance is not improved.

What we have described here is a bare-bones sketch of the principles of employee-assistance programs. There are numerous different adaptations within this framework. Companies interested in setting up such a program would be well advised to seek out people with knowledge and experience to aid in planning and implementing their program. Small companies might look to their neighboring small companies to explore the feasibility of a consortium arrangement. There are numerous routes possible to seek out consultants. Local councils on alcoholism often have EAP specialists available. A call to an area alcoholism-treatment facility may help track one down. Some health-maintenance organizations or group medical insurance plans have such consultants on staff. And of course, ALMACA, the Association of Labor Management Administrators and Consultants on Alcoholism (1800 North Kent Street, Suite 907, Arlington, VA 22209), is a major source of information on the subject.

This is a challenging and exciting time. Occupational programs have made significant progress in demonstrating that the "human approach" is good business.

■ *In closing*

As alcohol services expand, as alcohol knowledge grows, more attention is being paid to how treatment can best be provided to different groups of people. Recall the impact culture has on the development of alcohol problems. It also influences treatment. Culture influences where people turn for help and their ability to accept it. Culture will dictate the circumstances most likely to trigger a resumption of drinking. The culture will assign the degree of stigma to a member's having an alcohol problem.

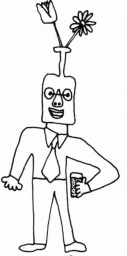

Portrait of a man who thinks he's clever when he's drunk

The United States is not a homogeneous collection of people. Age, sex, race, ethnic background, where one lives —these factors make a difference. They are forces that mold how we each think, behave, and feel.

When it comes to alcohol, persons from the same group are likely to share basic attitudes and face similar problems. Anyone who encounters an alcoholic clearly from different circumstances and who doesn't ask how this might alter treatment is ignoring some important information if they wish to help the person.

In reading this chapter, we hope you have been confronted with some new ideas. We hope this not only alters your thinking about alcoholics who are women, employed, adolescent, or elderly, but also prods you to find out more about other special populations. Further reading is one

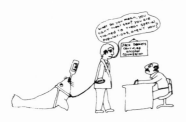

way, but not the only way, or even the best. Another is to put aside temporarily what you think you know, and approach it with fresh eyes. Go find someone from a particular group, and ask him what it is like to be a member of that ethnic, racial, religious, or minority group. And *listen.* Sitting in our little rural New England town, we do not presume to even attempt a description of the black, Chicano, Native American, urban, southern, or West Coast experiences. Also, we don't expect you necessarily to be knowledgeable about the Vermont Yankee farmer or the Franco-Americans. Wherever one finds oneself, there is some important homework to be done to improve our understanding of groups different from our own.

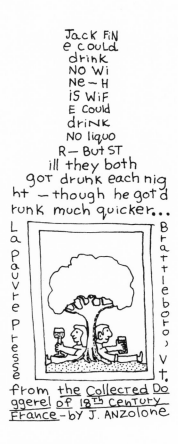

Jack FiN
e could
drink
NO Wi
Ne – H
iS WiF
E could
drinK
NO liquo
R – But ST
ill they both
goт drunk each nig
ht – though he got'd
runk much quicker...

La pauvre Presse

Brattleboro, Vt.

from the Collected Do
ggerel of 18ᵀᴴ CenTury
France – by J. Anzolone

Chapter 11

End papers

▪ *Points for reflection*

It is probably to anyone's advantage to give a little thought to alcohol use. How do *you* use alcohol? What are your attitudes toward drinking? How do you feel about drunkenness? Is it OK in some circumstances; if so, where is the dividing line? At what point is it offensive? Are you uncomfortable riding in a car when the driver has been drinking? Do you believe—wholeheartedly—that alcoholism is a disease, like pneumonia or arthritis, or does it seem somehow different; if so, what is different? There are no right or wrong answers to these questions. The point we are trying to make is that most of us do not even consider them. Alcohol is all around us, most people drink, the majority moderately and without problems—and drinking is for most a largely unconscious, unconsidered behavior. Yet it is this very fact that in part contributes to the atmosphere that is conducive to alcohol problems.

How might you begin to think about alcohol? One way is to look at how you use alcohol. Is it to celebrate, relax, go to sleep, turn off worries, let loose? In what settings do you typically drink: at home, out on the town, special occasions, with meals, with particular people, as part of your job? How much do you spend on alcohol during a week? Are there any notable exceptions? Are there any circumstances likely to result in a problem if you drink, such as medical conditions, medications, driving after imbibing? Are you at special risk for developing alcoholism—family history, culturally (e.g., being a drinker from a strict teetotaling family)? How would others describe your drinking?

Another method for really looking at your use of alcohol is to pick a time period, a week or two, and not drink. Conduct this little experiment without telling anyone. What are the occasions during that period when you would otherwise naturally have a drink? Are there particular times when not drinking seems like at least "a bit of a drag" and using alcohol would be nicer than not? Does anyone comment on your not drinking? Are there particular occasions or persons who don't accept an offhanded "No, thanks" at a drink offer? Are there any occasions when getting something nonalcoholic is a real accomplishment? Further, if you're out somewhere, how much are you charged for the cola or the tonic with a twist of lemon?

There's more to it, of course, than yourself. Drinking behavior and drinking problems occur in a climate that we all help create for one another. How do you serve alcoholic beverages in your home? Is serving drinks almost a must? How much energy do you devote to making sure you have alcohol on hand? At gatherings or parties in your home is it common or rare for people to become drunk? How do you handle that?

■ *Is there someone in your life whose drinking should be of concern?*

An emerging alcohol problem, for all the reasons discussed throughout this book, is sometimes hard to spot. So consider for a moment those closest to you.

Are there people in your life you constantly worry about in terms of their drinking—that maybe they'll drink too much, or maybe they'll make a scene, or maybe they shouldn't be driving?

If you don't routinely have a well-stocked bar, are there some people for whom you'd be sure you had something on hand?

In a circle of people picking something to do, is there someone who can be counted on to opt for the bar over the ice cream parlor following the movie?

Is there someone who regularly brings an extra bottle to a party so you don't run out, or would be the one to suggest going down to the package store to replenish the supplies?

Is there someone who talks about drinking a lot—having been here, there, or somewhere else, really "tying one on," or commenting because some place didn't serve drinks, or the wedding reception only had a fruit punch?

Is there anyone whom you'd particularly notice if they said no to an offer of a drink?

Is there someone who really counts on a drink for something special (e.g., to unwind after a hard day)?

What these questions are getting at is the relationship of the person to alcohol; is it casual or fairly central? How much organizing, whether conscious or unconscious, is going on to allow or provide for the presence of alcohol? To use the analogy of friendship, alcohol can be a lovely casual acquaintance, but it proves to be, over the long haul, a poor intimate friend.

If there is a person or persons who do come to mind as you reflect on these questions, this shouldn't be taken as a definitive diagnosis of alcoholism. Besides, that's ultimately a professional judgment. In fact, it is quite possible there is no alcohol problem. But these behaviors could be fertile ground for one to develop. Think about it; in most of the instances cited, other people's behavior doesn't challenge the drinking and actually can promote it. To consider your part—how much accommodation do you make for drinking, whether your own or someone else's? If a gooey fudge sundae makes your mouth water, after the movie are you going to settle for a beer and munchies at the bar because of someone else's preference? Is an essential ingredient of friendship being able to serve drinks? Is a bottle of wine with dinner sufficient, or do you have to provide a full cocktail hour and after-dinner aperitifs, routinely? Are you willing to voice your views on alcohol use?

■ *Where to turn for help*

Are you saying to yourself, look there's no question, I know that Jack, or Ann, or Tom, or Betty has a problem; what do I do, where can I turn for help? Hopefully, this book has helped you better understand what is going on, made it abundantly clear that the prognosis is bright indeed if someone seeks assistance, and there are far more resources than you had ever imagined.

If you've not a clue as to the alcohol services available, start by looking in the local telephone directory yellow pages under alcoholism, or the white pages under "Alcoholics Anonymous." Almost every community, no matter how small, has something, including AA and Al-Anon, as well as alcohol counselors. Although this may not be exactly what you are seeking, you will certainly be provided with a list of agencies, phone numbers, persons to contact. On the other hand, you may speak with your physician or call your local mental health center or hospital and ask for the names of alcohol resources. In large communities or metropolitan areas, you may be overwhelmed by the choices.

There are also places (listed at the end of this chapter) that you can write for further information about the disease or treatment resources.

If you wish to be in touch with a professional facility, in addition to AA or Al-Anon, what might you consider? The optimum would be a special alcohol or chemical dependency program, which may be affiliated with a hospital as a special unit or be a wholly separate agency. This is an appropriate place for a family member to turn to help sort out what's going on. Such programs are not only for the alcoholic. The advantage of such a program is that within one center there will be a mix of professional staff whose special expertise is alcoholism, which should provide a full range of services from inpatient to outpatient, for the alcoholic and family.

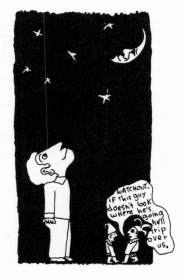

• • •

Alcoholism has been called the "lonely sickness." It is, for the alcoholic, the spouse, and the children particularly. There is an overwhelming sense of being the only person with such a problem. The statistics don't help. From the insider's point of view, the rest of the world seems unreachably "normal." It seems impossible to believe that anyone else ever shared such experiences.

This book has endeavored to share enough information to begin to dispel the "no one ever—" feelings. It can only play a tiny part, however. It is the deep hope of all concerned with the book that those who suffer from alcoholism, both directly and indirectly, will seek the help that is available and join the increasing ranks of the recovering and their families.

Sources for further information

Alcoholics Anonymous. General Services Organization (AA)
468 Park Avenue South
New York, NY 10016
(Box 459), Grand Central Station, New York, NY 10163)   212-686-1100
  To make contact in your local community, look under "Alcoholics Anonymous" in the white pages of the telephone directory.

Al-Anon Family Group Headquarters
PO Box 182
Madison Square Station
New York, NY 10010   212-686-1100
  To make a contact in your local community, look in the white pages of the telephone directory under Al-Anon.

National Clearinghouse on Alcohol Information (NCALI)
PO Box 2345
Rockville, MD 20852   301-468-2600
  This is a public information service of the National Institute on Alcohol Abuse and Alcoholism, a federal agency. Literature on a wide array of alcohol topics is available on request.

National Council on Alcoholism
733 Third Avenue
New York, NY 10017   212-986-4433
  This is a private national organization with a broad range of functions from public education to fostering professional associations. It has chapters in many communities that conduct educational programs, or provide referral services for alcoholism treatment, or offer consultation to groups.

Suggested reading

First person accounts

Allen, Chaney. *I'm Black, and I'm Sober.* CompCare Publications, 1978.
Burditt, Joyce R. *The Cracker Factory.* New York: Collier Books (The MacMillan Co.), 1977.
Brooks, Cathleen. *The Secret Everyone Knows.* San Diego, CA: The Kroc Foundation, 1980. Available on request from Operation Cork, 8939 Villa LaJolla Drive, San Diego, CA 92037.
  This pamphlet is written by a young woman whose parents were alcoholic. It is intended for children of alcoholics. It very nicely addresses a child's feeling of shame and loneliness in living with this "secret," and realistically describes how a child can seek help.
  Each of these relates a personal encounter with alcoholism, from the development of disease through the crisis period to treatment and recovery.

Others

Johnson, Vernon. *I'll Quit Tomorrow.* New York: Harper & Row, 1973.
  This offers both a highly readable and very understandable account of what a developing alcohol problem feels like for the alcoholic and how this looks and feels for those close to him. For those around the alcoholic it provides a way of understanding what is happening and what needs to be done in recovery.
Alcoholics Anonymous. New York: Alcoholics Anonymous World Services, Inc., 1955.
  This was first published in 1939. There are now over a million in print. It provides in members' own words how the AA fellowship came into being and how it works.

Index

Page numbers followed by *t* indicate tables.

Group work in treatment of alcoholism—cont'd
  educational, 166-167
  as fad, 168
  functions of, 167-168
  problem-solving, 167
  self-awareness, 167
  as therapy, 165-166
Guilt in recovery period, handling, 154
  clergy assistance in, 185-186

H

Habitual excessive drinking, definition of, 39
Hallucinosis, alcoholic, in alcohol withdrawal, 107
Health care, alcohol and, 23-24
Heart
  alcohol effects on, 80-81
  failure of, in alcoholism, 80
  holiday, in alcoholism, 81
  rhythm of, abnormalities in, in alcoholism, 81
Hematological system, alcohol effects on, 77-80
Hematoma, subdural, from alcoholism, 94-95
Hemolysis, abnormal, in alcoholism, 78
Hemorrhoids
  in alcoholic cirrhosis, 76
  in alcoholism, 73
Hepatic coma in alcoholic cirrhosis, 76-77
Hepatitis, alcoholic, 75
Hepatocerebral disease, chronic, in alcoholism, 93
Hepatorenal syndrome in alcoholism, 82-83
Heredity, alcoholism and, 54-57
Heterosexuality, becoming comfortable with, as task
    of adolescence, 238
Hodgkin's disease, alcohol use in, 96
Holiday heart in alcoholism, 81
Homicide, alcoholism and, 22, 23
Homosexuality, latent, alcoholism and, 60
Hormones
  alcohol effects on, 86
  sex, female, increased, in alcoholism, 83
Host in etiology of alcoholism, 54-65
  genetic factors of, 54-57
  psychological factors of, 57-65
Housewives, changing role of, 218-219
Hughes Act, 18
Hyperactivity in children of alcoholic families, 131
Hyperglycemia, alcohol intake and, 30
Hyperlipoproteinemia, Type IV, in alcoholism, 81
Hypertension in alcoholism, 82
Hypnotics, interaction of, with alcohol, 112t
Hypoglycemia from excessive alcohol intake, 30
Hypoglycemics, interaction of, with alcohol, 111t

I

Illness
  losses by elderly due to, 228
  psychiatric, 200-206; see also Psychiatric illness
Immunoglobulins, alcohol effects on, 80
Impotence in alcoholism, 83
Independence, struggle toward, as task of adolescence,
    239

Infant, effects of alcoholic family on, 132
Infection of joint space in alcoholism, 89
Insomnia, 101-102
  sleeping pills for, precautions for, 100-101
  treatment of, 101-102
Intestines, alcohol absorption from, 27
Intoxication, pathological, 91
Irish, alcoholism rates among, 66, 67
Iron-deficiency anemia in alcoholism, 78
Irritation, gastrointestinal, from alcohol, 73
Italy, drinking habits in, 67

J

Jaundice in alcoholic hepatitis, 75
Jews, alcoholism rates among, 67, 68
Job, effects of alcoholism on, 124-125
Joint space, infection of, in alcoholism, 89

K

Kidneys, alcohol effects on, 30
Korsakoff's psychosis in alcoholism, 91, 92

L

Lactic acidosis in alcoholism, 96
Learning theories, alcoholism and, 62-63
Leukocytes, alcohol effects on, 79
Librium
  for alcohol withdrawal, 209
  withdrawal from, 213
Life expectancy, alcoholism and, 22
Lithium carbonate, 208
Liver
  alcohol effects on, 30-31
  in alcohol metabolism, 28-29
  cancer of, in alcoholic cirrhosis, 77
  cirrhosis of, alcoholic, 75
  disease of, in alcoholism, 74-77
  fatty, in alcoholism, 75
Losses of elderly
  coping mechanisms for, 227-228
  nature of, 228-230
Lungs, alcohol effects on, 85

M

Magnesium, serum levels of, diminished, in alcoholism,
    96
Malabsorption in alcoholism, 73
Manic-depressive illness, 201-202
  alcoholism and, 96
Marchia-fava-Bignami disease in alcoholism, 93
Marital relationship of alcoholic, 124
Meditation in treatment of alcoholism, 191-192
Megaloblastic anemia in alcoholism, 78
Memory, loss of
  from alcohol abuse, 102-105
  in Korsakoff's psychosis, 92
Menstrual cycle, alcohol absorption and, 33